Dorsal Ventricular Ridge

WILEY SERIES IN NEUROBIOLOGY

R. Glenn Northcutt, Editor

DORSAL VENTRICULAR RIDGE: A TREATISE ON FOREBRAIN
ORGANIZATION IN REPTILES AND BIRDS
by *Philip S. Ulinski*

In Preparation:

COEXISTENCE OF NEUROACTIVE SUBSTANCES IN NEURONS

edited by Victoria Chan-Palay and Sanford L. Palay

DORSAL VENTRICULAR RIDGE

A Treatise on Forebrain Organization in Reptiles and Birds

Philip S. Ulinski
Department of Anatomy and
Committee on Neurobiology
The University of Chicago

A Wiley-Interscience Publication

JOHN WILEY & SONS

New York • Chichester • Brisbane • Toronto • Singapore

Copyright © 1983 by John Wiley & Sons, Inc.

All rights reserved. Published simultaneously in Canada.

Library of Congress Cataloging in Publication Data:

Ulinski, Philip S. (Philip Steven), 1943–
  Dorsal ventricular ridge.

  (Wiley series in neurobiology)
  "A Wiley-Interscience publication."
  Bibliography: p.
  Includes indexes.
  1. Dorsal ventricular ridge. 2. Brain—Localization
of functions. 3. Nervous system—Reptiles. 4. Nervous
system—Birds. I. Title. II. Series.

QL938.D65U44 1983   596'.048   83-3670
ISBN 0-471-87612-7

Printed in the United States of America

10 9 8 7 6 5 4 3 2 1

SERIES PREFACE

Neuroscience is a rapidly expanding interdisciplinary field that is yielding significant insights into the organization and function of nervous systems. An outgrowth of several more traditional disciplines—Animal Behavior, Comparative Biology, Cybernetics, Neuroanatomy, Neurochemistry, Neurophysiology, and Physiological Psychology—Neuroscience arose because of many reasons, but central to the focus of Neuroscience is the growing realization that no single approach or discipline can fully explain how nervous systems are organized; how they come into being ontogenetically, as well as phylogenetically; how a specific nervous system works; and what operational principles are applicable to most, if not all, nervous systems.

From subcellular organelles and processes to entire networks mediating behavior, the complexity and diversity exhibited by nervous systems is staggering. The goal of Neuroscience is to understand how these complex and diverse systems work as devices for information processing, control, and communication. Unlike artificial devices that are man-made and thus specifically designed to solve limited, well-defined sets of problems, nervous systems are the result of a historical process called evolution. Thus their analysis is further confounded by the fact that they have arisen opportunistically and without optimal design. Understanding how they have arisen, how they have adapted to solve problems that are virtually unlimited, is a challenge that can not be met by a single discipline. Although individual Neuroscientists will continue to focus on specific questions related to a particular facet of neural organization or a single species, achievement of the goals of Neuroscience demands an eclectic approach that is rapidly becoming its hallmark.

v

The Wiley Series in Neurobiology reflects this eclecticism, and the Series will present work ranging from subcellular to behavioral topics, from specialized monographs to contributions spanning several disciplines. As a forum in which nervous systems are viewed and analyzed from widely different perspectives, it is hoped that these offerings will not only provide information to researchers in all disciplines of Neuroscience, but will also provide further stimulation for an eclectic approach to the evolution, organization, and function of nervous systems.

R. Glenn Northcutt

Ann Arbor, Michigan
March 1983

PREFACE

The past two decades have seen an increasing interest in the neurobiology of nonmammalian vertebrates. It stems in part from the development of axonal tracing techniques that can be successfully applied to the unmyelinated fibers systems that dominate the brains of nonmammals. These techniques have led to a profusion of information on the basic anatomy of the brains of nonmammals. The interest also stems from the gradual acceptance and application of ethological approaches, particularly of "neuroethological" investigations, that seek to understand the neural bases of naturally occurring behaviors (e.g., Lorenz, 1981; Ewert, 1982). In contrast to physiological psychologists, many neuroethologists have focused on behaviors in nonmammalian vertebrates and, as their models have developed, have had a pressing need for more and better information about the neurobiology of the species they study.

Perhaps because of the pace and tempo of the activity, there has been relatively little time for the synthesis and integration of information. This has led to a situation in which neuroanatomists, on the one hand, often make little attempt at relating their findings to behavioral problems and neuroethologists, on the other hand, often find it difficult to use the complex and sometimes confusing information generated by neuroanatomists. The ideal is presumably to establish a framework of data and concepts that facilitates the easy incorporation of new facts and ideas into a growing body of information.

My goal in writing this book is to attempt a synthesis of this sort for a particular region of the forebrains of reptiles and birds. This region was originally called the "dorsal ventricular ridge" in reptiles, but the term has been gradually and informally extended to more or less specific regions of the brains of birds as well. Both anatomical and behavioral results implicate the dorsal ventricular ridge (DVR) in a variety of important behaviors. There is, however, no formal definition of DVR and no overall notion of the place that it plays in the organization of the forebrain. This is not to say that individuals working on DVR and related structures have not been converging on such an idea quite rapidly during the past few years, but only that it is nowhere explicated and critically related to the relevant data in a way that would be of general use to persons not actively involved in this field of research.

It seems to me that the appropriate format for the endeavor is that of a treatise, which Webster defines as "a systematic exposition or argument including a methodical discussion of the facts and principles involved and the conclusions reached." I believe that the establishment of an "argument" at this time is important as a framework for discussion that can either be emended by new data or overthrown in favor of a more accurate concept by future workers. The essence of the argument I am offering is that it is possible to achieve a definition of DVR that can adequately be applied to both reptiles and birds, and that DVR plays a particular role, that of a sensory linkage, in the generation of behavior in these animals. (I will explain what I mean by a sensory linkage in Chapter 1.) It seemed to me particularly important from the outset that there be a "discussion of the facts involved" because there is at this time no one place where all the relevant information is brought together. Much of Chapters 2 through 6 is thus filled with relatively specific accounts of data on the development, anatomy, and physiology of DVR. These sections may exceed in detail the taste of some readers (who will want to proceed quickly to Chapter 7), but I am unapologetic in feeling that an exposition of this sort is currently important to the field.

I was relatively slow to accept the need for a discussion of the "principles involved." However, a series of conversations at scientific meetings over the past few years and many, very useful discussions in my Department with Professor Larramendi have gradually convinced me that an examination of strategies and tactics is at least as important at this time as is a recitation of the facts of the matter. Chapter 7 is therefore principally concerned with applying the facts and elements of the argument that occupies the initial chapters to general problems in vertebrate biology and neurobiology. I think that a particularly important issue here is what strategy to use in comparing the results obtained on reptiles and birds to those obtained for other groups of vertebrates. The traditional approach used by neuroanatomists working on nonmammalian vertebrates has been to seek comparisons based on homology or commonality of ancestry, often being motivated by a desire to recreate or in some way understand the evolution of human brains. By contrast, neurobiologists studying invertebrates have tended to adopt more functional approaches and have been generally more successful in making contact with behavior. The last half of Chapter 7 is devoted to a discussion of these two approaches as applied to DVR and related structures. The general conclusion is that comparisons based on homology are difficult to apply to groups of animals that are as widely separated as are reptiles and birds versus mammals. The suggestion is that the concept of sensory linkages may be profitably used as a basis for comparisons of forebrain organization in the three groups of animals and that it can be more easily related to aspects of behavior.

As to the "conclusions reached," the major conclusion has to be that we are in our understanding of the forebrains of reptiles and birds at a level of understanding that was reached in studies of the cerebral cortex of mammals a hundred years ago: it is for the first time possible to accurately and more or less completely sketch out the general pattern of forebrain organization of reptiles and birds. The good news, so to speak, is that the technologies and ideas developed for studies on the brains of mammals can be borrowed wholesale and applied to studies on reptiles and birds. My prediction is that progress in understanding forebrain organization in these forms will advance significantly during the next two decades.

I am indebted to Drs. D. B. Newman and L. M. H. Larramendi for making available material that has been used in preparing this manuscript. Drs. Anton Reiner and Laura Bruce provided me with unpublished manuscripts. Professor Larramendi and Dr. Reiner also carefully read the manuscript and suggested many significant improvements in the final draft. Shirley Aumiller and Maryellen Kurek aided me in preparing many of the illustrations. Dorothy Crowder and Debra Randall were uncommonly patient in typing several "last" drafts of the manuscript. The National Institutes of Health and the National Science Foundation have funded aspects of my personal research that have contributed directly to many of the ideas expressed here.

Philip S. Ulinski

Chicago, Illinois
August 1983

CONTENTS

1. **What Is DVR?**   1

2. **Embryology and a Definition of DVR**   11

   2.1. Early Embryology   11
   2.2. Late Embryology   15
       Snakes   15
       Lizards   15
       Rhynchocephalians   17
       Turtles   18
       Crocodilians   19
       Birds   21
   2.3. An Embryological Definition of DVR   29

3. **Two Patterns of DVR Organization**   33

   3.1. Snakes   35
   3.2. Lizards   48
       ADVR in Type II Lizards   49
       ADVR in Type I Lizards   52
       BDVR in Lizards   56
       Striatum in Lizards   57
   3.3. Rhynchocephalians   60
   3.4. Turtles   60

3.5. Definition of the First Pattern of DVR Organization   71
3.6. Crocodilians   75
3.7. Birds   77
      ADVR in Birds   77
      BDVR in Birds   83
      Striatum in Birds   86
3.8. Definition of the Second Pattern of DVR Organization   88

4. **Sensory Afferents to DVR and Striatum:**
    First Steps in the Linkages   91

4.1. Thalamic Afferents   92
      Sensory Thalamic Nuclei   92
      Thalamic Nuclei Involved in Diffuse Projections   140
      The Problem of Thalamostriate Projections   142
4.2. Cortical Afferents to ADVR   143
      Lizards   143
      Turtles   143
      Birds   143
4.3. Afferents to BDVR   145
      Nonolfactory Afferents   145
      Olfactory Afferents   145
4.4. Modality Specific Areas in DVR   148

5. **Brainstem Afferents to DVR: A Digression**   151

5.1. Monoaminergic Systems   152
      Lizards   152
      Turtles   153
      Crocodilians   154
      Birds   154
5.2. Thick Caliber Systems   157
      Snakes   158
      Lizards   158
      Turtles   158
5.3. Parallel Pathways from the Brainstem   158

6. **Efferent Connections: Last Steps in the Linkages**   161

6.1. Efferents from ADVR   161
      Snakes   *162*
      Lizards   *162*
      Turtles   *164*
      Crocodilians   *166*
      Birds   *166*
6.2. Efferents from the Striatum   171
      Lizards   *171*
      Turtles   *171*
      Crocodilians   *172*
      Birds   *173*
6.3. Efferents from BDVR   176
      Snakes   *176*
      Birds   *177*
6.4. Sensory–Motor and Sensory–Hypothalamic Linkages   179

7. **Telencephalic Pattern and Function: Strategies
    of Comparison**   **183**

7.1. Structural Features of DVR   184
      Neuronal Structure   *184*
      Thalamic Afferents   *185*
      Modality Specific Areas   *186*
      Radial Organization   *189*
      Nonthalamic Afferents   *190*
      Efferent Projections   *191*
      Two Patterns of DVR Organization   *192*
7.2. Sensory–Motor and Sensory–Hypothalamic Linkages   194
7.3. Comparisons with the Forebrain of Mammals   200
      Comparisons Based on Homology   *200*
      Comparisons Based on Design   *212*
      Sensory Linkages in Reptiles, Birds, and Mammals   *229*

REFERENCES   235

AUTHOR INDEX   267

SUBJECT INDEX   275

Dorsal Ventricular Ridge

Chapter One

WHAT IS DVR?

The dorsal ventricular ridge (DVR) is a forebrain structure characteristic of the brains of reptiles and birds. From a structural viewpoint, it forms the lateral walls of the telencephalon and protrudes into the lateral ventricle. This is illustrated in Figure 1.1, which shows the position of DVR in the telencephalon of a turtle brain in lateral and dorsal views. DVR is the stippled mass that extends from the ventrolateral wall of the cerebral hemisphere into the lateral ventricle. It is divided by a sulcus (indicated by the arrow) into an anterior part called the anterior dorsal ventricular ridge (ADVR) and a more caudally situated part called the basal dorsal ventricular ridge (BDVR). DVR has the same general position in all reptiles and birds. It is always divisible into ADVR and BDVR, although BDVR is called the archistriatum in the literature on birds.

The central theme of this book is that, from a functional viewpoint, DVR forms a *linkage* between the principal sources of sensory information to the telencephalon and some of the brain structures that modulate behavior. In general, sensory linkages are definable sequences of neurons that carry information from sensory receptors to structures in the brain which modulate behavior. The simplest sensory linkages involve the projections of primary afferents that receive information from muscle spindles and terminate directly on motoneurons. Somewhat more complicated linkages carry information from peripheral mechanoreceptors to interneurons that can modulate the firing patterns of motoneurons. Still more complicated linkages involve sensory projections to brainstem structures, such as the optic tectum, that project to the reticular formation of the brainstem or to the other sources of the descending pathways that modulate the activity of motoneurons. The most complex sensory linkages involve components of the telencepha-

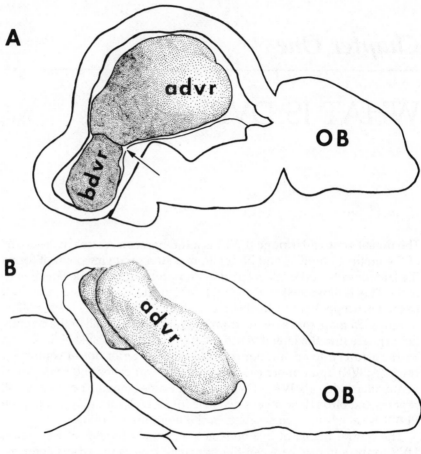

FIGURE 1.1.   Position of dorsal ventricular ridge. The position of dorsal ventricular ridge (DVR) in the telencephalon is illustrated in the case of the red-eared turtle, *Pseudemys scripta*. Lateral (A) and dorsal (B) views of the telencephalon are shown. DVR is the shaded mass that protrudes into the lateral ventricle. It is divided into two main parts, the anterior dorsal ventricular ridge (ADVR) and the basal dorsal ventricular ridge (BDVR), by a sulcus (arrow). *Abbreviation:* **OB,** olfactory bulb. From Balaban (1978a).

lon. Thus, ADVR receives information from the visual, auditory, and somatosensory systems and projects to the striatum, which lies in the basal forebrain and is a source of efferents to those descending pathways that modulate the activity of motoneurons (Fig. 1.2). It is thus likely that ADVR is part of a sequence of neuronal connections involved in the modulation of movement by sensory information. BDVR receives

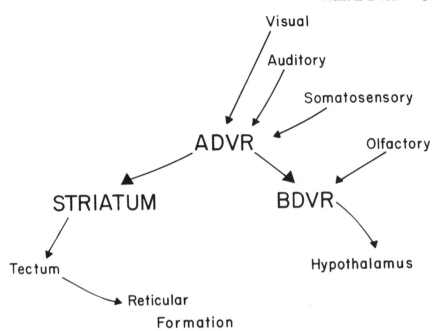

FIGURE 1.2. Sensory linkages. The roles of ADVR and BDVR as sensory linkages are summarized in this diagram. ADVR receives visual, auditory, and somatosensory projections from the thalamus and projects to BDVR. BDVR also receives chemical sensory information from the accessory or main olfactory bulbs. ADVR projects to motor systems in the reticular formation via the striatum and optic tectum. BDVR projects to the hypothalamus.

olfactory projections and is also in potential receipt of sensory information from ADVR. It projects, in turn, to the hypothalamus. It is thus likely that BDVR is involved in the modulation of hypothalamic activity by sensory information.

From an evolutionary viewpoint, DVR is one of several different elaborations of the telencephalon, each of which participates in sensory linkages. The telencephalon develops universally in vertebrates as a vesicle at the rostral end of the neural tube, but its subsequent development varies (Fig. 1.3). In bony fishes, the walls of the telencephalon fold back or evert (Nieuwenhuys, 1982). In other vertebrates, the walls of the telencephalon evaginate or pouch outwards to form cerebral hemispheres that contain lateral ventricles. In lungfishes and amphibians the walls of the cerebral hemispheres are relatively unmodified (Northcutt and Kicliter, 1980). In sharks, the hemispheric walls thicken and form a dorsally situated central nucleus (Northcutt, 1978b). In reptiles and in

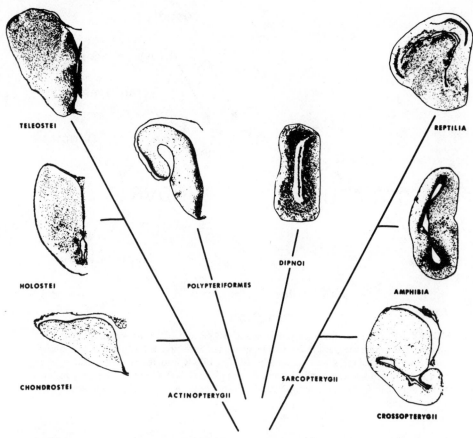

FIGURE 1.3.   Nonmammalian forebrains. Cross sections through the telencephalons of representatives of each of the major groups of nonmammalian vertebrates are shown. These can be compared to a similar cross section of the telencephalon of a mammal in Figure 1.4. From Northcutt (1981).

birds, DVR develops from the dorsolateral walls of the cerebral hemispheres and protrudes into the lateral ventricles. In mammals, the basal ganglia develop from the floor of the hemispheres and protrude into the lateral ventricles, whereas the roof of the telencephalon expands to form the laminated isocortex (Fig. 1.4). Regardless of which elaboration occurs, the telencephalon receives sensory information via projections from nuclei in the thalamus and gives rise to efferent projections that ultimately modulate both motoneurons and the hypothalamus (Northcutt, 1981).

An initial answer to the question posed by the title of this chapter is

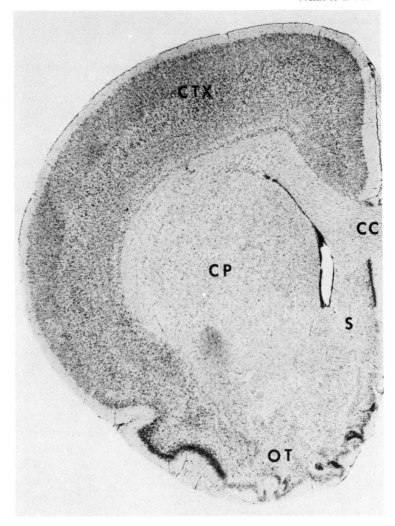

FIGURE 1.4. Mammal forebrain. A cross section through the telencephalon of a rat is shown to compare to those of the nonmammals in Figure 1.3. *Abbreviations:* **CC,** corpus callosum; **CP,** caudate-putamen; **CTX,** cortex; **OT,** olfactory tubercle; **S,** septum.

therefore that DVR is a component in one of several different variants of a basic, vertebrate pattern of brain organization: the telencephalon receives sensory information and projects to other regions of the brain in vertebrates. An overall understanding of the uses of sensory information in modulating vertebrate behavior must then rest ultimately on detailed accounts of each of the major variants of telencephalic structure and function, including DVR in the case of reptiles and birds. The information needed to provide a more detailed concept of DVR has accumulated slowly.

John Hunter, the English surgeon and comparative anatomist, first described DVR as an eminence in the lateral ventricle of a turtle brain that he dissected more than 200 years ago (Hunter, 1861). Owen (1866) restricted himself to noting the existence of similar eminences in other reptiles, but nineteenth century neuroanatomists such as Edinger, Meyer, and Ariëns Kappers devoted substantial effort to cytoarchitectural studies of DVR in a variety of reptiles and birds because of the structure's importance to theories of forebrain evolution (Ariëns Kappers, Huber, and Crosby, 1936). At this time, most authorities viewed DVR as homologous to the mammalian basal ganglia and described it using the term "striatum." The term "dorsal ventricular ridge" was coined by J. B. Johnston (1915) in a study of the forebrain of a turtle, *Terrapene carolina*. There were subsequent descriptions of DVR, most importantly by Crosby (1917) and Goldby (1934), but the experimental investigations of DVR's connections necessary to appreciate DVR's position in the brain were hampered without techniques for tracing the unmyelinated fibers that dominate the forebrains of nonmammals. The consensus in the mid-1960s was that neither DVR nor cortex receive direct thalamic, sensory projections in reptiles (Kruger and Berkowitz, 1960; Powell and Kruger, 1960) or birds (Powell and Cowan, 1961) and virtually nothing was known of its efferent projections.

This situation changed rapidly with the first applications of Nauta techniques for tracing axons in the sensory systems of nonmammals (Ebbesson, 1970). Karten (1967) showed that DVR receives direct projections from the auditory thalamus in pigeons. Karten and Hodos (1970) showed that DVR also receives direct projections from a visual nucleus in the thalamus of pigeons, and Hall and Ebner (1970b) reported analogous findings in the red-eared turtle, *Pseudemys scripta*. The application of tracing techniques based on axonal transport (Cowan and Cuénod, 1975) in the second half of the decade permitted studies of some connections of the striatal centers that lie under DVR, embedded in its afferent and efferent fiber systems, and that link DVR to the brainstem. Most recently, Golgi techniques have been applied to DVR in reptiles (e.g., Northcutt, 1970; Balaban, 1978a) and birds (Palacios, 1976) giving some idea of DVR's internal organization. These anatomical investigations were paralleled during the 1970s by physiological studies of the sensory systems that lead to DVR, principally in birds, and of the behavioral roles of DVR using the techniques of experimental psychology and psychophysics (e.g., Hodos, 1976) and of neuroethology (e.g., Greenberg, 1977, 1978).

The beginning of the 1980s is thus the first time since John Hunter's original observation that the minimal information necessary for a detailed appreciation of DVR and its place in the brains of reptiles and birds is available. What we know, in the broadest of terms, is that DVR is a telencephalic structure that can potentially link sensory information that reaches the forebrain via projections from thalamic sensory nuclei and from the olfactory system to regions of the brain that are directly implicated in modulating behavior. There has been, however, no attempt to synthesize the information that is available on the avenues by which sensory information reaches DVR, on the intrinsic organization of DVR, or on the organization of the pathways that carry information away from DVR to other brain regions.

What is needed is an account of the organization of DVR that is comparable to our current picture of the organization of the isocortex of mammals, whose position in the organization of mammalian brains is analogous to that of DVR in the brains of reptiles and birds. It is known, for example, that the isocortex develops by an outwards, radial migration of neuroblasts from the ventricular surface of the telencephalon (e.g., Sidman and Rakic, 1973; Jones, 1981b). These migrations result in a basic pattern of six cellular layers (e.g., Lorente de Nó, 1938) with regional variations that correspond to cortical areas defined by characteristic responses to sensory stimulation of the periphery (e.g., Woolsey, 1981a,b, 1982) or to electrical stimulation of cortical neurons (e.g., Phillips and Porter, 1977). The neurons in the isocortex include pyramidal cells in the third and fifth layers as well as several varieties of nonpyramidal neurons (e.g., Lund, 1981; Jones, 1981a). The nonpyramidal neurons are major targets for the thalamic afferents that carry sensory information to the isocortex (e.g., White, 1979). They are also involved in vertically aligned connections within the isocortex forming a partial substrate for the cortical columns or bands that seem to be a feature of each region of isocortex (e.g., Mountcastle, 1979). Pyramidal neurons are now known to receive sensory information directly from the thalamus (e.g., White, 1979) as well as via intracortical connections effected by the axons of nonpyramidal neurons (e.g., Peters and Regidor, 1981). They serve as the source of connections between isocortical regions and of efferent projections to other regions of the brain (e.g., Jones and Wise, 1977). These include projections to the superior colliculus, basal ganglia, spinal cord, and brainstem that certainly play indirect and direct roles in modulating the activity of motoneurons. In addition, isocortical projections to the amygdala (e.g., Turner, Mishkin, and Knapp, 1980) establish relations between the isocortex and the hypothalamus via amygdalar efferents to the hypothalamus. We therefore know that the isocortex is involved in linkages between sensory infor-

mation that is afferent to the telencephalon and descending telencephalic pathways, but we also know something of the design of each step
in the linkages.

The goal of this book is to go as far as is currently possible in elaborat-
ing a comparable picture of the organization of DVR in both reptiles and
birds. An analysis of this type should, of course, contribute significantly
to our understanding of the neural bases of behavior in reptiles and
birds by providing a general context for investigations of specific behaviors such as the control of song in birds and the generation of display
behaviors in lizards which are currently under way in many laborato-
ries. However, it is likely that a comprehensive understanding of DVR
organization will also help to better understand something of the general rules and principles that underlie the design of the nervous system,
particularly of the telencephalon.

The task of providing a cohesive account of DVR organization in
reptiles and birds is complicated by the substantial variation present in
the forebrains of these animals, presumably reflecting the fact that they
represent the endpoints of several evolutionary lines that developed and
radiated in parallel during the Mesozoic era. In addition, studies of the
various species of reptiles and birds have usually been conducted independently, with individual authors employing their own nomenclatures, so there is no consistent nomenclature or concept of DVR and
related structures. It is therefore necessary to delineate both the basic
pattern of DVR's structure and the variations that occur on this pattern.

The first step must be to establish a definition of DVR that holds for
all of the groups of reptiles and birds. This is achieved in Chapter 2,
which considers the embryology of DVR for each of the major groups. It
turns out that there is an embryological similarity underlying the variations of DVR structure that occur in adult brains that permits the formulation of a general definition of DVR. Chapter 3 is a survey of these
variations and tentatively defines two patterns of DVR organization.
One is characteristic of all of the reptiles except crocodilians; the other is
seen in crocodilians and in birds. The delineation of these patterns forms
the basis for a treatment of the pathways that carry information to DVR.
Chapter 4 considers the sources of sensory information to DVR and
identifies modality specific areas within DVR. Chapter 5 considers the
several, parallel brainstem projections to DVR and the striatum. Finally,
Chapter 6 completes the analysis by examining the efferent projections
from DVR that link it to those brainstem structures that modulate movement and to the hypothalamus. These four chapters review the data
available on each step in the flow of information to and from DVR and
provide the justification for considering DVR as a step in a set of sensory

linkages. Chapter 7 returns to some of the broader functional and evolutionary questions that surround DVR. It first summarizes the major features of DVR and then turns to a comparison of DVR to equivalent structures in the forebrains of mammals. The pros and cons of comparisons based on homology are evaluated. Comparisons based on the design of sensory linkages are then explored and the chapter concludes with a consideration of some of the functional similarities and differences between mammals and reptiles and birds.

Chapter Two

EMBRYOLOGY AND
A DEFINITION OF DVR

Fundamental insights can often be gained in comparative discussions by examining the embryology of the structure under consideration. In the case of DVR, the early embryology of the forebrain is the same in reptiles and birds and the major structural differences seen between adults of different species arise from differences that occur later in development. This chapter surveys the development of the dorsal telencephalon in each major taxonomic group of reptiles and birds. The basic similarity in developmental patterns that emerges from this discussion is then used to frame a definition of DVR that holds for both reptiles and birds and that can be used as the basis for comparisons of adult DVR structure in the next chapter.

2.1. EARLY EMBRYOLOGY

The early embryology of the brain (Fig. 2.1) is similar in snakes (Herrick, 1892; Källén, 1951), lizards (Tandler and Kantor, 1907; Hetzel, 1974; Källén, 1951; Senn, 1979), *Sphenodon* (Wyeth, 1924), turtles (Holmgren, 1925; Källén, 1951; Kirsche, 1972), crocodilians (Reese, 1910; Neumayer, 1914; Källén, 1951), and birds (Kamon, 1906; Rogers, 1960). The telencephalon forms by a bilateral evagination of the rostral neural tube, thus forming the interventricular foramina and lateral ventricles. The telencephalic walls are first composed entirely of neuroepithelial cells and are equally thick dorsally and ventrally.

11

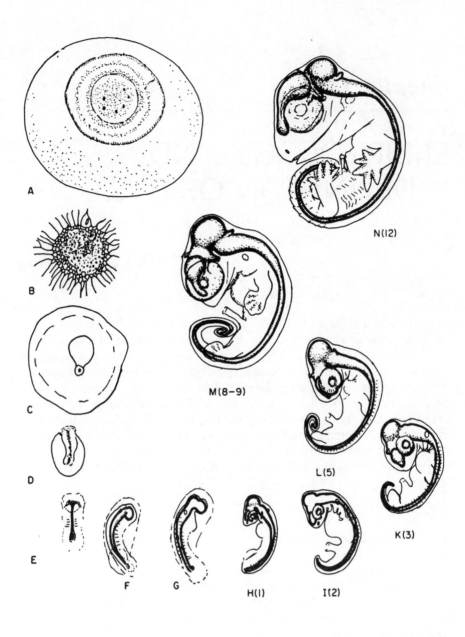

FIGURE 2.1. Overview of embryology. The overall pattern of the development of the brain is shown in the case of the lizard *Lacerta sicula*. A–F show the cleavage pattern of the egg and the extent of embryonic development within the oviduct. G is an embryo at

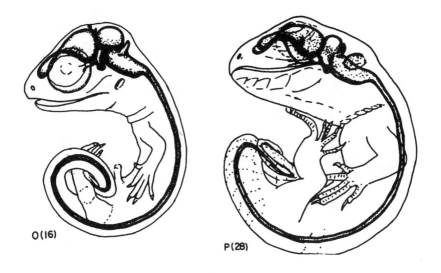

O(16)

P(28)

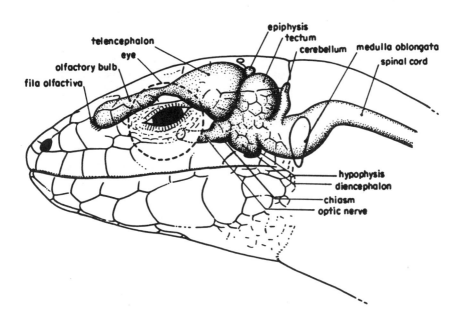

filo olfactiva
olfactory bulb
eye
telencephalon
epiphysis
tectum
cerebellum
medulla oblongata
spinal cord
hypophysis
diencephalon
chiasm
optic nerve

the time of oviposition. H–P show embryos between oviposition and hatching. Embryonic stages are indicated by numbers (in parentheses) of incubation days at 30°C. Q is a lateral view of an adult brain *in situ* showing major structures. From Senn (1979).

13

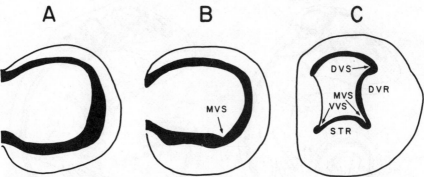

FIGURE 2.2. Early development of DVR. The stages of DVR development that are common to all species of reptiles and birds are summarized. (A) A section through the right telencephalic hemisphere shortly after its evagination. The dorsal hemispheric wall is thinner than is the ventral wall, but there are no ventricular sulci. (B) The middle ventricular sulcus (MVS) has appeared and separates the dorsally situated pallium from the ventrally situated striatum. (C) The dorsal ventricular sulcus (DVS) divides the pallium into the cortex (not labeled) and DVR. The middle ventricular sulcus (MVS) and the ventral ventricular sulcus (VVS) form the borders of the striatum (STR). The neuroepithelial layer is shown in black.

Differentiation continues as a consequence of the proliferation and growth of neuroblasts at particular regions of the neuroepithelium, leading to local thickenings of the telencephalic wall (Jacobson, 1978; Lund, 1978; Cooke, 1980). Transitions to regions in which other proliferations are occurring are marked by sulci or grooves on the ventricular wall. The results of these processes are common to all reptiles and birds (snakes: Warner, 1946; lizards: Källén, 1951; Hetzel, 1974; *Sphenodon:* Hines, 1923; turtles: Johnston, 1916; Holmgren, 1925; Källén, 1951; Kirsche, 1972; crocodilians: Källén, 1951; birds: e.g., Kuhlenbeck, 1938; Jones and Levi-Montalcini, 1958; Källén, 1962). They are shown diagrammatically in Figure 2.2, which illustrates four sections through the telencephalon shortly after the evagination of the cerebral hemispheres. In the earliest section (Fig. 2.2A), the walls of the ventral telencephalon are thickest because the proliferation of neuroblasts begins ventrally. A short time later (Fig. 2.2B), the lateral wall of the telencephalon is divided into dorsal and ventral components by a middle ventricular sulcus (MVS). Proliferation continues in the dorsal half of the telencephalon so that two major bulges are separated by three ventricular sulci (Fig. 2.2C). The dorsal ventricular sulcus (DVS) separates the cortex from the anlage of DVR. The middle ventricular sulcus (MVS) separates the DVR anlage from that of the striatum (STR). The ventral ventricular sulcus (VVS) forms the ventral border of the striatum.

2.2. LATE EMBRYOLOGY

Neuroblasts continue to migrate away from the neuroepithelium between the dorsal and middle ventricular sulci as development proceeds and thereby cause a progressive thickening of DVR. They invariably migrate in two pulses, consequently forming two masses of neuroblasts separated by a cell-poor zone called the zona limitans. However, the details of these processes vary between groups. In particular, reptiles show a developmental pattern in which DVR undergoes a relative ingrowth causing it to protrude into the lateral ventricle throughout its rostrocaudal extent. By contrast, DVR retains much of its embryonic position in birds, and the rostral extent of the lateral ventricle maintains a slit-like appearance. The details of these processes in individual groups of reptiles and birds will now be considered.

Snakes

Warner (1946) studied forebrain development in water snakes (*Natrix sipedon*) and water moccasins (*Agkistrodon piscivorus*) using 40 embryos that were described in terms of unspecified lengths. Källén (1951) studied 14 specimens of the grass snake (*Natrix natrix*). These studies show that DVR development in snakes conforms to the reptilian pattern. The hemisphere is divided into four sectors by ventricular sulci in Warner's 35-mm embryo (Fig. 2.3A) and the ventrolateral sector could be subdivided by a middle ventricular sulcus (sulcus interstriaticus) into a ventral and thicker striatum (paleostriatum) and a dorsal DVR (neostriatum). DVR is delimited dorsally by a dorsal ventricular sulcus. In 45-mm stages (Fig. 2.3B), DVR is a thick bulge protruding into the ventricle and bounded dorsally by lateral cortex. The same situation persists in 55-mm embryos (Fig. 2.3C), except that the zona limitans now lies ventrolateral to DVR. The mantle layer of DVR is continuous with that of lateral cortex. The fibers of the lateral forebrain bundle that carry thalamic afferents to DVR can be seen in a cell-poor zone ventral to DVR in 65-mm embryos. DVR essentially attains its adult form by 70-mm stages through a relative growth into the lateral ventricle. A cell-poor zone thus forms DVR's ventral border and the lateral cortex occupies its adult position on the lateral surface of the forebrain (Fig. 2.3D,E).

Lizards

Källén (1951) gives a brief treatment of development in *Lacerta* sp. and *Chamaeleo* sp., but Hetzel (1974) provides a more extensive treatment of

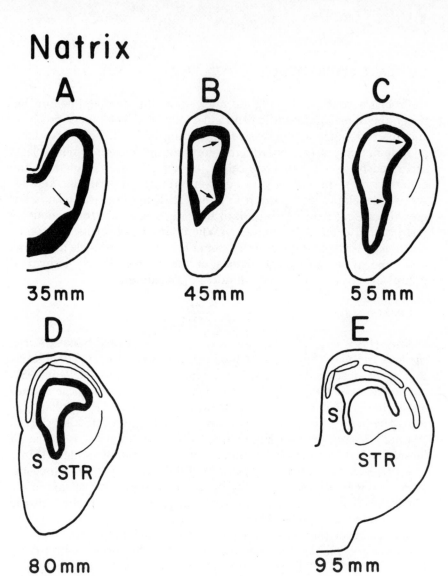

Natrix

A
35mm

B
45mm

C
55mm

D
80mm

E
95mm

FIGURE 2.3. DVR development in snakes. The development of DVR in the water snake (*Natrix sipedon*) is summarized from the work of Warner (1946). Embryonic stages are given in terms of unspecified lengths. (A) The middle ventricular sulcus (arrow) marks the boundary of the pallium and striatum. (B) The borders of DVR are marked by the dorsal ventricular sulcus (upper arrow) and middle ventricular sulcus (lower arrow). (C) DVR now bulges medially into the lateral ventricle and is separated from the lateral cortex by the zona limitans (thin line). (D) DVR has begun its rotation into the lateral ventricle. The zona limitans shifts ventrolaterally and separates DVR from the striatum (STR). (E) The rotation of DVR is complete. A cell-poor zone lies ventral to DVR and lateral cortex has its adult position. *Other abbreviation:* **S**, septum. The neuroepithelial layer is shown in black. The magnification was not indicated in Warner's figures.

Lacerta

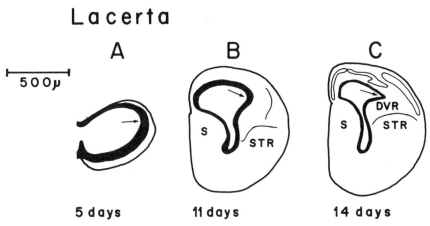

FIGURE 2.4. DVR development in lizards. The development of DVR in *Lacerta sicula* is shown based on the work of Hetzel (1974). (A) The middle ventricular sulcus (arrow) separates the pallium from striatum. (B) The dorsal ventricular sulcus (arrow) marks the dorsal boundary of DVR. DVR has begun to bulge into the ventricle. It is separated laterally from the lateral cortex by the zona limitans and ventrally from the striatum (STR) by a cell-poor zone. (C) DVR's rotation into the lateral ventricle continues. Lateral cortex has its adult position and the adult relationship between DVR and the striatum has been established. *Other abbreviation:* **S**, septum. The neuroepithelium layer is shown in black.

telencephalic development in *Lacerta sicula*. Eggs hatch 31 days after being laid, but some development takes place prior to laying. The hemispheric vesicle is formed by the third embryonic day. A middle ventricular sulcus (sulcus terminalis) appears during the fifth day. The later development of DVR is not described in detail, but its general features seem to resemble those seen in snakes (Fig. 2.4B,C).

Rhynchocephalians

Hines (1923) described telencephalic development in *Sphenodon* using 14 embryos from the collection prepared by Dendy (1899). She used Dendy's alphabetical designation of embryological stages. The telencephalic vesicle is not divided by ventricular sulci in stage N, but is divided into sectors by stage P (Fig. 2.5A) where a middle ventricular sulcus (sulcus interstriaticus) is present on the lateral wall of the vesicle. Above this sulcus, a zona limitans lies external to cells migrating from the ependyma. By stage PQ (Fig. 2.5B) a dorsal ventricular sulcus (sulcus superstriaticus) lies above DVR (neostriatum), which is bordered laterally by the zona limitans. Lateral cortex lies external to this zone. DVR increases in size through stage Q and protrudes markedly into the ventricle. DVR

Sphenodon

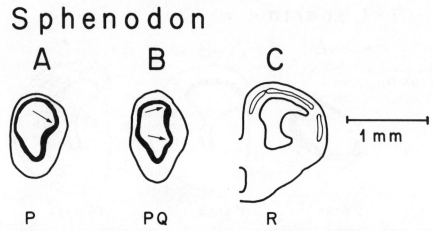

FIGURE 2.5.   DVR development in *Sphenodon*. The development of DVR in the tuatara (*Sphenodon punctatum*) is shown based on Hines's (1923) work. Embryological stages are designated alphabetically (P, PQ, R) according to Dendy (1899). (A) The middle ventricular sulcus (arrow) separates the pallium from the striatum, which bulges into the ventricle. (B) The borders of DVR are marked by the dorsal ventricular sulcus (upper arrow) and the middle ventricular sulcus (lower arrow). (C) DVR bulges into the lateral ventricle. The neuroepithelial layer is shown in black.

is somewhat larger in stage R (Fig. 2.5C), but it is not quite as pronounced as in adults.

Turtles

DVR development has been studied in two genera of turtles. It has been studied in painted turtles, *Chrysemys marginata* and *C. picta*, by Johnston (1916; three specimens), Holmgren (1925; 22 specimens) and Källén (1951; nine specimens). Ages can be designated by carapace length. Both Källén and Holmgren recognized dorsal and ventral components of the telencephalic vesicle (d and c migrations and dorsal and ventral areas, respectively), but Holmgren used the presence of a zona limitans as a boundary criterion and placed the division of the vesicle into components somewhat later in developmental time than did Källén. Both authors recognized that two major groups of neuroblasts migrate away from the neuroepithelium of the dorsal components. The first migration (secondary cortex or d^{I+II} migration) forms lateral cortex. Holmgren stressed that this first group of neuroblasts comes to lie lateral to the zona limitans. The second major migration comes to lie medial to the zona limitans. It is under way in animals with carapaces of about 6 mm (Holmgren, Källén), is bounded ventrally by the middle ventricular sulcus (sulcus a of Källén), and forms DVR. The dorsal ventricular sulcus (sulcus d of Källén) is not clear at 12- or 13-mm stages (Holmgren, Källén), but is present by 17- and 22-mm stages (Johnston, Källén). DVR expands and protrudes into the ventricle during later developmental stages.

Kirsche (1972) studied forebrain development in the tortoise *Testudo h. hermanni* using 23 embryos and provides particularly good photographs of forebrain sections. The development of the dorsal telencephalon is essentially as in *Chrysemys*. Neuroblasts begin migrating away from the neuroepithelium of the dorsal component by day 18. These cells form a distinct migration, separated from cells in a second migration by a zona limitans between days 23 (carapace length 6.5 mm; Fig. 2.6A) and 27 (carapace length 8.0 mm). A middle ventricular sulcus is present by day 30 (carapace length 10.5 mm; Fig. 2.6B) and the dorsal ventricular sulcus by day 34 (carapace length 13.0 mm; Fig. 2.6C). DVR (epistriatum) subsequently enlarges and protrudes into the ventricle, but the cytoarchitectonic areas of DVR (see Section 3.4) are not clear at 48 days (Fig. 2.6D), the latest stage illustrated.

Crocodilians

Källén (1951) studied 21 embryos of *Alligator mississippiensis*. A middle ventricular sulcus (sulcus a) is present in an 11-mm embryo (Fig. 2.7A). By 15 mm (Fig. 2.7B), DVR has formed, bounded below by the middle ventricular sulcus and above by the dorsal ventricular sulcus (sulcus d). DVR changes in contour with further growth. The middle ventricular sulcus becomes shallow and the dorsal ventricular sulcus becomes a deep fissure marking the lateral border of DVR. DVR begins to bulge into the ventricle by 24 mm (Fig. 2.7C). Källén identified four successive migrations of cells (d^I, d^{II}, d^{III}, and d^{IV}) between the two sulci. He felt that d^I and d^{II} contribute to cortical areas while d^{III} and d^{IV} fuse and form DVR. The striatum is derived from migrations ventral to the middle ventricular sulcus. The precise relation of lateral cortex to DVR is not clear from Källén's description.

In summary, differences in the timing of developmental events make it difficult to establish precise comparisons between species. However, the data available are sufficient to determine that there is a basic pattern of DVR development common to all of the reptiles.

Testudo

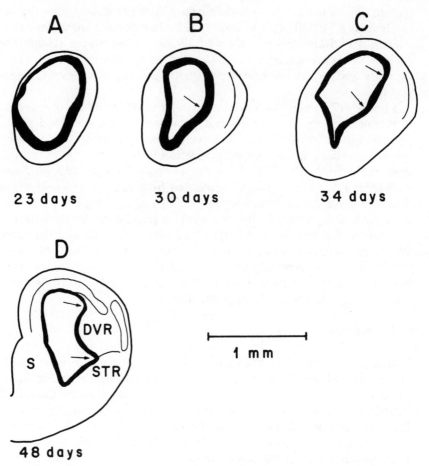

A

23 days

B

30 days

C

34 days

D

DVR

S

STR

48 days

1 mm

FIGURE 2.6. DVR development in turtles. The development of DVR in the tortoise, *Testudo hermanni*, is shown based on the work of Kirsche (1972). (A) The dorsal telencephalic wall is thinner than is the ventral wall. (B) The middle ventricular sulcus (arrow) separates the pallium from the striatum. The zona limitans (thin line) is forming in the lower pallium. (C) The dorsal ventricular sulcus (upper arrow) and the middle ventricular sulcus (lower arrow) mark the boundaries of DVR. DVR has grown wider so that the zona limitans is shifted laterally. (C) DVR has begun to rotate into the lateral ventricle. Lateral cortex has its adult position. A cell-poor zone separates DVR from the striatum (STR). *Other abbreviation:* **S,** septum. The neuroepithelial layer is shown in black.

Alligator

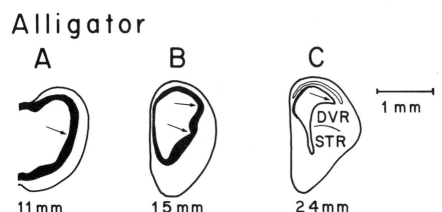

FIGURE 2.7. DVR development in crocodilians. The development of DVR in the American alligator (*Alligator mississippiensis*) is shown based on the work of Källén (1951). (A) The middle ventricular sulcus (arrow) separates the pallium from the striatum. (B) The dorsal ventricular sulcus (upper arrow) and the middle ventricular sulcus (lower arrow) mark the borders of DVR. (C) DVR has begun to rotate into the lateral ventricle. A cell-poor zone separates DVR from the striatum (STR). The neuroepithelial layer is shown in black.

Birds

The later stages of DVR development are somewhat different in birds. The majority of embryological studies of avian telencephalons have been conducted on chickens. Kuhlenbeck (1938) used 35 chick embryos and Källén (1962) used 27 embryos; both authors employed standard histological techniques. Jones and Levi-Montalcini (1958) used 78 embryos prepared with the DeCastro silver stain. Tsai, Garber, and Larramendi (1981a,b) used cumulative labeling with tritiated thymidine to determine birthdates and migration routes of telencephalic neurons. The ages of embryos have been designated either in days or in Hamburger–Hamilton stages (Hamburger and Hamilton, 1951).

Källén, Jones and Levi-Montalcini, and Tsai et al. provide descriptions of the overall pattern of telencephalic ontogenesis that are essentially identical. The lateral wall of the telencephalon is divided into dorsal and ventral parts by the proliferation of neuroblasts ventrally by the fifth day (H–H stages 25–27). Källén recognized two migrations (c^I and c^{II}) in the dorsal part of the ventral area. By day 6 (H–H stages 28–29), a fiber layer separates the dorsal and ventral components of the lateral hemispheric wall. Two successive migrations (d^I and d^{II}) can now be recognized in the dorsal component. By day 7 (H–H stages 30–32), a

Gallus

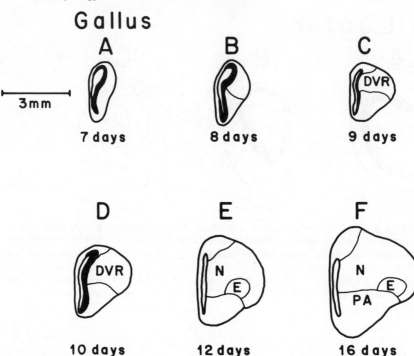

FIGURE 2.8. DVR development in birds. The development of DVR in the domestic chicken (*Gallus domesticus*) is shown based principally on the work of Tsai, Garber, and Larramendi (1981a,b). (A) The dorsal telencephalic wall is thin and the striatum bulges into the ventricle ventrally. (B) The dorsal medullary lamina (thin line) separates DVR (above) from the striatum (below). (C) DVR is bounded above by the frontal medullary lamina and below by the dorsal medullary lamina. (D) DVR continues to expand by a lateral migration of neuroblasts. (E) The ectostriatum (E) and neostriatum (N) can be distinguished in DVR. (F) DVR and the striatum have thin adult configurations. *Other abbreviation:* **PA,** paleostriatum augmentatum.

third migration (d^{111}) is visible in the ventrolateral dorsal component (Fig. 2.8A). The dorsal component shows its major expansion on day 8 (H–H stages 33–34; Fig. 2.8B). There is a strong development of the third migration and the lamina hyperstriatica, an adult fiber layer, is present. The adult configuration of nuclear groups is achieved at least superficially by the ninth day (H–H stages 35–36; Fig. 2.8C), although some important late migrations occur. Notice that the distinct ingrowth of DVR into the lateral ventricle that is characteristic of reptiles does not occur in birds.

There has also been a consensus concerning the origin of specific

DVR and striatal structures. However, it is necessary to comment on the nomenclature of avian DVR before their embryology can be described. Three terminologies have been used to designate the components of avian DVR. Rose (1914) recognized a number of fields that he designated by letters. Kuhlenbeck (1938) recognized a number of nuclei. The most widely used nomenclature is that of Ariens Kappers, Huber, and Crosby (1936). The relation between the terminology of Ariens Kappers, Huber, and Crosby and that of Rose and of Kuhlenbeck is summarized by Karten and Hodos (1967) and Pearson (1972). Atlases include those for pigeons (Karten and Hodos, 1967), chickens (van Tienhoven and Juhasz, 1962), and canaries (Stokes, Leonard, and Nottebohm, 1974).

As in reptiles, DVR in birds contains both ADVR and BDVR. ADVR is divided into several major subdivisions (Figs. 2.9 and 2.10). The hyperstriatum dorsale and hyperstriatum ventrale (HV) constitute the most dorsal subdivision. The hyperstriatum is bordered dorsally by the fibrous frontal medullary lamina (LFM). The hyperstriatum ventrale is bordered ventrally by the lamina hyperstriatica (LH). The neostriatum lies below the lamina hyperstriatica. It is the largest component and contains three parts. Neostriatum frontale (NF) is situated rostrally, neostriatum intermediale (NI) is centrally placed, and neostriatum caudale (NC) is situated caudally. A specific region in the neostriatum caudale is designated as field L (L) using Rose's terminology. The third subdivision of ADVR is the ectostriatal complex (E) which lies between the neostriatum and dorsal medullary lamina (LMD) in rostrolateral ADVR. Nucleus basalis (BAS) lies dorsal to the dorsal medullary lamina rostral to the ectostriatum. The temporo-parieto-occipital area covers the lateral aspect of the neostriatum. BDVR is called the archistriatum in birds. It is situated ventrolateral to ADVR and caudal to the anterior commissure.

The cortical component of the pallium is generally poorly developed in birds. However, many birds show an enlargement of a dorsal region of the pallium that forms a distinct swelling. It is referred to by its German name, the Wulst. The Wulst contains the hyperstriatum accessorium and intercalatus. These structures lie above the ventricle caudally, but are separated from the hyperstriatum dorsale by the lamina frontalis suprema rostrally.

Since birds do not have a well-developed lateral cortex, the first cells generated in the dorsal component of the telencephalon contribute instead to the external segments of the hyperstriatum that form the Wulst in adults. Autoradiographic studies (Tsai, Garber, and Larramendi, 1981a,b) indicate that these cells are born on days 5–9 (Figs. 2.11 and 2.12). They initially migrate laterally from the neuroepithelium and oc-

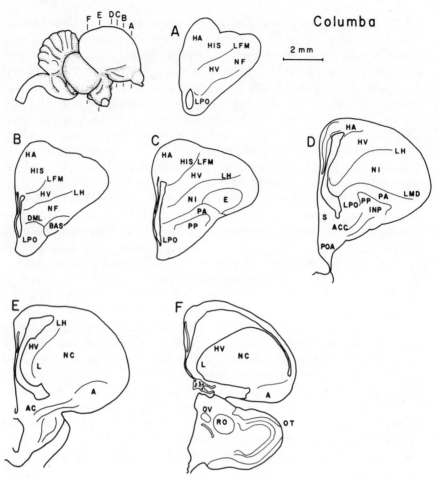

FIGURE 2.9. Schematic summary of subdivisions of avian DVR. The major components of the telencephalon in birds is diagrammed on a series of sections through the brain of a pigeon. DVR is bounded dorsally by the frontal medullary lamina (LFM) and the caudal extent of the lateral ventricle. It is bordered ventrally by the dorsal medullary lamina (LMD). Rostrally (sections A and B), DVR contains the hyperstriatum ventrale (HV), the frontal neostriatum (NF), and nucleus basalis (BAS). At intermediate levels (sections C and D), DVR contains the hyperstriatum ventrale (HV), the intermediate neostriatum (NI), and the ectostriatum (E). At caudal levels (sections E and F), DVR contains the hyperstriatum ventrale (HV) and the caudal neostriatum (NC). Field L is a subdivision of the caudal neostriatum. *Other abbreviations:* **A,** archistriatum; **AC,** anterior commissure; **ACC,** nucleus accumbens; **Ha,** hyperstriatum accessorium; **HIS,** hyperstriatum intercalatus superioris; **INP,** intrapeduncular nucleus; **LH,** lamina hyperstriatica; **LPO,** parolfactory lobe; **OT,** optic tectum; **OV,** nucleus ovoidalis; **PA,** paleostriatum augmentatum; **PP,** paleostriatum primitivum; **POA,** preoptic area of hypothalamus; **RO,** nucleus rotundus; **S,** septum.

24

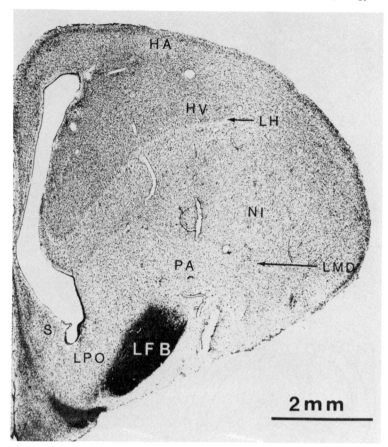

FIGURE 2.10.   ADVR in pigeon. Subdivisions of avian ADVR are shown in a cross section through the telencephalon of a pigeon. The level of the section corresponds to that of
section D in Figure 2.9. *Abbreviations:* **HA,** hyperstriatum accessorium; **HV,** hyperstriatum
ventrale; **LFB,** lateral forebrain bundle; **LH,** lamina hyperstriatica; **LMD,** dorsal medullary
lamina; **LPO,** parolfactory lobe; **NI,** neostriatum intermediale; **PA,** paleostriatum augmentatum; **S,** septum.

cupy a position in the lateral telencephalic wall adjacent to the ectostriatum. This point is of some interest because both populations of
neurons receive visual projections. Cells generated subsequently migrate laterally and separate the cells that form the Wulst from those that
form the ectostriatum. These cells with later birthdates form the neostriatum in the adult. The result of this sequence of migrations is that cells
destined to form the Wulst are shifted dorsomedially and come to lie on

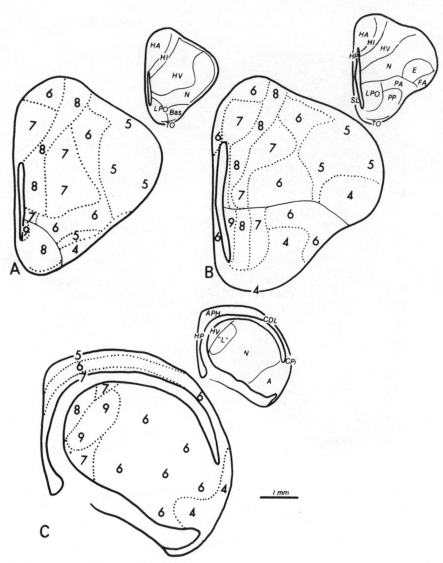

FIGURE 2.11. Isochrone birthdate maps of 16-day embryonic chick telencephalon. Dotted lines separate zones containing neurons with different birthdates. Since the range of birthdates can vary from 1 to several days, numbers represent the embryonic days on which 50% of the neurons were born. *Abbreviations:* **A,** archistriatum; **APH,** parahippocampal area; **BAS,** nucleus basalis; **CDL,** area corticalis dorsolateralis, **CPi,** piriform cortex; **E,** ectostriatum; **FA,** frontoarchistriatal path; **HA,** hyperstriatum accessorium; **HI,** hyperstriatum intercalatus; **HV,** hyperstriatum ventrale; **HP,** hippocampal area; **L,** field L; **LPO,** parolfactory lobe; **N,** neostriatum; **PA,** paleostriatum augmentatum; **PP,** paleostriatum primitivum; **SL,** septum; **TO,** olfactory tubercle. From Tsai, Garber, and Larramendi (1981a).

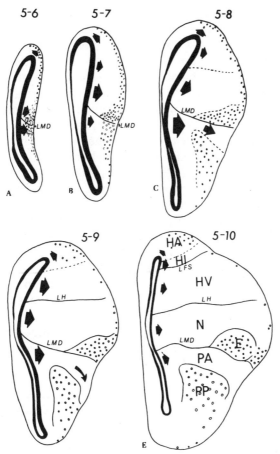

FIGURE 2.12. Tracings from autoradiographs of midtelencephalic sections of embryos fixed on days 5 through 10. Unlabeled cells are shown as open circles. They represent neurons generated before day 5. *Abbreviations:* **E,** ectostriatum; **HA,** hyperstriatum accessorium; **HI,** hyperstriatum intercalatus; **HV,** hyperstriatum ventrale; **LFS,** lamina frontalis suprema; **LH,** lamina hyperstriatica; **LMD,** dorsal medullary lamina; **PA,** paleostriatum augmentatum; **PP,** paleostriatum primitivum. From Tsai, Garber, and Larramendi (1981b).

the dorsal surface of the hemisphere. The neostriatum and ectostriatum develop from migrations that proceed laterally from the neuroepithelium. The cells situated laterally in the neostriatum are generally the first generated, so the structure shows an overall "outside-in" pattern, but some intermixing of cells with different birthdates does occur. Neurons in the ectostriatum are generated on days 4 and 5, conforming to an overall ventrodorsal gradient in birthdates.

Field L shows a particularly interesting developmental pattern. Its neurons are generated very late, on days 8 and 9 (Tsai, Garber, and Larramendi, 1981a,b). They migrate into their adult position by two separate migrations. The first originates in the ependyma of the dorsal component of the telencephalon, but the second originates from ependyma in the ventral component close to that which forms the parolfactory lobe. These neuroblasts migrate into field L in a stream that can be visualized in Golgi (Tsai, 1977) and silver (Jones and Levi-Montalcini, 1958) preparations. They reach field L by the twelfth day.

The striatum develops from neuroepithelium located ventral to the middle ventricular sulcus. Its principal parts are the paleostriatum primitivum, the paleostriatum augmentatum, and the lobus parolfactorius. Neurons in paleostriatum primitivum are generated on day 4 and move laterally in Källén's migration c^I. They initially lie next to the neostriatal and ectostriatal neurons of the dorsal component. However, neurons in the paleostriatum augmentatum are generated later, on days 4–7, and move laterally in Källén's migration c^{II}. In so doing, they move between the ectostriatum and paleostriatum primitivum and result in the adult configuration of ectostriatum, paleostriatum augmentatum, and paleostriatum primitivum, in dorsoventral sequence. The parolfactory lobe is generated on days 6–9 in the ventral component.

Jones and Levi-Montalcini (1958) report that the afferent fibers of the forebrain bundles are present on day 6. The efferent components seem to be generated on days 10–12.

Results obtained on other species of birds are less detailed, but are generally consistent with the developmental patterns seen in chickens. Källén (1953) studied nine pigeon embryos. Dorsal and ventral components are present in the lateral wall by a 7-mm stage (96 hours). Initial proliferations lead to d^I and d^{II} migrations in the dorsal component by a 9-mm stage. The third, d^{III}, migration is present in the dorsal component by a 12-mm stage and the ventral component shows c^I and c^{II} migrations. The d^{III} migration forms the neostriatum, ectostriatum, and field L. The c^I migration forms the paleostriatum primitivum; the c^{II} migration forms the paleostriatum augmentatum. Durward (1934) studied nine sparrows (*Passer domesticus*) that were designated in head lengths. The telencephalon is evaginated in a 5-mm stage. Dorsal and ventral components are formed in the lateral telencephalic wall by a 7-mm stage. The dorsal component contains inner and outer migrations. The dorsal medullary lamina separates the dorsal and ventral components by 8.0- and 8.5-mm stages. The paleostriatum is formed in a 14.5-mm stage. Haefelfinger (1958) describes telencephalic development in parakeets.

2.3. EMBRYOLOGICAL DEFINITION OF DVR

The overall similarity of telencephalic development in reptiles leads to a definition of DVR as the component of the telencephalon which grows into the lateral ventricle between the dorsal and middle ventricular sulci. This is shown in Figure 2.13 in the developmental sequence A,B,C. Comparison of this sequence to those in Figures 2.3–2.7 shows that this idea holds easily for all of the taxa of reptiles.

The term DVR is now also generally applied to the forebrains of birds. The developmental sequence A,B',C' in Figure 2.13 shows that the same definition holds at least as a first approximation for birds. However, some difficulties arise in achieving a precise definition of ADVR in birds. First, the absence of an ingrowth of DVR into the ventricle leads to some ambiguity in defining ADVR's lateral boundary in birds. This is not a difficulty in reptiles because the lateral recess of the lateral ventricle separates ADVR from the overlying cortex. However, ADVR is essentially continuous with the cortex dorsorostrally in birds. Thus, some parts of the "hyperstriatum" of Ariens Kappers, Huber, and Crosby (1936) are usually included as components of ADVR (hyperstriatum ventrale and dorsale), whereas others (hyperstriatum intercalatus, and accessorium) are usually included as components of the Wulst. However, it is necessary to trace the hyperstriatum ventrale caudally before it is evident that it lies below the lateral ventricle.

Further complications arise from other embryological considerations. The studies of Tsai, Garber and Larramendi (1981a,b) demonstrate that at least some of the neurons in the hyperstriatum accessorium originate from neuroepithelial cells near the middle ventricular sulcus. They, therefore, originate from the same region of the neuroepithelium as do ADVR neurons. However, they are shifted dorsomedially over the surface of the hemisphere to a final position in the Wulst. The studies of Jones and Levi-Montalcini (1958) and of Tsai (1977) show that at least some of the neurons in field L of the neostriatum originate by a late migration from neuroepithelium adjacent to the parolfactory lobe. Thus the neuroepithelium between the dorsal and middle ventricular sulci gives rise to some neurons that are not included in DVR, and DVR includes some neuronal populations that are generated in the ventral telencephalon. With these difficulties in mind, ADVR in birds will be defined here to include the hyperstriatum dorsale and ventrale, neostriatum, ectostriatum, nucleus basalis, and the temporo-parieto-occipital area. These are the structures that are topographically located between the dorsal and middle ventricular sulci in adults.

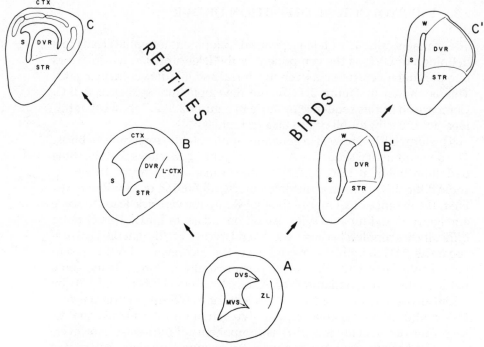

FIGURE 2.13. DVR development in reptiles and birds. Differences in the later stages of DVR development between reptiles and birds are summarized. (A) The stage depicted is slightly later than stage (C) of Figure 2.2. Two waves of neuroblasts have originated from the neuroepithelium bordered by the dorsal ventricular sulcus (DVS) and the middle ventricular sulcus (MVS). They are separated by the cell-poor zona limitans (ZL). Those lying external to the zona limitans contribute to the cortical component (lateral cortex in the reptiles; Wulst in birds) of the pallium. Those lying internal to the zona limitans contribute to DVR in both reptiles (B, C) and birds (B', C'). (B) The zona limitans separates DVR from lateral cortex (L-CTX). (C) The lateral cortex retains its external position and DVR has undergone a relative rotation into the lateral ventricle. It thus is bordered both laterally and medially by recesses of the lateral ventricle and is positioned dorsal to the striatum (STR). (B') Neuroblasts situated external to the zona limitans have shifted dorsomedially into the Wulst (W) and a cell-poor layer separates DVR from the striatum (STR). (C') The formation of the Wulst is almost completed and DVR has expanded in width by virtue of a continued, lateral migration of neuroblasts. Notice that the orientation of DVR has not changed from the embryonic orientation shown in (A). *Other abbreviations:* **CTX,** cortex; **S,** septum.

Subject to these qualifications, the basic developmental pattern seen in the forebrains of different groups of reptiles and birds is sufficiently similar to universally define DVR as the part of the telencephalon that develops between the dorsal and middle ventricular sulci. Equipped with this definition, the nature of DVR in adult reptiles and birds can now be considered in Chapter 3.

Chapter Three

TWO PATTERNS OF DVR ORGANIZATION

Chapter 2 established that DVR's basic form is a product of its early embryology and is, from a topological point of view, similar in all reptiles and birds. There are, however, striking interspecific differences in both the size and neuronal structure of adult DVRs that presumably reflect their subsequent histogenesis. Figure 3.1 provides an overview of the size and shape differences that occur in DVR. It shows drawings of transverse sections through ADVR from representatives of each of the major groups of reptiles and of birds.

The sections are all drawn to the same scale and therefore give some impression of the variation in size which occurs in DVR. Such differences in size must contribute significantly to the greater brain weight to body weight ratios of birds (Jerison, 1973), although there have not been adequate quantitative studies of this point. There is also variation in the relative size of the cerebral hemispheres within both the reptiles (e.g., Platel, 1979) and birds (e.g., Portmann and Stingelin, 1961). The general impression is that the hemispheres (and probably DVR) are larger in species with greater body weights, but that DVR in some species is larger than would be predicted solely as a function of body weight. This point has been established directly for lizards by Platel (1980a,b) who determined the variation in the volumes of the telencephalon and DVR per unit body weight for a series of lizards and showed that arboreal or highly visual forms tend to have relatively larger DVRs.

Variations in forebrain size occur within other vertebrate radiations such as sharks (Ebbesson and Northcutt, 1976; Northcutt, 1977), bony

33

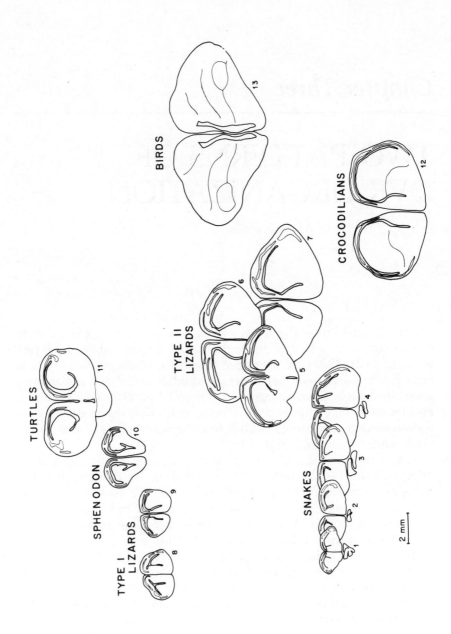

BIRDS

CROCODILIANS

TURTLES

TYPE II
LIZARDS

SPHENODON

TYPE I
LIZARDS

SNAKES

2 mm

34

fishes (Northcutt and Braford, 1980), and mammals (e.g., Jerison, 1973), but their precise significance is not known. One suggestion (e.g., Jerison, 1973) is that the concomitant increase in the number of neurons contained in the structure is an important factor and, although neuronal counts have not been carried out on DVR, it seems certain that there is some increase in the numbers of neurons present in larger DVRs. It has been speculated that large numbers of neurons allow greater computational complexity (e.g., Jacobson, 1975), increased intelligence (e.g., Jerison, 1973), or increased learning ability (e.g., Bonner, 1980). The difficulties associated with the objective measures of concepts such as complexity, intelligence, or learning have encumbered the testing of hypotheses (e.g., Radinsky, 1982), but Hahn, Jensen, and Dudek (1979) review the current status of these ideas. A second possibility is that the size of a neural structure is related to the number of neural maps of sensory surfaces that they embody and the relative magnification of the sensory surfaces within these maps (Jerison, 1977).

In addition to size variations, DVR shows interspecific differences in the nature and distribution of its neuronal populations. The major task of this chapter is to establish the basic patterns and variations that occur in the neuronal structure of DVR. The strategy is to begin with a description of the ADVR and striatum of snakes. The discussion will then be broadened to include other groups of reptiles and eventually birds to determine if the same general pattern of ADVR organization is present in these groups. The conclusion is that there are at least two major patterns of ADVR organization. The *first pattern* is seen in snakes, lizards, *Sphenodon*, and turtles. The *second pattern* is seen in crocodilians and in birds.

3.1. SNAKES

DVR in snakes is divided (Senn and Northcutt, 1973) into a rostrally situated anterior dorsal ventricular ridge (ADVR) and a caudally situated basal dorsal ventricular ridge (BDVR). In colubrid snakes, ADVR ex-

---

FIGURE 3.1. Size and shape of DVR. Variations in DVR are summarized by sections through the forebrains of several reptiles and birds. Code to species: 1, garter snake (*Thamnophis sirtalis*); 2, water snake (*Natrix sipedon*); 3, blue racer (*Coluber constrictor*); 5, desert iguana (*Dipsosaurus dorsalis*); 6, tegu lizard (*Tupinambis* sp.); 7, monitor lizard (*Varanus* sp.); 8, Moorish gecko (*Tarentola maurentania*); 9, alligator lizard (*Gerrhonotus multicarinattus*), 10, tuatara (*Sphenodon punctatum*); 11, red-eared turtle (*Pseudemys scripta*); 12, caiman (*Caiman sclerops*); 13, pigeon (*Columba livia*).

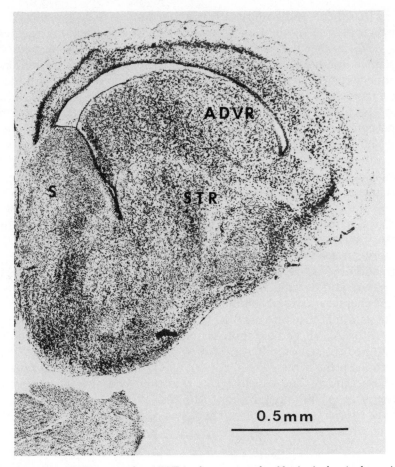

FIGURE 3.2.   ADVR in a snake. ADVR in the water snake, *Natrix sipedon*, is shown in a cross section through the telencephalon. *Abbreviations:* **ADVR,** anterior dorsal ventricular ridge; **S,** septum; **STR,** striatum.

tends caudally to cover BDVR. In boid snakes, it forms only the rostral face of BDVR (Ulinski, 1976). An example of a section through ADVR in a snake is shown in Figure 3.2. It is an eminence that protrudes vertically into the lateral ventricle, but it varies somewhat in absolute and relative size between species (Masai, Takatsuji, and Sato, 1980). For example, ADVR is about 0.8 mm wide in the vine snake (*Oxybelis aeneus*) and about 1.0 mm wide in garter snakes (*Thamnophis sirtalis*) and boa constrictors (*Constrictor constrictor*). However, these snakes vary markedly in body weight so ADVR is relatively large as compared to body weight in light-bodied arboreal snakes such as *Oxybelis* and other advanced snakes (the Caenophidia: Underwood, 1967), but relatively small as compared to body weight in the boid snakes such as *Constrictor*.

The structure of ADVR in snakes has been studied by Ulinski (1976, 1978a). Earlier, less detailed studies are referenced in these papers. ADVR contains oval or round neurons whose somata are about 10–20 μm in diameter (Fig. 3.3). Although the somata contain most of the organelles common to neurons, they lack large stacks of rough endoplasmic reticulum. Neurons are scattered throughout ADVR, but frequently occur in clusters of two to six neurons with touching somata (Fig. 3.4A). Lines of appositions most frequently involve the direct contact of plasma membranes without obvious membrane specializations (Fig. 3.4B). However, rows of specialized junctions are sometimes seen between two apposed somata (Fig. 3.4C). These are about 0.5 μm long and consist of two electron-dense bands about 50 Å wide separated by a 40-Å electron-lucent space. The absence of paramembrane specializations suggests that these junctions are not desmosomes or other adhesive contacts. It is possible that they resemble gap junctions in forming a substrate for electrotonic synapses (Ulinski, 1976). Clusters of apposed neurons are most frequent around ADVR's periphery.

ADVR neurons fall into three categories based on the properties of their dendritic trees (Ulinski, 1978a). The first are juxtaependymal cells that are positioned adjacent to the ventricular surface (Fig. 3.5). They have dendrites that extend concentric with the ventricular surface for up to 250 μm bearing a moderate to dense cover of dendritic spines. As is usual, the spines of ADVR neurons are postsynaptic to terminals with round synaptic vesicles and asymmetric active zones (Ulinski, 1976). Neurons in the second and third categories have stellate dendritic fields, bear dendritic spines, and have dendritic field diameters of 300–400 μm. Those in the second category are heavily covered with spines and occur preferentially around ADVR's periphery (Fig. 3.6). Since this region contains large numbers of neuronal clusters, many of these neurons probably participate in clusters. This can be verified when clusters of neurons are occasionally impregnated in Golgi preparations (Ulinski, 1976). The axons of these neurons bear large varicosities. Axon terminals of similar size and shape contain spherical synaptic vesicles and have asymmetric active zones (Fig. 3.7; Ulinski, 1976). Neurons in the third category are also stellate, but bear only a moderate population of dendritic spines and occur preferentially in central ADVR (Fig. 3.8). Their axons usually collateralize with vertically oriented components. Those neurons situated near the ventral border of ADVR frequently have axons that can be traced into the striatum below ADVR.

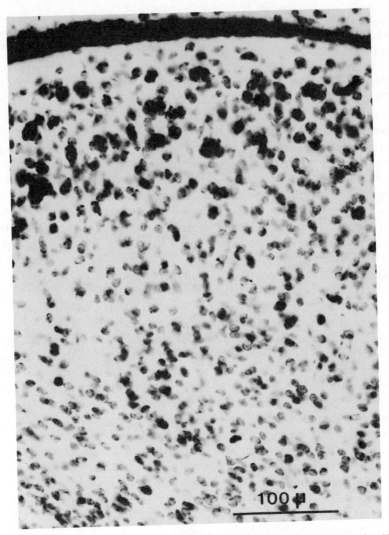

FIGURE 3.3. Zones in snake DVR. The outer region of ADVR in the water snake (*Natrix sipedon*) is shown in a Nissl stain to illustrate the zonal organization of snake DVR. Zone A is the cell-poor zone immediately beneath the ependymal layer. Zone B contains many clusters of apposed somata. Zone C contains more isolated neurons and fewer clusters. Zone D is located deeper in and is not shown. It resembles zone C in Nissl preparations.

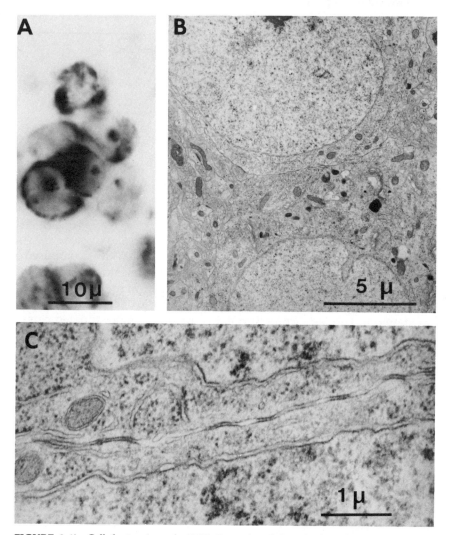

FIGURE 3.4. Cell clusters in snake DVR. Examples of clusters of touching neurons from ADVR of the water snake (*Natrix sipedon*) are shown in light and electron microscopic preparations. (A) Light photomicrographs of ADVR neurons including a cluster of several apposed somata. (B) Electron micrograph of two somata with apposed plasma membranes. (C) Enlarged view of two apposed plasma membranes showing a view of membrane specializations.

VENTRICLE

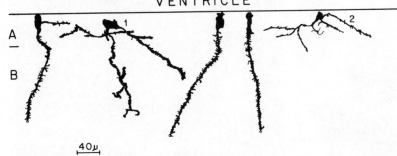

FIGURE 3.5. Juxtaependymal cells. Two examples (1 and 2) of juxtaependymal cells in Golgi preparations are shown. They can be compared to the tanycytes whose processes extend through zones A and B and into the deeper regions of ADVR. From Ulinski (1978a).

This information leads to the concept that snake ADVR is composed of a series of four zones arranged concentric with the ventricular surface (Fig. 3.9; Ulinski, 1978a). Zone A lies directly adjacent to the ventricular ependyma. It contains primarily fibers and the juxtaependymal cells (not shown in Fig. 3.9). Zone B contains the peripherally situated clusters of heavily spinous stellate cells. Zone C contains the majority of the centrally situated, less spinous stellate cells. Zone D contains those cells at ADVR's ventral border that project to the striatum.

Golgi preparations indicate that intrinsic connections interconnect the four zones (Ulinski, 1976, 1978a). This is an important point because the

VENTRICLE

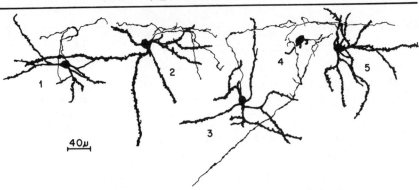

FIGURE 3.6. Zone B spiny cells. Examples of spiny cells from Golgi preparations are shown. Neurons 1, 2, 3, and 5 are drawn to show the dendritic trees. The dendrites are omitted in neuron 4 to give a better view of the axon. From Ulinski (1978a).

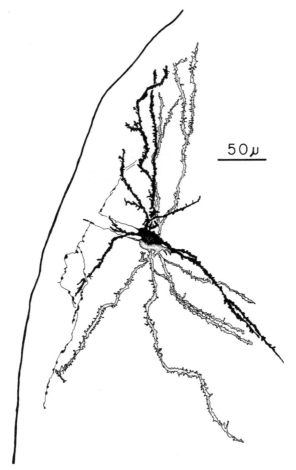

50 µ

FIGURE 3.7. Neurons in a cell cluster. Two spiny neurons from a zone B cluster are shown from a Golgi preparation. From Ulinski (1978a).

existence of such radial connections within ADVR will emerge as a general feature of the structure. The axons of spiny neurons in zone B typically ascend into zone A, run some distance concentric with the ventricle, and then recurve into zones B and sometimes C. The axons of neurons in zone C either ascend, descend, or ramify into several branches that may include both ascending and descending collaterals (Fig. 3.10). As mentioned above, the axons of cells in zone D tend to course out of ADVR and into the striatum. These observations are consistent with orthograde degeneration experiments in which small lesions were placed in ADVR (Fig. 3.11; Ulinski, 1978a). Lesions placed in

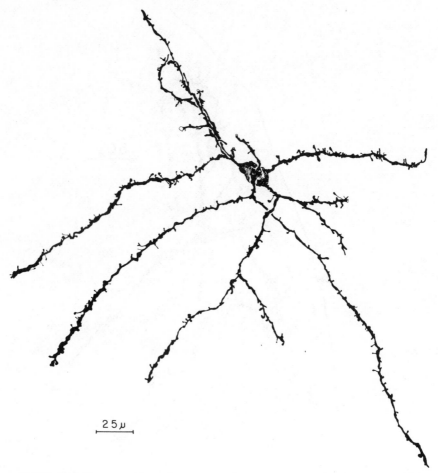

25 μ

FIGURE 3.8. Neuron with moderate spine density. An example of a neuron with a moderate density of dendritic spines from the center of ADVR is shown in a Golgi preparation. From Ulinski (1978a).

zones A, B, or C produce degeneration restricted to a relatively confined region within ADVR, whereas lesions that encroach on zone D produce degenerated axons that can be traced out of ADVR and into the subjacent striatum (see Section 6.1).

BDVR contains three nuclei in snakes (Fig. 3.12). The posterior dorsal ventricular ridge (PDVR) is a wedge-shaped group of neurons situated laterally in BDVR. It is bordered medially by nucleus sphericus, which is a cup-shaped aggregation of neurons. The ventromedial nucleus lies ventromedial to nucleus sphericus in some species but is not present in

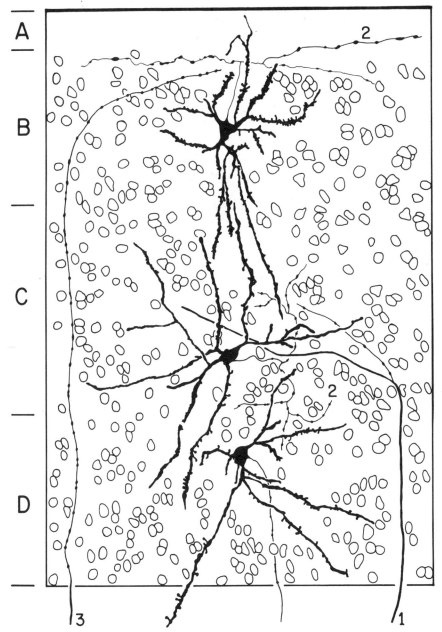

FIGURE 3.9. Zonal organization of snake ADVR. The zonal organization of snake ADVR is depicted in this drawing of a segment of ADVR. Zone A lies adjacent to the ventricle and contains juxtaependymal cells (which are not shown). Zone B contains clusters of spiny neurons with apposed somata. Zones C and D contain a greater population of neurons with a moderate density of dendritic spines. Those in zone D have axons that course ventrally into the striatum. From Ulinski (1978a).

43

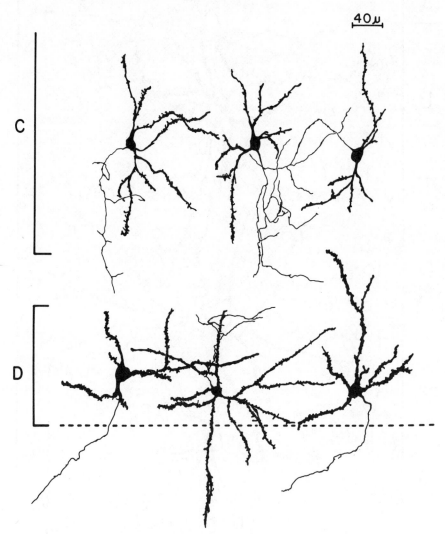

FIGURE 3.10.   Neurons in zones C and D. Examples of neurons in zones C and D are shown in Golgi preparations. From Ulinski (1978a).

others. There are significant variations in the relative development of each of these nuclei between species of snakes (Senn and Northcutt, 1973; Northcutt, 1978a).

Only nucleus sphericus has been studied in detail. It appears as a clump of neurons in embryonic brains (Warner, 1946). This clump gradually differentiates into a cup-shaped aggregation with its mouth or

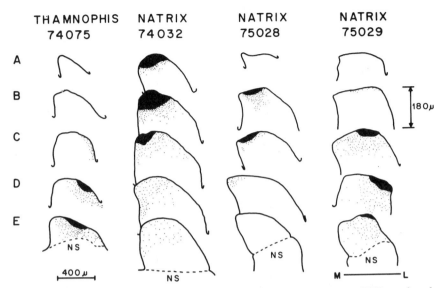

THAMNOPHIS 74075	NATRIX 74032	NATRIX 75028	NATRIX 75029

FIGURE 3.11. Intrinsic projections in snake ADVR. Small lesions in ADVR produced degeneration restricted to ADVR in Fink–Heimer preparations. Each case is depicted by a series of five sections with A being the most rostral. The black shows the extent of the lesion. From Ulinski (1978a).

hilus facing rostrally. The accessory olfactory tract, which carries information from the vomeronasal or Jacobson's organ via the accessory olfactory bulb, enters the hilus of nucleus sphericus. Ulinski and Kanarek (1973) recognized three layers in nucleus sphericus of boa constrictors, *Constrictor constrictor*. These layers appear to be present in all snakes and each layer contains a distinct population of neurons (Fig. 3.13). The hilar layer comprises the center of the nucleus and contains multipolar neurons. The walls of the nucleus are formed by densely packed neurons, the mural cells, whose spiny dendrites extend into both the hilar layer and the marginal layer. The marginal layer surrounds the mural layer and contains scattered marginal cells whose dendrites bear a moderate population of dendritic spines and ramify concentric with the mural layer.

A common feature of BDVR is that some of its neurons concentrate sex hormones. In garter snakes of the genus *Thamnophis*, the ventromedial nucleus and nucleus sphericus concentrate estradiol and testosterone (Halpern, Morrell, and Pfaff, 1982). Labeled neurons are found particularly along the medial wall of nucleus sphericus.

The striatum in snakes has been described by Ulinski (1978a). It contains three major nuclei (Fig. 3.14). The medial striatal nucleus (MS) is a

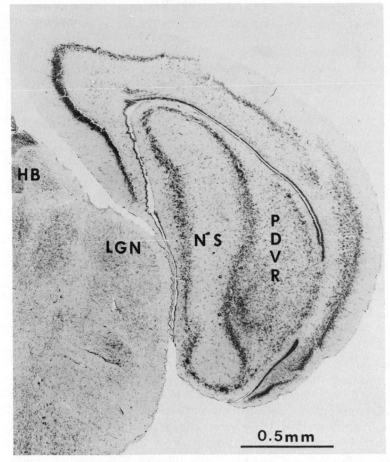

FIGURE 3.12. BDVR in a snake. BDVR in the python, *Python reticularis*, is shown in a cross section through the caudal telencephalon. Nucleus sphericus (NS) and the posterior dorsal venricular ridge (PDVR) are components of BDVR. *Abbreviations:* **HB,** habenula; **LGN,** lateral geniculate nucleus.

group of densely packed neurons that lies lateral to nucleus accumbens and below the medial recess of the lateral ventricle. The intrapeduncular nucleus (IP) consists of large neurons situated within the fibers of the lateral forebrain bundle as they approach ADVR's ventral border. The perifascicular complex (PF) consists of neurons that surround the accessory olfactory tract (a bundle of fibers carrying axons from the accessory olfactory bulb to nucleus sphericus; A0T).

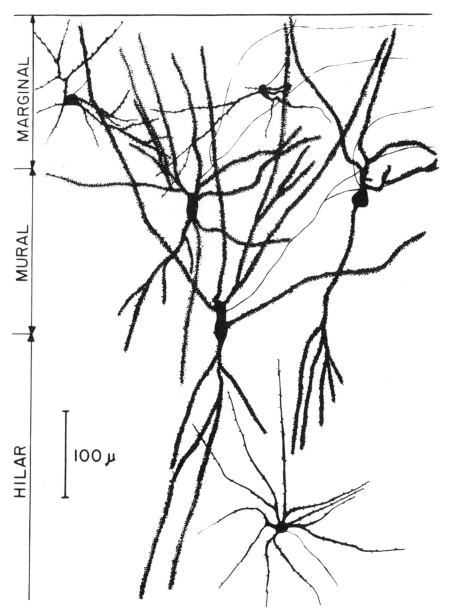

FIGURE 3.13. Nucleus sphericus. Neurons in nucleus sphericus are shown as they appear in rapid Golgi preparations in the boa constrictor, *Constrictor constrictor*. The nucleus has three layers (hilar, mural, and marginal). Each layer contains a distinct population of neurons. From Ulinski and Kanarek (1973).

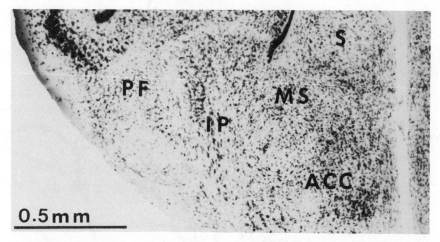

FIGURE 3.14. Striatum in snakes. The striatum of a water snake (*Natrix sipedon*) is shown in a Nissl preparation. A cell-poor zone separates the striatum from the overlying ADVR. The striatum contains the medial striatal nucleus (MS), the intrapeduncular nucleus (IP) and the perifascicular complex (PF). *Other abbreviations:* **ACC,** nucleus accumbers; **S,** septum.

Using these descriptions as a starting point, the next section examines DVR in lizards to determine if it conforms to the pattern that is seen in snakes.

3.2. LIZARDS

As in snakes, DVR in lizards is divided into an anterior dorsal ventricular ridge and a basal dorsal ventricular ridge (Senn and Northcutt, 1973; Ulinski and Peterson, 1981). The term ADVR replaces older terms such as hyperstriatum anterius or neostriatum. There is substantial variation in the structure of ADVR between lizards, and Northcutt (1972, 1978a), following the work of Senn (1970, 1974), has divided lizards into two groups on the basis of several features of forebrain organization, including that of ADVR. Type I or lacertomorph lizards include the families Gekkonidae, Scincidae, Lacertidae, Anguidae, and Helodermatidae as well as some smaller families. Type II or dracomorph lizards include the families Teidae, Varanidae, Agamidae, Iguanidae, and Chamaeleonidae. ADVR in Type II lizards is discussed first because it most closely resembles that in snakes.

ADVR in Type II Lizards

The shape of ADVR in lizards resembles that seen in snakes and, as in snakes, varies in size between species. Variations in the size of ADVR in Type II lizards has been studied by Platel (1980b) who determined the volumes of ADVR and other constituents of the telencephalon in 10 species. The volume of ADVR varies as a power function of body weight ($V = kS^\alpha$). The coefficient of allometry is relatively small ($\alpha = 0.523$), but the points for Type II lizards lie above the regression line of log (ADVR volume) versus log (body weight) calculated for six lacertid lizards chosen for reference. This indicates that Type II lizards have ADVRs that are relatively large per unit body weight.

Some information on ADVR is included in general accounts of lizard forebrain anatomy (e.g., Meyer, 1893; Shanklin, 1930), but the most detailed descriptions of ADVR in Type II lizards have been of the tegu lizards, *Tupinambis teguixin* or *T. nigropunctatus* (Curwen, 1938; Hoogland, 1977), and the green iguana, *Iguana iguana* (Northcutt, 1967; Bruce, 1982). An example of ADVR in a Type II lizard is shown in Figure 3.15. ADVR in these lizards resembles that in snakes in that neurons are scattered relatively evenly throughout the structure (Fig. 3.16A). Clusters of touching neurons also occur throughout ADVR, but they are more frequent and larger within a band that is situated concentric to the ventricle and immediately deep to the thin, periventricular cell poor zone. ADVR in Type II lizards can thus be divided into zones that resemble those seen in snakes. The first zone is the cell-poor periventricular zone. The second is the cell cluster zone. Third is the central zone that contains smaller and less frequent cell clusters. Observations of Golgi preparations in the iguanid lizards *Iguana iguana* (Northcutt, 1967) and *Dipsosaurus dorsalis* (Ulinski, unpublished observations) indicate that neurons within the cell cluster and central zones are multipolar, vary in their dendritic branching patterns from stellate to double pyramidal, and bear a moderate cover of dendritic spines. They have dendritic fields that are about 250 μm in diameter. Detailed studies of the intrinsic connections of ADVR in Type II lizards have not been carried out. However, Hoogland (1977) used stereotaxic lesions and Fink–Heimer techniques to show that neurons deep in ADVR project to superficial ADVR.

Bruce (1982) studied the cytoarchitecture of ADVR in the green iguana, *Iguana iguana*. There are three major areas defined on the basis of the specific cytoarchitectonic characteristics within each of the zones. The areas are named the medial, caudolateral, and rostrolateral areas

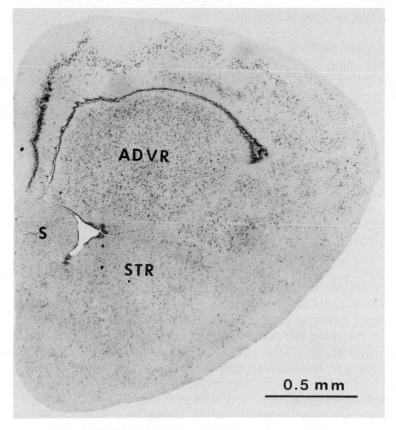

FIGURE 3.15.   ADVR in a Type II lizard. ADVR in the monitor lizard (*Varanus benegalensis*) is shown in a cross section through the telencephalon. *Abbreviations:* **ADVR,** anterior dorsal ventricular ridge; **S,** septum; **STR,** striatum.

based on their positions. All three areas contain a zone 2, which is filled with single and clustered neurons. Zone 4 is slightly less dense than zone 2. The transition between the two zones is gradual, with zone 3 poorly distinguished. In the medial area, clusters of neurons are present in zone 2 with about three or four neurons per cluster. There is a tendency for neurons to be lined in rows perpendicular to the ventricular surface. Caudally, zone 2 becomes more diffuse but otherwise the same cytoarchitectonic characteristics are present. Zone 2 is about 0.1 to 0.2 mm thick. In the caudolateral area, neurons in zone 2 are occasionally organized in clusters of two or three, but they are not common. The rostrolateral area has a more distinct zone 2. Clusters of two to eight

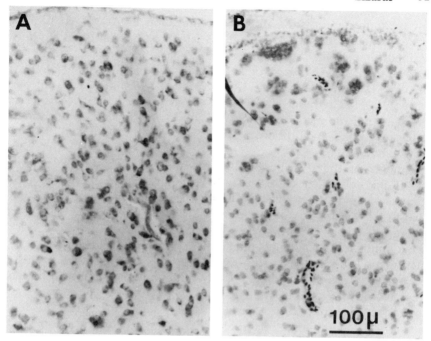

FIGURE 3.16.   Cell clusters in lizard DVR. The cytology of DVR neurons is shown in a Type II lizard (*Tupinambis*, A) and a Type I lizard (*Gerrhonotus multicarinnatus*, B). In *Tupinambis*, cell clusters are smaller and less frequent. In *Gerrhonotus*, large cell clusters occur frequently near the ventricle.

neurons are present and the shift from zone 2 to zone 4 is more apparent than in other areas because there are fewer clusters and smaller numbers of neurons within the clusters in zone 4.

Histochemical preparations stained for the mitochondrial enzyme succinic dehydrogenase (SDH) also display inhomogeneities within DVR. SDH is a relatively nonspecific stain because mitochondria are distributed extensively in neurons, and the cellular basis for the patches of high SDH activity is not certain. However, there is some reason to believe that patches of SDH activity represent the terminal fields of thalamic afferents within DVR. Northcutt (1978a) points out that the positions of SDH positive patches in *Iguana* correlate with the positions of thalamic terminal fields. Pritz and Northcutt (1977) were able to compare the positions of SDH positive patches in *Caiman* to the positions of terminal fields in animals with nucleus rotundus or nucleus reuniens lesions and showed that the patches of SDH activity correspond closely to the terminal fields. Thus, the distribution of SDH is of potential interest in understanding the internal organization of ADVR. In lizards, Baker-Cohen (1968) observed that the lateral part of ADVR is strongly stained for SDH in the common anole, *Anolis carolinensis*, and in the horned toad, *Phrynosoma cornutum*. There is also a weakly stained medial area in ADVR in both species. Northcutt (1978a) identified four patches of high SDH activity in ADVR of the green iguana, *Iguana iguana* (Fig. 3.17). Lateral and medial patches correspond roughly to those identified by Baker-Cohen. In addition, patches are present in central ADVR and at its lateral edge.

Studies of the distribution of different neurotransmitters within ADVR and related structures are only beginning. However, such investigations are potentially valuable because they can provide information that is very useful in working out the intrinsic organization of ADVR. There have been a few studies of the distribution of the peptides methionine and leucine enkephalin in the brains of lizards. These substances are believed to be neurotransmitters that are the natural agonists for opiate receptors (e.g., Snyder and Childers, 1979). Their distribution has been investigated in the common anole (*Anolis carolinensis*) using immunocytochemical techniques (Naik, Sar, and Stumpf, 1981). A few neurons that show enkephalin-like immunoreactivity are found scattered through ADVR.

ADVR in Type I Lizards

Platel (1980b) studied forebrain variation in 14 Type I lizards. The coefficient of allometry for ADVR is larger ($\alpha = 0.679$) than for Type II lizards, but the points for Type I lizards tend to fall below the regression line for lacertids. This indicates that Type I lizards have relatively small ADVRs per unit body weight.

ADVR in Type I lizards contains a band of neuronal clusters that is concentric with the ventricle (Fig. 3.18). In contrast to the cell cluster band in snakes and Type II lizards, the cell cluster band in Type I lizards is quite distinct and is separated from the central zone by a cell-poor layer (Fig. 3.16B). The nature of the band of clusters varies significantly between species (Northcutt, 1978a; Senn and Northcutt, 1973). In the tokay gecko, *Gekko gecko*, the cell cluster band is relatively uniform, but is broken into three mediolateral areas. The cells within a cluster are not uniform and a cluster may contain a single giant cell surrounded by a wreath of small cells. In *Lialis burtoni* (Pygopodidae) and *Xantusia vigilis* (Xantusidae), the zone is asymmetric in that the medial band consists of densely packed small cells. Giant cells sometimes occur outside of the clusters. The asymmetry in the zone can be greater in lacertids and

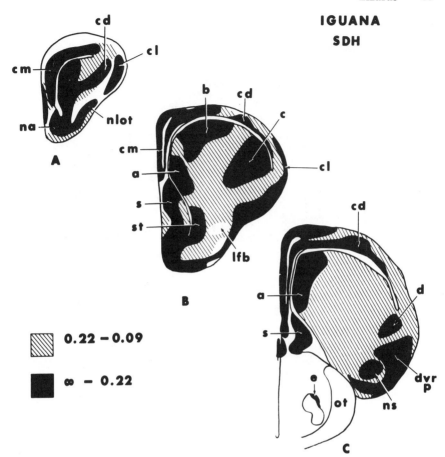

IGUANA

SDH

0.22 – 0.09

∞ – 0.22

FIGURE 3.17. Succinic dehydrogenase activity in *Iguana* telencephalon. The activity of the enzyme succinic dehydrogenase (SDH) is plotted on three transverse sections through the telencephalon of an iguana. Black areas indicate regions of high SDH activity. Notice that ADVR contains four patches (a, b, c, and d) of high SDH activity. *Abbreviations:* **cd,** dorsal cortex; **cm,** medial cortex; **cl,** lateral cortex; **e,** entopeduncular nucleus; **dvrp,** posterior dorsal ventricular ridge; **lfb,** lateral forebrain bundle; **na,** nucleus accumbens; **nlot,** nucleus of the lateral olfactory tract; **ot,** optic tract; **ns,** nucleus sphericus; **s,** septum; **st,** striatum. From Northcutt (1978a).

scincids in that the medial edge of the zone is about one-half the thickness of the lateral edge. Finally, in anguids such as *Gerrhonotus*, the lateral edge of the zone can be five times thicker than the medial edge of the zone and giant cells are particularly obvious in the lateral part of the zone.

The only Golgi observations on Type I lizards are by Ramón (1896) on

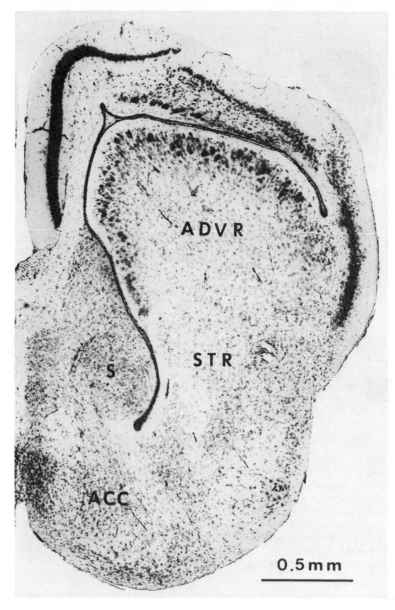

FIGURE 3.18. ADVR in a Type I lizard. ADVR is shown in a cross section through the forebrain of a tokay gecko (*Gekko gecko*). *Abbreviations:* **ACC,** nucleus accumbens; **ADVR,** anterior dorsal ventricular ridge; **S,** septum; **STR,** striatum.

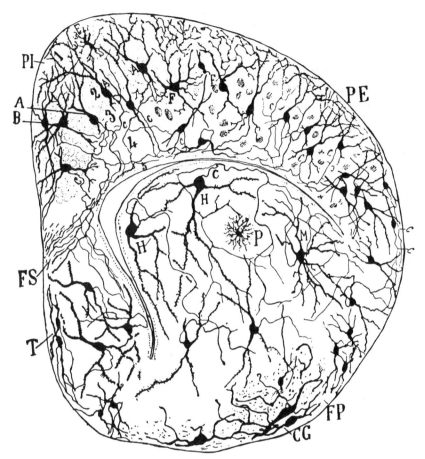

FIGURE 3.19. ADVR in a Type I lizard. Neurons in ADVR of the lizard *Lacerta* are shown as they appear in Golgi preparations. The neurons designated "H" are spiny neurons in the cell cluster zone. The neuron designated "M" is an aspiny neuron deep in ADVR. From Ramón (1896).

Lacerta sp. He shows two spiny cells (Fig. 3.19) with somata in the cell cluster zone (Goldby, 1934). Their axons ascend into the cell-poor zone and then recurve into the central zone. A spiny cell located dorsally in the central zone has an axon that collateralizes within the central zone and then ascends into the cell cluster zone. Neurons located ventrally in the central zone have axons that descend from ADVR into the striatum. Thus, the zonal organization in *Lacerta* generally resembles that seen in snakes in that the intrinsic connections interconnect the zones and the most ventral cells project to the striatum. Similarly, lesions of superficial

ADVR in the tokay gecko (*Gekko gecko*) produce terminal degeneration in deep ADVR (Butler, 1976).

ADVR in the tokay gecko, *Gekko gecko*, contains three cytoarchitectonic areas comparable to those present in *Iguana* (Bruce, 1982). The medial, caudolateral, and rostrolateral areas are separated from each other by shallow sulci. In the medial area, zone 2 consists of a thin plate of neurons that are quite densely packed rostrally but become more diffuse caudally where clusters of about six neurons are present. The caudolateral area contains enormous clusters of neurons in zone 2; these include as many as 25 neurons. The clusters are organized into columns arranged perpendicular to the ventricular surface. The rostrolateral area is characterized by a very thick zone 2. Clusters are organized in columns about three neurons wide. The neurons are densest at the ventricular surface and gradually become more diffuse in deeper ADVR, so that it is very difficult to distinguish between zones 2 and 4. A cell-poor zone 3 is not at all apparent. Zone 4 consists of scattered neurons in all three areas.

BDVR in Lizards

BDVR in lizards (Fig. 3.20) contains the same three nuclei as it does in snakes (Senn and Northcutt, 1973; Northcutt, 1978a; Ulinski and Peterson, 1981). Of these, only nucleus sphericus has been studied. It varies dramatically in size and its degree of differentiation as a function of the size of the accessory olfactory bulbs (Rudin, 1974) and of the behavioral emphasis that a particular species places on chemoreception. Thus, the microsmatic anoles of the genus *Anolis* have poorly developed olfactory structures and nucleus sphericus is represented by a solid nuclear group in BDVR, rather than its more typical cup-shaped configuration (Armstrong, Gamble, and Goldby, 1953). Nucleus sphericus has its cup-shaped configuration in other iguanid lizards such as *Iguana iguana* (Northcutt, 1967) and *Dipsosaurus dorsalis* (Ulinski and Peterson, 1981). Golgi preparations (Fig.3.21) on the latter species show that mural and hilar cells can be identified (Ulinski and Peterson, 1981), but that the mural cells are more multipolar than they are in snakes. In macrosmatic lizards such as *Tupinambis, Varanus,* and *Helodermata,* nucleus sphericus is a large, cup-shaped structure (Northcutt, 1978a). The mural layer may be convoluted, as in *Helodermata,* and the hilar cells may form a series of shelf-like arrays in the hilus, as in *Varanus*. These modifications are apparently related to the presence of a bifid tongue that is used in a variety of chemosensory behaviors in many of these genera (e.g., Auffenberg, 1978).

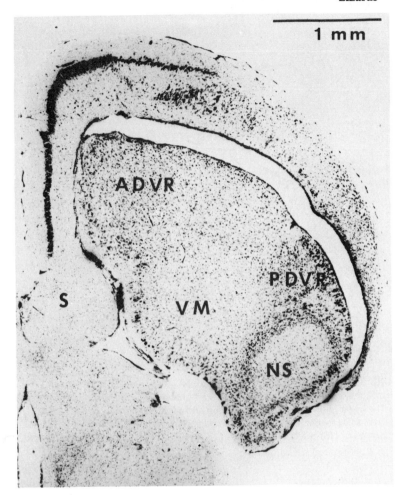

FIGURE 3.20.   BDVR in a lizard. BDVR is shown in a cross section through the telencephalon of the desert iguana (*Dipsosaurus dorsalis*). BDVR contains nucleus sphericus (NS), posterior dorsal ventricular ridge (PDVR), and the ventromedial nucleus (VM). *Other abbreviations:* **ADVR,** anterior dorsal ventricular ridge; **S,** septum.

As in snakes, the ventromedial nucleus of BDVR concentrates estradiol and testosterone in *Anolis carolinensis* (Martinez-Vargas, Keefer, and Stumpf, 1978; Morrell et al., 1979).

Striatum in Lizards

Several different terminologies have been applied to the striatum of lizards (Platel, 1972). The striatum of the tegu lizards (Fig. 3.22) has been

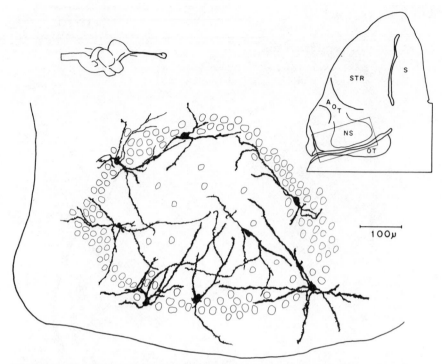

FIGURE 3.21. Nucleus sphericus in a lizard. Neurons in nucleus sphericus of the desert iguana (*Dipsosaurus dorsalis*) are shown in a horizontal section through a Golgi preparation. The insets show the plan of the section and a low-power view of the section. The area in the rectangle is magnified in the main part of the figure. *Abbreviations:* **AOT**, accessory olfactory tract; **NS**, nucleus sphericus; **OT**, optic tract; **S**, septum; **STR**, striatum. From Ulinski and Peterson (1981).

the best studied. Curwen (1938) provided an early description of the striatum in *Tupinambis*, but the nomenclature of Hoogland (1977) is in current usage. The striatum (his ventral striatum) is separated from ADVR (his dorsal striatum) by a cell-poor area and contains a small-celled part medial to the lateral forebrain bundle and a large-celled part lateral to the bundle. The lateral border of the striatum is formed by the nucleus of the lateral olfactory tract. The large cells of the nucleus in-trapeduncularis are situated within the most ventrally positioned fibers of the lateral forebrain bundle.

Comparison of tegu and snake materials suggests that a common nomenclature could be applied to both lizards and snakes. Thus, the small-celled ventral striatum of Hoogland corresponds to the medial striatal nucleus of snakes. The nucleus intrapeduncularis of Hoogland

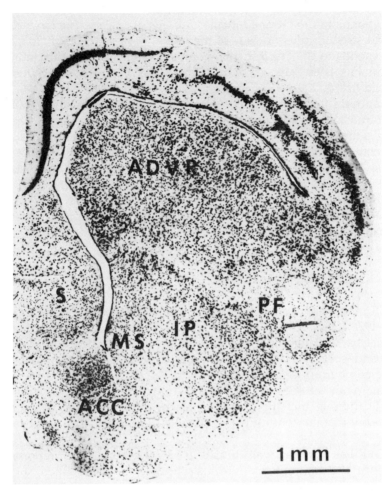

FIGURE 3.22. Striatum in tegu lizard. The cytoarchitecture of the striatum in *Tupinambis* is illustrated in a transverse section through the rostral telencephalon. The small-celled part of the striatum or medial striatal nucleus (MS) lies lateral to the ventricle. The intrapeduncular nucleus (IP) lies embedded in the fibers of the lateral forebrain bundle. The large-celled part of the striatum or perifascicular complex (PF) lies lateral to the major contingent of forebrain fibers. *Other abbreviations:* **ACC,** nucleus accumbens; **ADVR,** anterior dorsal ventricular ridge; **S,** septum.

corresponds to the intrapeduncular nucleus of snakes. The large-celled ventral striatum plus nucleus of the lateral olfactory tract of Hoogland corresponds to the perifascicular complex of snakes. A similar nomenclature has been suggested by Ulinski and Peterson (1981) for the iguanid lizard *Dipsosaurus dorsalis*.

It appears that the striatum is associated with a particular profile of neurotransmitters and enzymes associated with transmitters. One of these is the enzyme acetylcholinesterase (AChE). DVR generally shows low activities of AChE while the striatum typically has high AChE levels. AChE activity has been studied in *Lacerta muralis* by Contestabile and DiPardo (1976) and in the green iguana, *Iguana iguana* (Fig. 3.23), by Northcutt (1978a). AChE activity was high in the striatum and nucleus accumbens in both species. The striatum contains neurons with enkephalin-like immunoreactivity in *Anolis* (Naik, Sar, and Stumpf, 1981).

3.3.   RHYNCHOCEPHALIANS

ADVR in *Sphenodon* resembles that of snakes and lizards in form (Cairney, 1926; Durward, 1930). Like that of Type I lizards, it contains a distinct band of neuronal clusters just below the ventricle (Fig. 3.24). The band is relatively uniform in structure and is sharply delimited from scattered neurons deeper in ADVR. The cell cluster zone is continuous laterally with the second layer of the cortex. Hines's (1923) Figures 12 and 13 indicate that this band is present at stage R; the description points out that the continuity is established secondarily, late in development.

BDVR has not been well studied in *Sphenodon*. Northcutt reports the presence of a ventromedial nucleus, but not of a well-defined nucleus sphericus. The striatum of *Sphenodon* generally resembles that of lizards (Cairney, 1926; Durward, 1930).

3.4.   TURTLES

DVR in turtles can also be divided into an ADVR and a BDVR (Balaban, 1978a). ADVR has been most extensively studied in the cryptodiran turtles *Chrysemys picta* (Northcutt, 1970) and *Pseudemys scripta elegans* (Balaban, 1978a). Earlier work is cited in these papers. The general character of ADVR (Fig. 3.25) seems to be constant between turtles, including the pleurodiran turtle *Podocnemis unifilis* (Riss, Halpern, and Scalia, 1969). It is typically an eminence that protrudes deeply into the

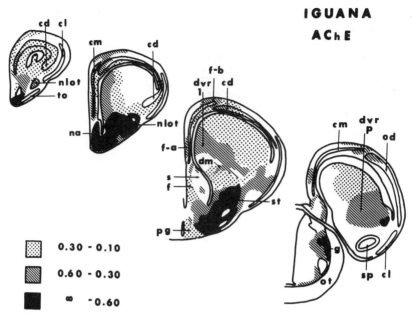

IGUANA
AChE

FIGURE 3.23. Acetylcholinesterase activity in *Iguana* forebrain. The distribution of the enzyme acetylcholinesterase (AChE) is shown in four sections through the forebrain of an iguana. Black indicates high concentrations of AChE. Notice that the striatum contains high levels of AChE. *Abbreviations:* **cd,** dorsal cortex; **cl,** lateral cortex; **cm,** medial cortex; **dvr 1,** medial zone of the anterior dorsal ventricular ridge; **dvr p,** posterior division of the dorsal ventricular ridge; **f,** fornix; **f–a,b,** areas of moderate AChE density in dorsal and ventral components of medial cortex; **g,** ventral division of lateral geniculate nucleus; **na,** nucleus accumbens; **nlot,** nucleus of the lateral olfactory tract; **ot,** optic tract; **pg,** preoptic periventricular gray; **s,** septal nuclei; **sp,** nucleus sphericus; **st,** striatum; **to,** olfactory tubercle. From Northcutt (1978a).

lateral ventricle. There are variations in its relative size, but these have not been systematically studied.

Neurons in turtle ADVR resemble those in other reptiles (Balaban, 1978a). Large neuronal clusters occur frequently near the ventricle; small clusters occur less frequently within ADVR (Fig. 3.26). ADVR neurons fall into three groups in Golgi preparations. Juxtaependymal cells have discoidal dendritic fields up to 400 μm in diameter and 60 μm thick that are oriented concentric with the ventricle (Fig. 3.27). Their dendrites bear a moderate cover of spines. Spiny neurons are the most frequent type in ADVR. They all have dendritic field diameters of about 300 μm and bear a heavy cover of spines, but differ in the morphology of their dendritic trees. Superficial spiny neurons have relatively flat dendritic

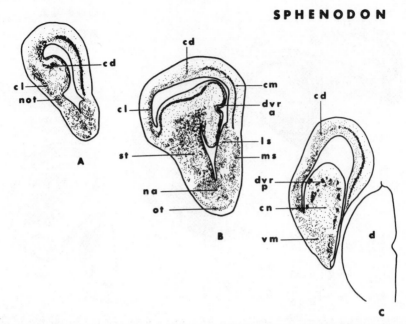

SPHENODON

FIGURE 3.24.   DVR in *Sphenodon*. ADVR and PDVR are shown in cross sections through the forebrain of *Sphenodon*. *Abbreviations:* **cd**, dorsal cortex; **cm**, medial cortex; **cl**, lateral cortex; **dvra**, anterior dorsal ventricular ridge; **dvrp**, posterior dorsal ventricular ridge; **d**, dorsal thalamus; **ls**, lateral septal nucleus; **ms**, medial septal nucleus; **na**, nucleus accumbens; **not**, nucleus of the lateral olfactory tract; **ot**, optic tract; **st**, striatum; **vm**, ventromedial nucleus.

trees and participate in neuronal clusters (Fig. 3.28). Their axons initially proceed toward the ventricle and branch in the periventricular cell-poor zone. The branches bear varicosities and then recurve into ADVR. Deep spiny neurons have dendritic fields that vary in shape from stellate to double pyramidal (Fig. 3.29). Finally, there is a population of aspiny neurons scattered throughout ADVR (Fig. 3.30). They have stellate dendritic fields composed of up to nine, spine-free dendrites and are about 200 μm in diameter. They are impregnated only infrequently.

The ultrastructure of turtle ADVR has been studied by Weiss (1982). Observations on the dorsal area (see below) of *Pseudemys* indicate that the majority of synaptic contacts involve axon terminals that contain clear, round synaptic vesicles and form asymmetric junctions. A minority of terminals contain clear, pleomorphic vesicles and form symmetric junctions, whereas only a few terminals contain small granular vesicles. Most synaptic contacts are on dendritic spines, a small proportion occur

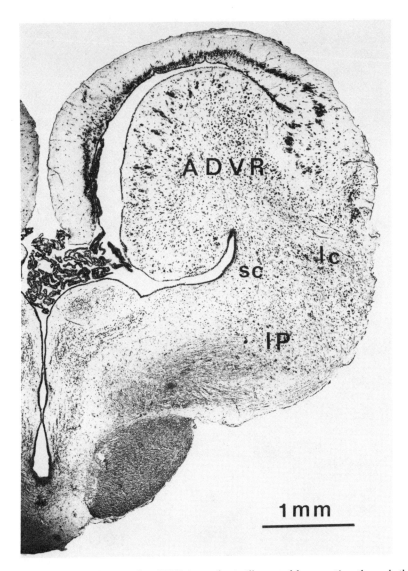

FIGURE 3.25. ADVR in turtle. ADVR in turtles is illustrated by a section through the forebrain of a red-eared turtle (*Pseudemys scripta*). *Abbreviations:* **ADVR,** anterior dorsal ventricle ridge; **IP,** intrapeduncular nucleus; **lc,** large-celled striatum; **sc,** small-celled striatum.

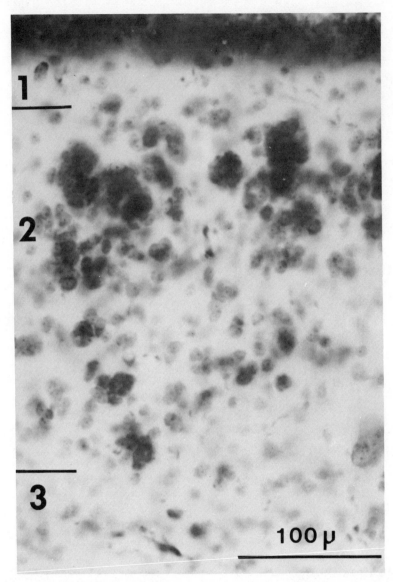

FIGURE 3.26. Zones in turtle ADVR. The zonal pattern of turtle ADVR is shown in the outer part of medial area of ADVR in a Nissl preparation from *Pseudemys*. Zone 1 contains the somata of a few, scattered juxtaependymal cells. Zone 2 contains large clusters of opposed somata. Zone 3 is a thin, cell-poor space. Zone 4 (not shown) contains primarily isolated somata and relatively few clusters. Compare this figure to Figure 3.34, which shows the same region in Golgi preparations.

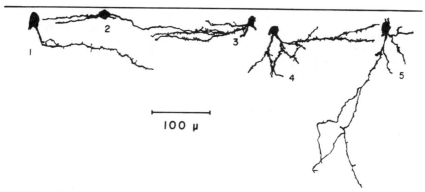

FIGURE 3.27. Juxtaependymal cells. Four examples on juxtaependymal neurons from ADVR of *Pseudemys* are shown in a Golgi preparation. From Balaban (1978a).

on dendritic shafts, and a few contacts are found on somata. Somata of neurons involved in cell clusters form frequent casual appositions with neighboring somata, but there is no clear evidence for gap junctions (Fig. 3.31). This stands in contrast to the situation in snakes where membrane specializations occur between neurons in clusters. Somatic membranes within clusters of neurons that are not involved in casual appositions are covered by glial sheaths or occasionally contacted by axon terminals. The glial sheaths probably include the velate processes of tanycytes whose cell bodies are in the ependymal layer.

ADVR in *Pseudemys* and *Chrysemys* can be divided into four concentric zones (Fig. 3.32) based on the distribution of the four types of neurons (Balaban, 1978a). Zone 1 is a cell-poor periventricular zone. It contains the juxtaependymal cells. Zone 2 is characterized by relatively large neuronal clusters. These contain spiny neurons whose dendrites extend toward the ventricle into zone 1 and deeper into ADVR into zone 3. Zone 3 is a relatively distinct cell-poor zone. Zone 4 is the largest zone. It extends from zone 3 to ADVR's ventral border and contains predominantly spiny neurons.

Golgi preparations indicate that there are radial connections between zones 2 and 4 (Balaban, 1978a). The axons of zone 2 spiny neurons recurve into zone 4 and the collateral systems of zone 4 spiny neurons contain radial components that extend into zone 2. Similarly, lesions superficial in ADVR in *Chrysemys* (Northcutt, 1970) and *Pseudemys* (Balaban, 1978a) produce degeneration deep in ADVR, whereas deep lesions produce degeneration superficial in ADVR (Northcutt, 1970).

The four zones extend throughout ADVR, but there are marked variations in the cytology of the zones that permit the delineation of four

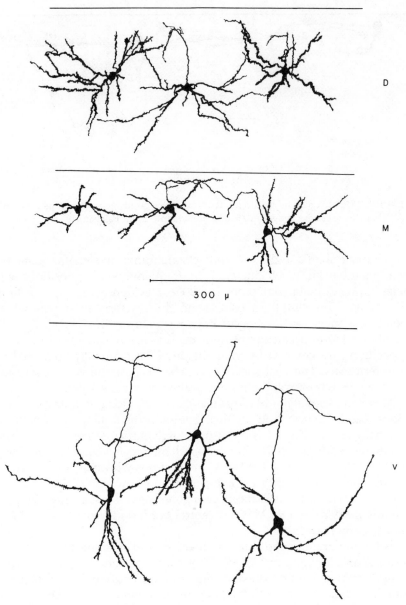

D

M

300 µ

V

FIGURE 3.28. Zone 2 spiny neurons. Examples of spiny neurons from the cell cluster zones of dorsal (D), medial (M), and ventral (V) areas in *Pseudemys* are shown from Golgi preparations. From Balaban (1978a).

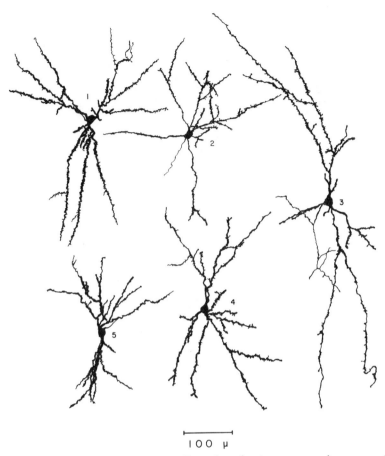

100 μ

FIGURE 3.29. Zone 4 spiny neurons. Examples of spiny neurons from zone 4 in *Pseudemys* are shown from Golgi preparations. From Balaban (1978a).

cytoarchitectonic areas within ADVR (Balaban, 1978a). One of these areas, central area, consists of neurons embedded within the fibers of the lateral forebrain bundle as they enter ADVR. The other three areas lie between central area and the ventricular surface. Dorsal area is a crescent-shaped region situated laterally in ADVR (Fig. 3.33). Medial area is situated in the center of ADVR and is characterized by particularly large neuronal clusters in zone 2 (Fig. 3.34). Ventral area is situated in the most medial region of ADVR (Fig. 3.35). Although the thalamic afferents to ADVR will be discussed in Section 4.1, it is worth noting here that dorsal area, medial area, and ventral area each receive projections from a particular thalamic nucleus (Balaban and Ulinski, 1981a).

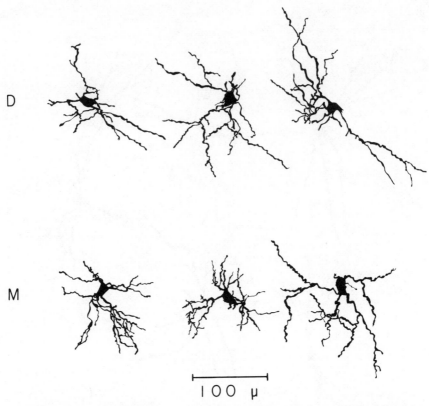

FIGURE 3.30. Aspiny neurons. Examples of aspiny neurons from ADVR of *Pseudemys* are shown from Golgi preparations. From Balaban (1978a).

The SDH activity in turtle ADVR has been studied for several species (*Pseudemys scripta, Chrysemys picta picta, C. p. belli,* and *Testudo graeca*) by Baker-Cohen (1968) and by Contestabile and DiPardo (1976). Dorsal area shows a strong activity while the neuropiles of the remaining areas are weakly stained. The large cell clusters in medial area are active.

BDVR lacks nuclei with sharp boundaries in turtles (Fig. 3.36), although various authors have identified one or more nuclei, usually designating them as amygdaloid nuclei (Johnston, 1915; Hewitt, 1967; Carey, 1970; Northcutt, 1970; Balaban, 1978a). Northcutt (1970) reports that BDVR in *Chrysemys* contains "pyramidal" neurons, small projection neurons, and stellate neurons in Golgi preparations. Neurons scattered along the ventricular surface of BDVR concentrate estradiol in *Pseudemys* (Kim, Stumpf, and Sar, 1981).

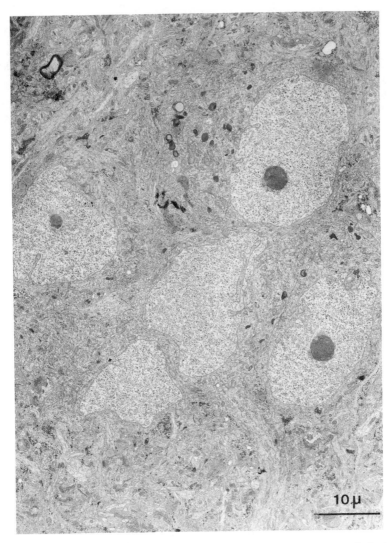

10 μ

FIGURE 3.31. Neuronal clusters. An electron micrograph shows a neuronal cluster in dorsal area of *Pseudemys* ADVR. Notice that several somata are in direct apposition without membrane specializations.

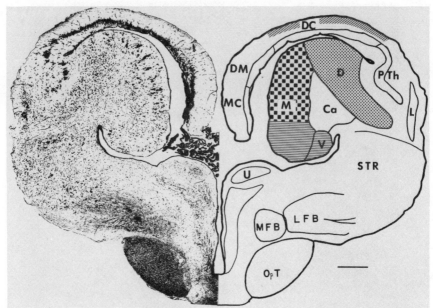

FIGURE 3.32. Areas in turtle DVR. The four cytoarchitectonic areas of turtle ADVR are diagrammed in this figure. The left side of the figure is a photograph of a section through the forebrain of *Pseudemys*. The boundaries of dorsal area (D), medial area (M), ventral area (V), and central area (Ca) are shown on the right. The pattern of thalamic projections to ADVR is also summarized. Dorsal area receives projections from nucleus rotundus (stipple). Medial area receives projections from nucleus caudalis (checkered pattern). Ventral area and the ventral part of medial area receive projections from nucleus reuniens (stripes). Scale equals 500 μm. From Balaban and Ulinski (1981b).

The striatum of turtles has been described by Humphrey (*Chelydra serpentina*; 1894), Johnston (*Terrapene carolina*; 1915), Carey (*Terrapene carolina*; 1967), Hewitt (*Testudo graeca*; 1967), Northcutt (*Chrysemys picta belli*; 1970), and Balaban (*Pseudemys* and *Chrysemys*; 1979). Although there are substantial variations in nomenclature, it seems possible to recognize three major groups of cells (Fig. 3.25). The first is a dorsolateral large-celled group that corresponds to the nucleus lentiformis of Johnston (1915). The second is a dorsomedial small-celled group (the nucleus caudatus of Johnston). The third are large cells embedded in the lateral forebrain bundle (the globus pallidus of Johnston).

The striatum has a high AChE activity in the turtles *Chrysemys picta* (Parent and Olivier, 1970/1971) and *Pseudemys scripta* (Contestabile and DiPardo, 1976; Kusunoki, 1971). The distribution of the peptide substance P (e.g., Nicoll, Schenker, and Leeman, 1980) in *Pseudemys* has

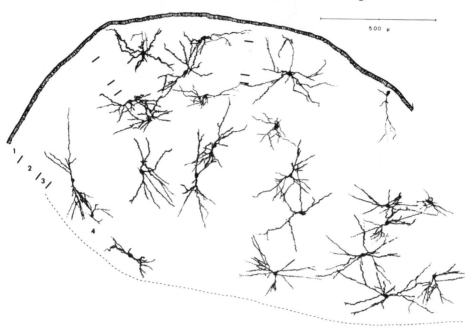

500 μ

FIGURE 3.33.   Dorsal area. Neurons in dorsal area of ADVR are shown as they appear in Golgi preparations of *Pseudemys*. From Balaban (1978a).

been studied using immunocytochemical techniques by Reiner, Karten, and Korte (1980). They found substance P-like immunoreactivity in the striatum.

3.5.   DEFINITION OF THE FIRST PATTERN OF DVR ORGANIZATION

To summarize the argument up to this point, DVR is readily divisible into a rostrally placed ADVR and a caudally placed BDVR in all of the taxa discussed so far. The intrinsic organization of ADVR in snakes, lizards, *Sphenodon*, and turtles can be viewed as variations on a common theme that will be called the *first pattern* of DVR organization. It is summarized diagrammatically in Figure 3.47, which shows segments taken from ADVR in representatives of each of the major taxa. This pattern is characterized by a zonal organization of ADVR defined in terms of variations in the cytology and distribution of neurons. The first zone is a relatively narrow, cell-poor zone immediately subjacent to the

300 μ

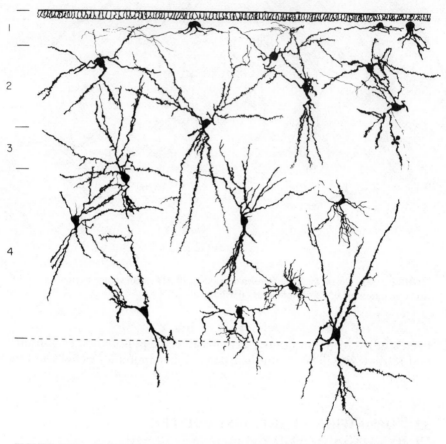

FIGURE 3.34.   Medial area. Neurons in medial area of ADVR are shown as they appear in Golgi preparations of *Pseudemys*. From Balaban (1978a).

ventricular surface of ADVR. It contains neurons (juxtaependymal cells) whose dendrites extend concentric with the ventricular surface. The second zone contains a relatively large number of clusters of neurons with touching somata. The number of such clusters and the number of their constituent neurons vary significantly between species. The remainder of ADVR consists of a third zone of scattered individual neurons and occasional clusters of touching neurons. The neurons in

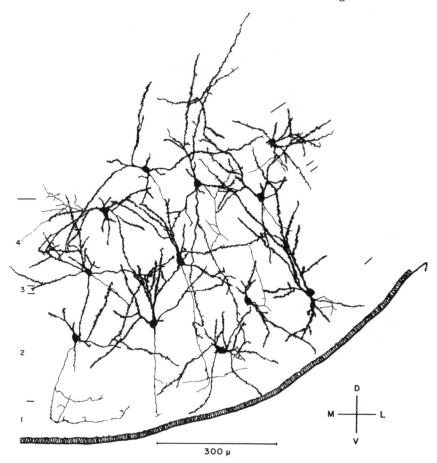

FIGURE 3.35. Ventral area. Neurons in ventral areas of ADVR are shown in Golgi preparations in *Pseudemys*. From Balaban (1978a).

the second and third zones are stellate neurons that are either spine laden or relatively aspiny. An important feature is that the axons of ADVR neurons have a pronounced radial orientation and interconnect the zones. Thus, stellate neurons in the second zone typically have axons that extend into the third zone and vice versa.

BDVR has not been sufficiently studied to describe an overall pattern. It tends to contain several nuclear groups. In squamate reptiles (snakes and lizards), it contains nucleus sphericus, which is a cup-shaped aggregation of cells that receive afferents from the accessory olfactory bulbs.

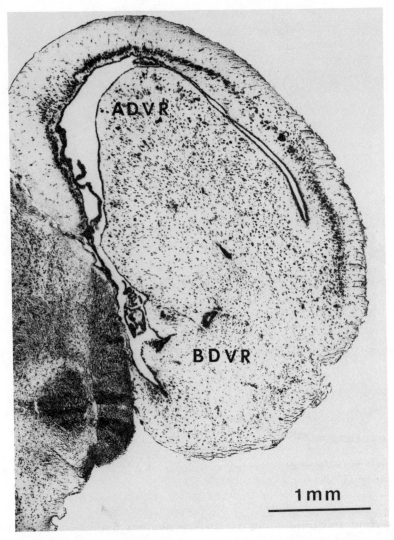

FIGURE 3.36. BDVR in a turtle. BDVR in the red-eared turtle, *Pseudemys scripta,* is shown in a cross section through the caudal telencephalon. *Abbreviations:* **ADVR,** anterior dorsal ventricular ridge; **BDVR,** basal dorsal ventricular ridge.

3.6. CROCODILIANS

ADVR in crocodilians and birds contains clusters of neurons scattered throughout the structure's extent. It thus lacks a zonal organization of the type present in other reptiles. Radially oriented connections are, however, present and interconnect regions that differ in the nature of their cell clusters.

Within the crocodilians, ADVR has been well studied only in *Alligator mississippiensis* and two species of *Caiman*, all members of the family Alligatoridae. However, illustrations of ADVR in *Crocodilus palustris* (Rose, 1923) suggest that it is comparable in the family Crocodylidae. It forms a relatively large, vertically oriented protrusion into the lateral ventricle in crocodilians, but does not show distinct zones (Fig. 3.37). Rose (1923) divided crocodilian DVR into nuclear fields that were designated by letters, and Riss, Halpern, and Scalia (1969) divided the forebrain of *Caiman* into a series of numbered zones (that are not zones in the sense used here). However, the most influential study is that of Crosby (1917). She referred to most of ADVR in *Alligator* as the dorsolateral area (DLA). An intermediolateral area (ILA) was recognized along the ventral border of ADVR rostrally. These areas are separated by relatively indistinct cell poor laminae. Clark and Ulinski (1982) restudied the cytoarchitecture of ADVR in *Alligator* and identified four areas. Their dorsolateral and intermediolateral areas correspond to those of Crosby. In addition, they recognized a dorsomedial area that is situated dorsally and medially to the rostral part of DLA and contains relatively large clusters of neurons and a lateroventral area that corresponds to the nucleus of the lateral olfactory tract identified by Crosby.

Clark and Ulinski (1982) studied the cytology of ADVR in *Alligator* using Nissl and Golgi techniques. Neurons in *Alligator* ADVR are similar to those of other reptiles in that clusters of small numbers of neurons are frequent (Fig. 3.38). Large clusters, such as those seen in some lizards, are not found. There is a tendency for clusters to form a periventricular zone within the dorsomedial area but not in the other areas. Three major types of neurons are present in Golgi preparations. Juxtaependymal neurons have dendrites that extend concentric with the ventricular surface (Fig. 3.39). Spiny neurons have stellate shaped dendritic fields that bear a variable number of dendritic spines (Fig. 3.40). Aspiny neurons have a large number of curly dendrites; they almost completely lack dendritic spines. Information on ADVR's intrinsic connections is not available for crocodilians.

Patches of SDH activity are seen in *Caiman* ADVR. Baker-Cohen (1968) and Contestabile and DiPardo (1976) report a strongly stained

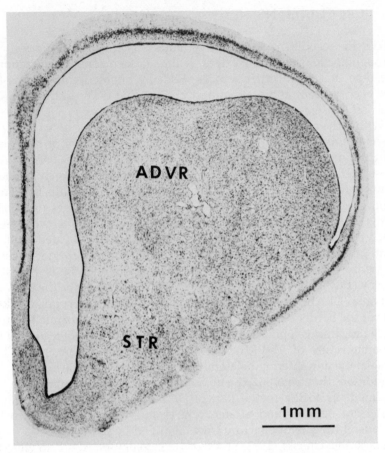

FIGURE 3.37. Crocodilian ADVR. ADVR in crocodilians is illustrated by a section through a Nissl preparation of *Alligator. Abbreviations:* **ADVR,** anterior dorsal ventricular ridge; **STR,** striatum.

oval patch in lateral dorsolateral area. Pritz and Northcutt (1977) found two patches, one laterally placed and one medially placed. They correspond to the position of terminal fields from nucleus rotundus and nucleus reuniens in the thalamus, respectively.

BDVR has been briefly described in *Alligator mississippiensis* (Crosby, 1917) and *Caiman sclerops* (Riss, Halpern, and Scalia, 1969). The striatum has been described in *Alligator* (Crosby, 1917) and *Caiman* (Riss, Halpern, and Scalia, 1969; Brauth and Kitt, 1980). Crosby's nomenclature is the most widely used and can be applied to both *Alligator* and *Caiman*. The striatum is referred to as the ventrolateral area (VLA) in this ter-

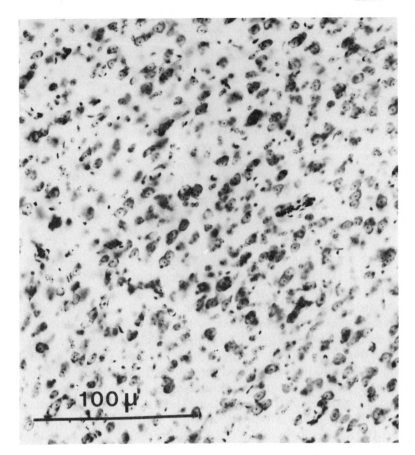

FIGURE 3.38. Clusters in *Caiman* ADVR. The cytology of neurons in *Caiman* ADVR is illustrated in a photomicrograph of neurons in the dorsolateral area of ADVR. Notice that clusters of neurons are scattered throughout the region depicted.

minology (Fig. 3.37). The small-celled VLA lies medial to the lateral forebrain bundle. The large-celled VLA consists of cells lying within the fibers of the forebrain bundle. Contestabile and DiPardo (1976) report strong AChE activity in the ventrolateral area of *Caiman*.

3.7. BIRDS

ADVR in Birds

The embryonic ingrowth of ADVR in reptiles leads to a situation in which the lateral ventricle surrounds DVR on three sides throughout its

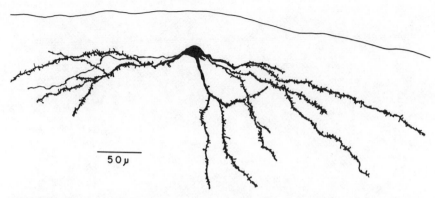

FIGURE 3.39.   Juxtaependymal neuron. A juxtaependymal neuron from a Golgi–Kopsch preparation of *Alligator* is shown.

rostrocaudal extent. By contrast, the absence of such an ingrowth in birds leads to a situation in which the lateral ventricle forms only the medial surface of rostral ADVR in adults. There is substantial variation, and in the hummingbirds *Chrysolampis mosquitus* (Craigie, 1928) and, to a lesser extent in *Lampornis mango* (Craigie, 1932), the ventricle extends laterally dorsal to ADVR in the rostral hemisphere. In other ratite (Craigie, 1935a,b, 1936, 1939) and carinate (e.g., Stingelin, 1958) birds, the lateral ventricle maintains its embryonic position as a vertically aligned slit in the rostral telencephalon. There is, however, a substantial variation in the position of ADVR within the hemisphere. In species such as the kiwi, *Apteryx australis*, DVR is elaborated mediolaterally and curves around onto the lateral surface of the brain (Durward, 1932; Craigie, 1930, 1935a).

The cytology of ADVR neurons has been studied by Stingelin (1958; see Pearson, 1972, for an English summary of Stingelin's work) who recognized nine types of neurons in the forebrains of birds. Generally speaking, isolated neurons are either small, round, or oval neurons that have little basophilic material in their cytoplasm or larger, multipolar neurons with some Nissl substance (Fig. 3.41). Clusters of neurons occur frequently and vary greatly in size. Electron microscopic observations (Saini and Leppelsack, 1977) in starlings (*Sturnus vulgaris*) indicate that the plasma membranes of neurons within cell clusters in field L are in direct contact. Specialized junctions are generally not seen, but there are some junctions that consist of dark patches in which the plasma membranes are separated by about 80 Å and the cytoplasmic faces both show electron-dense material. As in crocodilians, neuronal clusters oc-

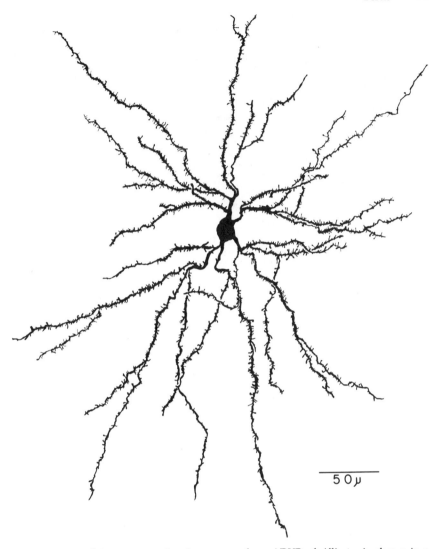

FIGURE 3.40. Spiny neuron. A spiny neuron from ADVR of *Alligator* is shown in a Golgi–Kopsch preparation.

cur throughout all of ADVR, so that there is no distinct cell cluster zone near the ventricle. There are variations both in the number of neurons present in the cluster and of the sizes of neurons present in a cluster (Stingelin, 1958). Nucleus basalis in mallard ducks (*Anas platyrhynchos*) is divided into dorsal and ventral parts (Dubbeldam, Brauch, and Don, 1981). Neurons in the dorsal part form columns of tightly packed

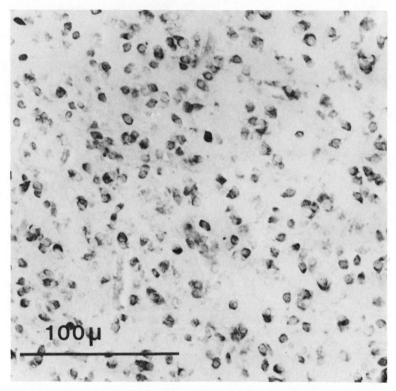

FIGURE 3.41. Neuronal clusters in avian ADVR. The cytology of neurons in avian ADVR is illustrated in this photograph of neostriatum in pigeon. Notice that clusters of neurons extend throughout the region depicted.

neurons that are separated by fascicles of fibers. Such columns are not present in the ventral part.

The majority of neurons in ADVR (Fig. 3.42) have stellate-shaped dendritic trees and bear dendritic spines (Ramón y Cajal, 1955, Fig. 26; Palacios, 1976; Saini and Leppelsack, 1977; Katz and Gurney, 1981; Dubbeldam, Brauch, and Don, 1981; Dobrokhotova, 1981). Axons tend to collateralize within the vicinity of the cell's dendritic tree as well as bearing radially oriented collaterals (Fig. 3.43; Palacios, 1976; Katz and Gurney, 1981). Saini and Leppelsack (1981) have studied neurons in the caudal neostriatum of starlings (*Sturnus vulgaris*) in some detail and recognize four types. Long-axon neurons with spiny dendrites are the most numerous and tend to be impregnated in clusters of touching neurons. Their somata are pear-shaped or triangular and measure 9–12

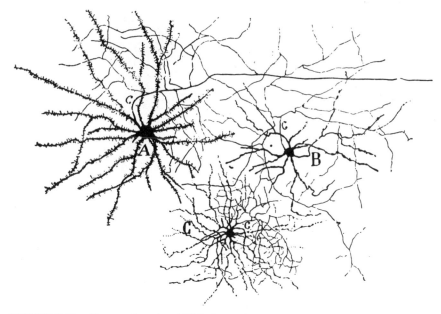

FIGURE 3.42. Neurons in avian ADVR. Examples of a spiny (A) and aspiny (B and C) neurons from avian ADVR is shown in Golgi preparations. From Ramón y Cajal (1955).

μm in diameter. They have three to four dendrites that are heavily covered with dendritic spines. Axons of these neurons tend to follow a straight or oblique course away from the somata and bear frequent collaterals. Long axon neurons with spine-poor dendrites also impregnate in groups. They tend to be found in the rostral and dorsal neostriatum close to the lamina hyperstriatica. Their somata are slightly smaller, measuring 7–10 μm in diameter. They have three to four thin dendrites that lack dendritic spines. Their axons can be routinely traced for long distances. Some bifurcate and form ascending and descending branches. The axons tend to bear frequent collaterals. The remaining two types of neurons are rarely impregnated. Short-axon neurons have dendrites with a few, irregularly scattered dendritic spines. Their axons bifurcate after a short distance and could not be followed far from the somata. Microneurons are scattered in the fascicles of fibers afferent to field L. They have small somata 5–7 μm in diameter and four short, smooth dendrites.

Radially oriented connections have been documented in two regions of avian ADVR using axonal tracing techniques. First, Karten and Hodos (1970) suggested that neurons deep in ectostriatum of pigeons project to

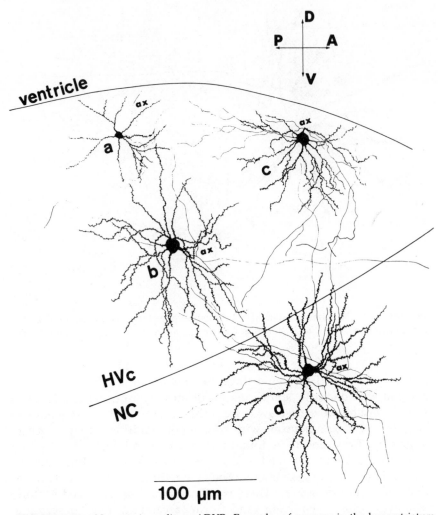

FIGURE 3.43.   Neurons in auditory ADVR. Examples of neurons in the hyperstriatum ventrale pars caudalis and the neostriatum caudalis that were filled with HRP are shown from preparations of zebra finch. From Katz and Gurney (1981).

a band of cells, the periectostriatal belt (E_p), that surrounds ectostriatum. Further, lesions in E_p produce terminal degeneration in a longitudinally oriented column within the overlying lateral neostriatum intermediale (NIL) (Ritchie and Cohen, 1977). This terminal field extends rostrocaudally from the caudal ectostriatum and caudal archistriatum. Also, injections of HRP into NIL label cells in dorsal E_p. These experiments suggest the following sequence of radial connections: $E \rightarrow E_p \rightarrow NIL$. In addition, injections of HRP in the temporo-parieto-occipital area lateral to the neostriatum retrogradely label neurons in E_p, indicating the existence of an additional radial projection from the ectostriatal complex.

The second set of radial connections involves field L. Kelly and Nottebohm (1976) showed with autoradiographic tracing techniques in canaries (*Serinus canarius*) that axons from field L ascend vertically and collect along the border of hyperstriatum ventrale. Since neurons in hyperstriatum ventrale have stellate dendritic fields (Katz and Gurney, 1981), the dendrites of those hyperstriatal neurons situated at the structure's border with the neostriatum should extend into the terminal field of axons ascending from field L. Similarly, Bonke, Bonke, and Scheich (1979) showed that field L in the guinea fowl (*Numida meleagris*) projects to the overlying neostriatum (Fig. 3.44). However, some field L projections in guinea fowl cross the lamina hyperstriatica and terminate in the hyperstriatum ventrale. These axons have been visualized in starlings by Saini and Leppelsack (1981) who could follow the axons of aspiny stellate cells in field L toward the hyperstriatum. The axons collateralized heavily along the ventral border of the lamina hyperstriatica prior to piercing it and arborizing within the hyperstriatum.

The distribution of SDH in birds has been studied by Baker-Cohen (1968) in parakeets (*Melopsittacus undulatus*), by Kusunoki (1969) in finches (*Uroloncha domestica*) and ducks (*Anas platyrhynchos*), and by Minelli (1970) in quail (*Coturnix coturnix*). The ectostriatum and paleostriatum augmentatum are always strongly stained. In addition, Kusunoki reports SDH activity in dorsomedial neostriatum and Baker-Cohen finds activity in a layer of neuropile between neostriatum and hyperstriatum, in caudal neostriatum, and in paleostriatum primitivum. The large neurons in the lateral forebrain bundle stain in all species.

BDVR in Birds

The archistriatum in birds corresponds in position to the basal dorsal ventricular ridge of reptiles in that it lies in the lateral, basal hemisphere caudal to the anterior commissure. Zeier and Karten (1971) recognized four major subdivisions of the archistriatum in pigeons (Fig. 3.45). These are the archistriatum anterior, intermediale, posterior, and mediale. Each division has different connections and can itself be subdivided into additional cytoarchitectural regions. Nottebohm, Stokes, and Leonard (1976) identified a discrete subdivision of the archistriatum, named the nucleus robustus archistriaticus, in canaries. This nucleus had been previously outlined in the red-winged blackbird, *Agelaius phoeniceus*, and

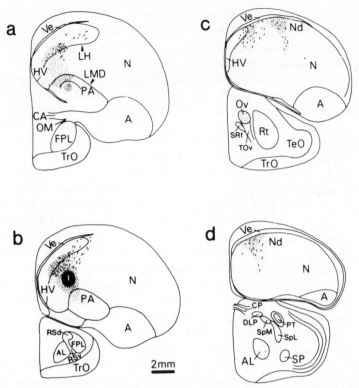

FIGURE 3.44. Projections of field L. The efferent projections of field L in a guinea fowl are shown following an injection of triated traces into field L. *Abbreviations:* **A**, archistriatum; **CA**, anterior commissure; **DLP**, nucleus dorsolateralis posterior; **AL**, ansa lenticularis; **CP**, posterior commissure; **FPL**, lateral forebrain bundle; **HV**, hyperstriatum ventrale; **LH**, lamina hyperstriatica; **LMD**, dorsal medullary lamina; **N**, neostriatum; **Nd**, neostriatum dorsale; **OM**, occipitomesencephalic tract; **Ov**, nucleus ovoidalis; **PA**, paleostriatum augmentatum; **PT**, pretectum; **Rt**, nucleus rotundus; **RSd**, nucleus reticularis superior, pars dorsalis; **RSv**, nucleus reticularis superior, pars ventralis; **SpM**, nucleus spiriformis medialis; **SpL**, nucleus spiriformis lateralis; **SRt**, nucleus subrotundus; **TrO**, optic tract; **Ve**, lateral ventricle. From Bonke, Bonke, and Scheich (1979).

Steller's jay, *Cyanocitta stelleri*, (Brown, 1971, 1973) and has been subsequently identified in the zebra finch, *Poephilla guttata*, (Gurney, 1981) and a variety of oscine songbirds (Nottebohm, 1980a). Its relation to the subdivisions of the archistriatum in pigeons is not certain, but its connections suggest that nucleus robustus corresponds to at least part of the intermediate archistriatum in pigeons. Golgi preparations of the nucleus robustus in canaries (DeVoogd and Nottebohm, 1981) and zebra finches (Gurney, 1981) demonstrate both spiny and aspiny stellate cells.

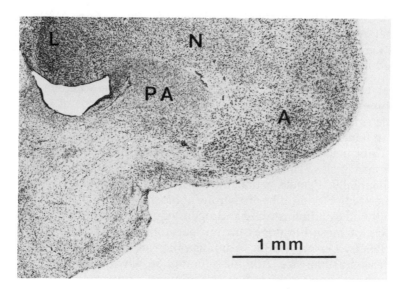

FIGURE 3.45.   Archistriatum. The archistriatum (A) is shown in a caudal section through the telencephalon of a chicken. *Other abbreviations:* **N**, neostriatum; **L**, field L; **PA**, paleostriatum augmentatum.

An interesting feature of certain nuclei in the DVR and striatum of songbirds is that they are sexually dimorphic. These nuclei include the hyperstriatum ventrale, area X of the parolfactory lobe, and nucleus robustus of the archistriatum, all of which have been implicated in the neural control of song (see Section 7.2). Only adult, male birds normally sing and the production of song is known to be under hormonal control (Nottebohm, 1980a). Autoradiographic observations on the nuclei involved in song control following the injection of tritiated testosterone indicate that their neurons concentrate hormones (Arnold, 1979, 1980; Arnold and Saltiel, 1978; Arnold, Nottebohm, and Pfaff, 1979) and that males contain a larger number of neurons that concentrate hormones (Arnold, 1980). The mechanisms underlying the action of the hormones are unknown. There are, however, morphological differences between males and females. The first is that the volumes of area X, hyperstriatum ventrale pars caudalis, nucleus robustus, and the hypoglossal motor nucleus are larger in males than in females in both canaries (Nottebohm and Arnold, 1976) and zebra finches (Gurney, 1981). Further, Nottebohm (1980b) has shown that the total volumes of hyperstriatum ventrale pars caudalis and nucleus robustus in 25 male canaries were correlated with the number of syllables in their songs. Volumes of hyperstriatum ventrale and nucleus robustus are correlated with the size of song repertoires (Canady, Kroodsma, and Nottebohm, 1981) in long-billed marsh wrens (*Cistothorus palustris*).

At least in the case of nucleus robustus, these variations in total volume seem to reflect two factors. First, the number of neurons in nucleus robustus of male zebra finches is approximately twice the number in females. Second, both the soma diameters (Gurney, 1981) and the dendritic field sizes (DeVoogd and Nottebohm, 1981) are larger in males than in females. These morphological features can be manipulated experimentally. Female zebra finches that are exposed to testosterone, 17β-estradiol, or 5α-dihydrosterone at hatching can be caused to sing in adulthood by administering androgens (Gurney and Konishi, 1980). The effects of these hormones on nucleus robustus was studied in zebra finches by Gurney (1981). Administration of 17β-estradiol leads to an increase in soma size. Administration of 5α-dihydrosterone leads to an increase in the number of neurons in nucleus robustus. Administration of testosterone causes increases in both neuronal number and neuronal size. Similar results have been obtained in canaries (Nottebohm, 1980a). Finally, the sizes of the hyperstriatum ventrale and nucleus robustus in male canaries vary seasonally in concert with the annual relearning of song (Nottebohm, 1981).

Striatum in Birds

Of the several nomenclatures available for the striatum of birds (e.g., Edinger, Wallenberg, and Holmes, 1903; Rose, 1914; Kuhlenbeck, 1938), that of Ariens Kappers, Huber, and Crosby (1936) is most widely used. They recognized two groups of cells (Fig. 3.46). The paleostriatum augmentatum (PA) is a broad band of cells which is separated from the overlying DVR by the dorsal medullary lamina (LMD). It forms a cap that overlies the paleostriatum primitivum (PP), which consists of cells lying within the fibers of the lateral forebrain bundle just below the paleostriatum augmentatum. In addition to the paleostriatal complex, two additional structures have been included in the striatum by other authors. The intrapeduncular nucleus (IP) consists of large cells embedded in the fibers of the lateral forebrain bundle ventral to the paleostriatum primitivum (Karten and Dubbeldam, 1973). The parolfactory lobe (LPO) of Edinger, Wallenberg, and Holmes (1903) lies between the paleostriatum augmentatum and the lateral ventricle. Songbirds have a

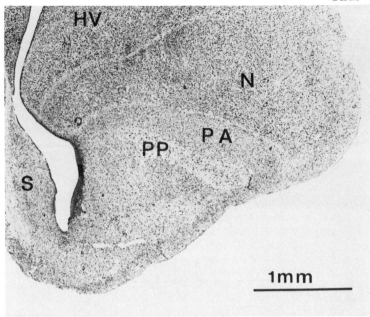

FIGURE 3.46. Striatum in birds. The cytoarchitecture of the striatum in birds is illustrated by a section through the forebrain of a chicken from a Nissl preparation. The paleostriatum augmentatum (PA) is continuous with the parolfactory lobe and lies below the cell-poor dorsal medullary lamina. The paleostriatum primitivum (PP) is situated ventral to the paleostriatum augmentatum. The intrapeduncular nucleus consists of neurons embedded ventral to the paleostriatum primitivum in the lateral forebrain bundle. *Other abbreviations:* **HV**, hyperstriatum ventrale; **N**, neostriatum; **S**, septum.

distinct region of the parolfactory lobe that is not seen in other birds; it has been named area X (Nottebohm, Stokes, and Leonard, 1976) and is implicated in the neural control of song (see Section 7.2).

Golgi preparations of chicken brains (Palacios, 1976) show that neurons in the paleostriatum augmentatum generally resemble the spiny stellate cells seen in the overlying neostriatum and ectostriatum. By contrast, neurons in the paleostriatum primitivum and intrapeduncular nucleus have relatively long, isodendritic dendrites with fewer dendritic spines (Fox et al., 1966; Palacios, 1976). Electron microscopic observations indicate that the dendrites of these neurons are densely covered with synaptic boutons (Fox et al., 1966).

All of the studies of AChE activity in birds (Karten and Dubbeldam, 1973; Minelli, 1970; Kusunoki, 1969; Parent and Olivier, 1970/1971; Dubé and Parent, 1981) report strong AChE activity in the paleostriatum augmentatum, intrapeduncular nucleus, and parolfactory lobe. The paleostriatum primitivum is low in AChE activity. High concentrations of

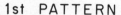

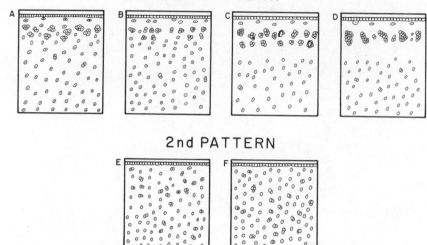

FIGURE 3.47. Zones in ADVR. These diagrams represent sections through ADVR which summarize the distribution of neurons in ADVR. Sections A through D show the first major pattern of ADVR organization in which a cell cluster zone is separated from the ependyma by a cell-poor periventricular zone. Sections E and F represent the second pattern in which cell clusters are spread evenly throughout DVR. (A) Snake; (B) Type II lizard; (C) Type I lizard; (D) turtle; (E) crocodilian; (F) bird.

enkephalin-like immunoreactivity are present in the paleostriatum and parolfactory lobe of pigeons (Bayon et al., 1980) and chicks (de Lanerolle et al., 1981).

3.8. DEFINITION OF THE SECOND PATTERN
OF DVR ORGANIZATION

In summary, DVR in crocodilians and birds can also be divided into an ADVR and a BDVR, although BDVR is traditionally called the archistriatum in birds. The intrinsic organization of ADVR in crocodilians and birds differs from that in squamates, *Sphenodon*, and turtles and shows a *second pattern* of DVR organization (Fig. 3.47). This pattern is characterized by the absence of a distinct periventricular cell cluster zone in ADVR. Isolated neurons and clusters of touching neurons are, instead, scattered throughout ADVR. BDVR in crocodilians has not been extensively studied, so that it is not possible to relate its organization to that of either BDVR in other reptiles or to the archistriatum in birds.

Some of the data discussed in this chapter raise the possibility that a feature common to both the first and second patterns of ADVR organization is the existence of radially oriented connections. This is seen in the first pattern by axons that ramify with vertical components that interconnect the zones. Similarly, in birds, radially oriented axons interconnect field L and the hyperstriatum ventrale and connect the ectostriatum with overlying structures. Such connections are of interest because they could serve to spread information that is carried to ADVR within radially oriented sectors. This idea will be considered further after the sources of sensory information to ADVR have been considered.

Chapter Four

SENSORY AFFERENTS TO DVR AND STRIATUM

First Steps in the Linkages

Having dealt with the basic structure of DVR, it is now possible to consider the relation of sensory pathways to DVR. This is important to the central argument of the treatise because it is these pathways that establish the initial steps in the sensory linkages through DVR. It should be stressed, however, that DVR in fact receives projections from many regions of the brain, only a fraction of which are obvious conduits of sensory information. The total set of brain structures that carry information to DVR can be determined by injecting large amounts of horseradish peroxidase (HRP) into DVR and cataloging those brain structures that contain retrogradely labeled neurons. This procedure has been carried out for ADVR in turtles (Belekhova et al., 1979; Balaban and Ulinski, 1981a) and lizards (Bruce and Butler, 1979; ten Donkelaar and De Boervan Huizen, 1981b) and shows that three major groups of structures project to ADVR: (1) thalamic nuclei, (2) cortical structures, and (3) brainstem structures. The first two groups of structures include some that carry sensory information to ADVR. Comparable experiments have not been executed for BDVR, but the available information is that BDVR receives sensory information via two sources. These sensory afferents to ADVR and BDVR will be treated in this chapter; brainstem projections to DVR and the striatum are the subject of Chapter 5.

4.1. THALAMIC AFFERENTS

Thalamic nuclei that project to ADVR can be divided into two groups (Balaban and Ulinski, 1981a). The first are nuclei that project to discrete areas of ADVR. Many of these are known or suspected to be sensory relay nuclei. The second are nuclei that give rise to widespread or diffuse projections to the forebrain.

Sensory Thalamic Nuclei

The projections of sensory thalamic nuclei to ADVR are best considered in the context of the major sensory pathways. This section therefore summarizes the organization of the (a) visual, (b) auditory, and (c) somatosensory pathways in reptiles and birds. The pathways that carry sensory information are first outlined in each case. The nature of the thalamic projection to ADVR are then considered. It is possible in a few cases to trace the flow of sensory information from the periphery to ADVR.

(a) Visual Pathways

1. *General Features of Visual Pathways.* Two thalamic nuclei carry visual information to the forebrain in reptiles and birds. The first is nucleus rotundus, which is located centrally in the thalamus and receives visual information via the optic tectum. The projection of the retina to the optic tectum is entirely crossed in *Sphenodon* (Northcutt, Braford, and Landreth, 1974), crocodilians (Braford, 1973; Repérant, 1975), birds (e.g., Repérant, 1973), and some lizards (e.g., Repérant et al., 1978), but is bilateral in snakes (Northcutt and Butler, 1974; Halpern and Frumin, 1973), other lizards (e.g., Repérant et al., 1978), and turtles (Bass and Northcutt, 1981). The factors determining the extent of crossing are unknown, but the degree of binocular overlap in the frontal visual fields does not seem to be involved (Northcutt and Butler, 1974; Repérant and Rio, 1976). Retinotectal projections are retinotopically organized (snakes: Terashima and Goris, 1975; *Iguana:* Stein and Gaither, 1981; *Alligator:* Heric and Kruger, 1965; turtles: Guselnikov, Morenkov, and Pivovarov, 1970; pigeons: Hamdi and Whitteridge, 1954; Clarke and Whitteridge, 1976). The optic tectum projects bilaterally to nucleus rotundus. Nucleus rotundus then projects to the ipsilateral ADVR in all of the species that have been studied.

The second thalamic nucleus that carries visual information to the forebrain is usually called the dorsal lateral geniculate nucleus or the principal optic complex. It is situated laterally, just medial to the optic tract, and receives direct projections from the retina (snakes: Halpern and Frumin, 1973; Repérant, 1973; Northcutt and Butler, 1974; lizards: e.g., Cruce and Cruce, 1978; *Sphenodon:* Northcutt, Braford, and Landreth, 1974; *Caiman:* Repérant, 1975; Braford, 1973; turtles: e.g., Hall and Ebner, 1970a; Bass and Northcutt, 1981; birds: e.g., Repérant, 1973). As in the retinotectal projection, there are interspecific variations in the extent of the ipsilateral projection. The retinogeniculate projection is known to be topographically organized in turtles (Ulinski, 1980) and birds (Pettigrew, 1979). The geniculate projects to a region situated immediately lateral to ADVR in all reptiles that have been studied. This projection has been reported in snakes (Wang and Halpern, 1977), tegu lizards (Lohman and van Woerden-Verkley, 1979) and iguanas (Bruce, 1982) in HRP experiments. The geniculate projects to the lateral edge of the dorsal cortex in turtles (e.g., Hall and Ebner, 1970b). The geniculate projections appear to be different in birds in that they terminate in the Wulst (e.g., Repérant, Raffin, and Miceli, 1974; Miceli, Peyrichoux, and Repérant, 1975). However, neurons in the Wulst are originally situated lateral to ADVR in chick embryos and are subsequently shifted to the dorsomedial corner of the pallium (Tsai, Garber, and Larramendi, 1981a,b), so that the same basic pattern may hold for both reptiles and birds.

The following sections consider the organization of the visual pathways from retina to ADVR in each group of reptiles and birds.

2. *Snakes.* The nature of nucleus rotundus in snakes has been the subject of some confusion. Northcutt and Butler (1974) identified a small group of cells in the thalamus as nucleus rotundus in the water snake, *Natrix sipedon.* However, Ulinski (*Natrix;* 1977a) and Schroeder (*Crotalus;* 1981) could not unequivocally identify a tectorecipient nucleus in central thalamus. More recently, Dacey and Ulinski (1983) have been able to identify nucleus rotundus in the caudal thalamus of the garter snake, *Thamnophis sirtalis* (Fig. 4.1). It both receives tectal afferents and projects to the forebrain (Fig. 4.2). Lesions involving the central, caudal zone of dorsal thalamus that contains rotundus produce terminal degeneration in the full extent of rostral ADVR (Ulinski, 1978a). Degenerated axons ascend vertically through the striatum and into ADVR. Particulate degeneration is scattered within ADVR and extends over the cell clusters in zone B, but not into the cell-poor zone A (Fig. 4.3). These data indicate that tectofugal visual information reaches ADVR in snakes. The existence of projections from the dorsal lateral geniculate nucleus to ADVR have been suggested in snakes (Wang and Halpern, 1977).

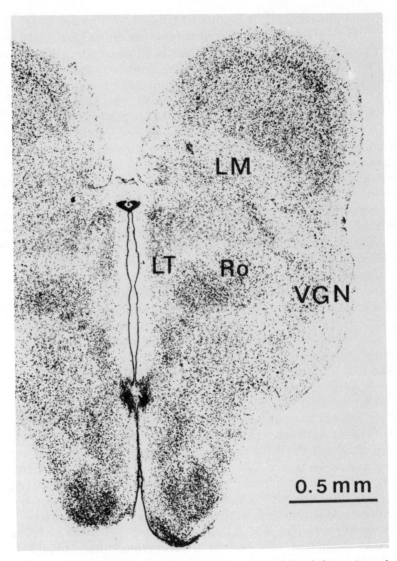

FIGURE 4.1. Thalamus in snakes. The cytoarchitecture of the thalamus in snakes is illustrated in this section through the caudal thalamus of a water snake, *Natrix sipedon*. Nucleus rotundus (Ro) lies in the central thalamus. The caudal tip of the ventral lateral geniculate nucleus (VGN) is seen laterally. *Other abbreviations:* **LM,** nucleus lentiformis mesencephali; **LT,** nucleus lentiformis thalami.

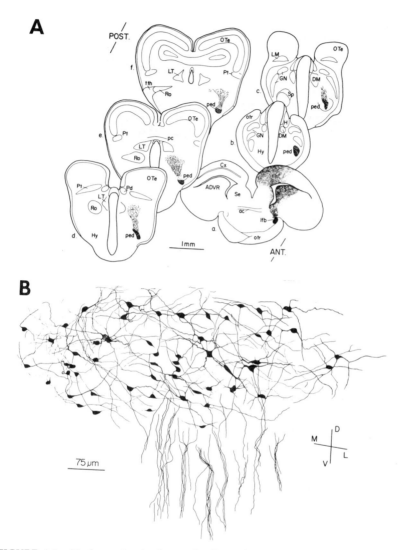

FIGURE 4.2. Nucleus rotundus in a snake. Rotundus is demonstrated in a garter snake (*Thamnophis sirtalis*) by retrograde labeling with HRP. (A) An injection of HRP in ADVR labels neurons in rotundus. The injection site is shown in the most rostral section (a), Labeled axons can be followed caudally to nucleus rotundus (Ro) in sections (d) and (e). (B) Retrogradely labeled neurons in nucleus rotundus. *Abbreviations:* **ADVR,** anterior dorsal ventricular ridge; **AC,** anterior commissure; **DM,** dorsomedial nucleus; **GN,** geniculate complex; **Hy,** hypothalamus; **H,** habenula; **lfb,** lateral forebrain bundle; **LM,** nucleus lentiformis mesencephali; **LT,** nucleus lentiformis thalami; **OTe,** optic tectum; **otr,** optic tract; **pc,** posterior commissure; **pd,** nucleus posterodorsalis; **ped,** dorsal peduncle of the lateral forebrain bundle; **Pt,** pretectal nucleus; **tth,** tectothalamic tract. From Dacey and Ulinski (1983).

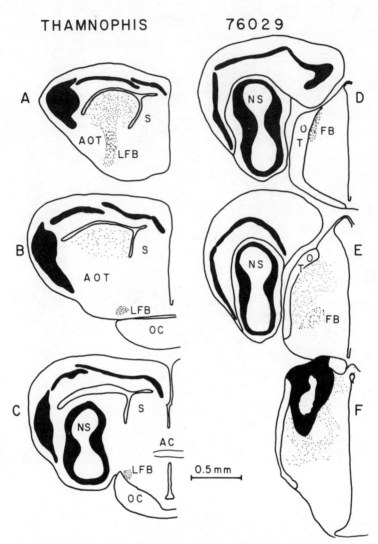

FIGURE 4.3. Thalamic projections to DVR in a snake. The extent of thalamic projections to ADVR in the garter snake *Thamnophis sirtalis* are shown following a large thalamic lesion (section F). The resulting degeneration is plotted in a Fink–Heimer preparation. Notice that the particulate degeneration extends over the area occupied by zone B at some points in sections (A) and (B). *Abbreviations:* **AC,** anterior commissure; **AOT,** accessory olfactory tract; **FB,** forebrain bundles; **LFB,** lateral forebrain bundle; **NS,** nucleus sphericus; **OC,** optic chiasm; **OT,** optic tract; **S,** septum. From Ulinski (1978a).

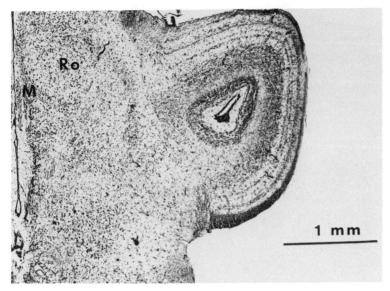

FIGURE 4.4. Thalamus in lizards. The pattern of thalamic nuclei in lizards is illustrated by a section through the caudal thalamus in the green iguana, *Iguana iguana*. The section passes through nucleus rotundus (Ro) and nucleus medialis (M).

Using the 2-deoxyglucose technique, Kubie and Allen (1978) demonstrated that neurons in ADVR show increased activity following visual stimulation.

3. *Lizards.* Nucleus rotundus is well developed in most lizards (Fig. 4.4) and in the amphisbaenian *Amphisbaenia darwinii* (Quiroga, 1979b). The limited information available on the morphology of rotundal neurons in lizards (*Lacerta*, Ramón, 1896) and in *Amphisbaenia* (Quiroga, 1979b) indicates that rotundal neurons have relatively large, stellate dendritic fields.

The tectum projects bilaterally to rotundus (Fig. 4.5) in *Iguana* (Butler and Northcutt, 1971) and the tokay gecko, *Gekko gecko* (Butler, 1978). Also, injections of HRP in nucleus rotundus of the monitor lizard, *Varanus exanthematicus*, retrogradely label neurons in the central gray of the tectum (Hoogland, 1982). An organization has been reported within the tectorotundal projection in *Gekko*. Unilateral tectal lesions produce patches or rods of degeneration bilaterally in rotundus that are separated by degeneration-free areas. Bilateral tectal lesions completely fill rotundus with terminal degeneration. These experiments suggest that there is some segregation of information from the two sides of the tec-

Iguana

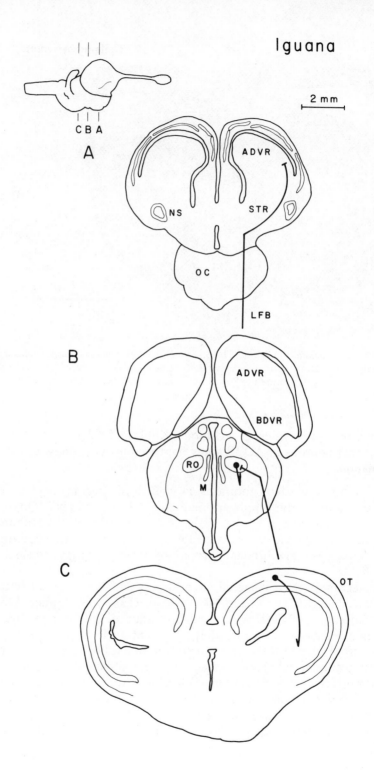

2 mm

tum within rotundus in *Gekko*. However, the large size of rotundal dendritic trees makes it likely that a given rotundal neuron receives information from both sides of the tectum.

It is known that nucleus rotundus projects to ipsilateral ADVR in iguanas (Fig. 4.5), monitor lizards, tegu lizards, and the tokay gecko. Injections of HRP into ADVR retrogradely label rotundal neurons in *Iguana* (Bruce and Butler, 1979; Bruce, 1982) and tegus (Lohman and van Woerden-Verkley, 1978). Large thalamic lesions in *Iguana* produce two disjunct patches of terminal degeneration in ADVR (Butler and Ebner, 1972). The position of the lateral patch corresponds to the rotundal projection field in other species. Lesions involving nucleus rotundus in tegu and monitor lizards produce degeneration in ADVR (*Varanus benegalensis:* Distel and Ebbesson, 1975; *Tupinambis:* Lohman and van Woerden-Verkley, 1978). Terminal degeneration extends into the central region of ADVR, but does not reach the cell cluster zone. Rotundal lesions produce terminal debris in ADVR in *Gekko* (Butler, 1976). The only electrophysiological study of ADVR in lizards is that of Peterson and Rowe (1976) who recorded evoked potentials from ADVR following flashes of light in the iguanid lizard, *Dipsosaurus dorsalis*. The potentials reversed in rostral, central ADVR and could be recorded directly inside of the ventricle.

Exposure to light caused an increase in uptake of 2-deoxyglucose in ADVR of *Anolis carolinensis* (Crews and Greenberg, 1981).

4. *Turtles.* The most extensive work on the tectofugal pathway in reptiles has been done on the turtles *Chrysemys, Pseudemys,* and *Emys,* and a general picture of the properties of each link in the pathway is available for these species (Fig. 4.6). These data will be summarized here because they provide some indication of the role that DVR plays in processing visual information.

Retinal ganglion cells in *Pseudemys* can be divided into at least two classes on the basis of soma size (Peterson and Ulinski, 1982) and physiological properties (Marchiafava and Weiler, 1980; Marchiafava and

---

FIGURE 4.5.   Tectofugal pathway in *Iguana*. The optic tectum (OT) receives visual information from the contralateral retina. Tectal cells project to nucleus rotundus in the thalamus (RO). The projection is bilateral, but the sparse contralateral projection is not shown. Rotundal neurons project via the lateral forebrain bundle (LFB) to the anterior dorsal ventricular ridge (ADVR), probably terminating in its lateral part. *Other abbreviations:* BDVR, basal dorsal ventricular ridge; OC, optic chiasm; M, nucleus medialis; NS, nucleus sphericus; STR, striatum. Based on studies by Butler and Northcutt (1971), Butler and Ebner (1972), and Bruce and Butler (1979).

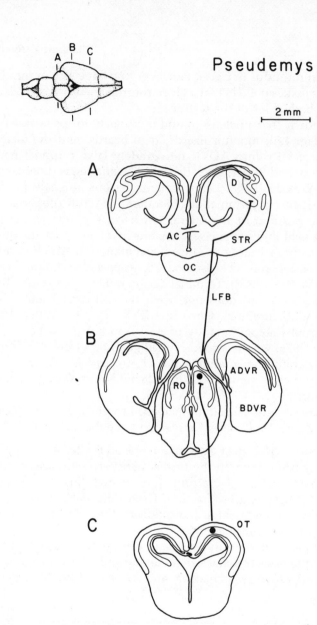

Pseudemys

FIGURE 4.6. Tectofugal pathway in turtles. The optic tectum (OT) receives bilateral retinal projections in the red-eared turtle, *Pseudemys scripta*. The tectum projects to nucleus rotundus (RO) in the thalamus. This projection is bilateral, but only the ipsilateral projection is shown. Nucleus rotundus projects through the lateral forebrain bundle (LFB) to dorsal area (D) of the anterior dorsal ventricular ridge. *Other abbreviations:* **AC,** anterior commissure; **BDVR,** basal dorsal ventricular ridge; **OC,** optic chiasm; **STR,** striatum. Based on studies by Hall and Ebner (1970a,b), Rainey and Ulinski (1982b), Balaban and Ulinski (1981b), and others.

Wagner, 1981). In general (Lipetz and Hill, 1970; Schwartz, 1973; Fulbrook and Granda, 1977; Bowling, 1980; Fulbrook, 1982), ganglion cells are sensitive to moving stimuli at about 9°/sec, are often directionally selective and are sometimes velocity tuned (Fulbrook, Granda, and Maxwell, 1980). Receptive fields are about 3°–10° in diameter and often have an inhibitory surround. Both size classes of ganglion cells project to the tectum (Peterson, 1978). The ganglion cells project bilaterally to the superficial layers of the optic tectum (Bass and Northcutt, 1981).

The properties of tectal units have been studied in *Pseudemys* (Robbins, 1972) and in *Agrionemys* and *Emys* (Boiko and Goncharova, 1976). Boiko and Goncharova found that 82% of their units lacked spontaneous background activity; Robbins found that units in the stratum fibrosum et griseum superficiale lack spontaneous activity while those in the stratum griseum periventriculare show high spontaneous rates of discharge. The latencies of responses vary from 75 to 500 msec as a function of stimulus intensity. Robbins reported on, off, and on–off responses. Boiko and Goncharova found small receptive field sizes (5°–10°) in the superficial layers and larger receptive field sizes (31°–110°) in the deeper layers. Units with small field sizes have circular receptive fields; units with larger fields tend to be elliptical in shape with their long axes parallel to the horizontal meridian. Boiko and Goncharova found that 10% of their units showed directional selectivity with vertical preferences being most common. Robbins found that his deep units often showed directional selectivity with horizontal movements in the temporal to nasal direction being most effective. Superficial units are color sensitive with spectral sensitivity curves that varied in shape, but usually peaked between 600 and 700 nm.

The tectum projects bilaterally to nucleus rotundus (Figs. 4.6 and 4.7), which is a large and well demarcated structure in turtles (Rainey, 1979; Rainey and Ulinski, 1982a). The rotundal border is formed by a monolayer of neurons whose dendrites extend into the core of the nucleus (Fig. 4.8). Rotundal neurons are morphologically homogeneous and have stellate-shaped dendritic fields that extend up to two-thirds of the nucleus' diameter. Injections of HRP into the lateral forebrain bundle retrogradely label at least 99% of the neurons in rotundus. It thus appears likely that all of the neurons in rotundus project to the forebrain.

The nature of the tectorotundal projection has been studied with several anatomical techniques. Tectal lesions produce terminal degeneration bilaterally in rotundus (Hall and Ebner, 1970a; Rainey and Ulinski, 1982b). Each tectal lesion produces degeneration scattered throughout rotundus. The quantity of degeneration increases with the size of the lesion. The nature of the tectorotundal projection can be more fully

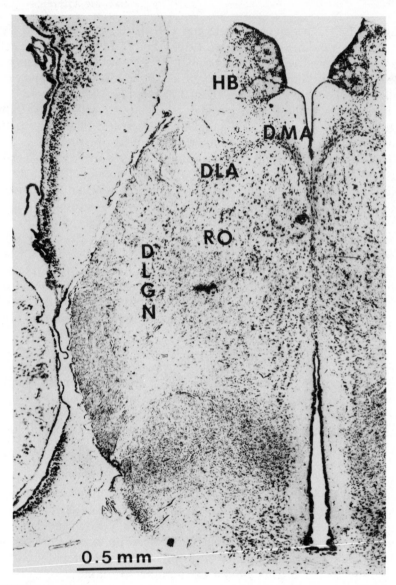

FIGURE 4.7. Thalamus in turtles. The pattern of thalamic nuclei in turtles is illustrated by a section through the diencephalon of the red-eared turtle, *Pseudemys scripta*. The section passes through the habenula (HB), the dorsomedial anterior (DMA) and dorsolateral anterior (DLA) nuclei of the perirotundal group, the dorsal lateral geniculate nucleus (DLGN), and nucleus rotundus (RO).

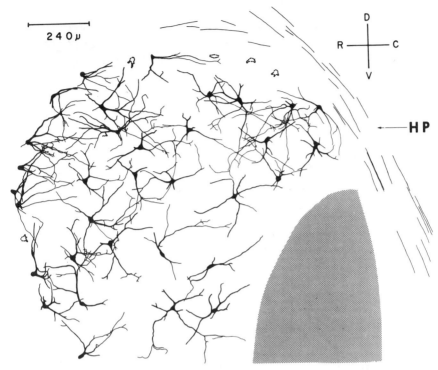

240µ

D

R —— C

V

←—— H P

FIGURE 4.8. Nucleus rotundus in a turtle. Neurons in nucleus rotundus of the red-eared turtle *Pseudemys scripta* are shown in a parasagittal section from a Golgi–Cox preparation. *Abbreviation:* **HP,** habenulopeduncular tract. From Rainey (1979).

visualized using the orthograde transport of HRP (Rainey and Ulinski, 1982b). Following a relatively restricted injection of HRP in the tectum, a fascicle of labeled axons can be followed from the tectum to the ventrolateral surface of the ipsilateral rotundus (Figs. 4.9 and 4.10). Individual fibers turn into rotundus and often bear at least one collateral. Such collaterals together form a fan of fibers that extends throughout most of rotundus. Each collateral usually bears several varicose branches. Axon terminals that have clear, round synaptic vesicles and form asymmetric active zones degenerate following tectal lesions (Kosareva et al., 1973; Tumanova and Ozirskaya, 1973; Rainey and Ulinski, 1982b). They are presynaptic to dendrites, primarily those with relatively small dendritic shafts. These experiments suggest that information from a restricted region of visual space reaches postsynaptic elements throughout rotundus. The projection of the tectum to nucleus rotundus has been confirmed physiologically by electrical stimulation of the tectum and the

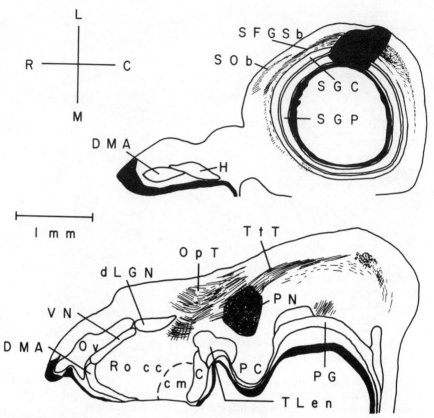

FIGURE 4.9. Tectorotundal projection in a turtle. These two semischematic sections depict the mesencephalic part of the tectorotundal projection in *Pseudemys*. They are sketches of efferent tectal axons that were solidly filled after an iontophoretic injection of HRP into the tectum. The upper drawing depicts a horizontal section through the ventral part of the tectal injection site. The lower drawing depicts a section through the subtectal and pretectal parts of the tectothalamic tract. Labeled axons within rotundus are not drawn. Axons in the SFGSb can be traced as a population into the tectothalamic tract when intermediate sections are examined serially. *Abbreviations:* C, caudal nucleus; cc, central core subregion of rotundus; cm, caudomedial core subregions of rotundus; dLGN, dorsal lateral geniculate nucleus; DMA, dorsomedial anterior nucleus; H, habenula; OpT, optic tract; Ov, ovalis complex; PC, posterior commissure; PG, pericentral gray; PN, pretectal nucleus; SFSGb, sublamina b of stratum fibrosum et griseum superficiale; SGC, stratum griseum centrale; SGP, stratum griseum periventriculare; SOb, sublamina b of stratum opticum; TLen, thalamic lentiform complex; VN, ventral nucleus. From Rainey and Ulinski (1982b).

recording of evoked potentials in rotundus (Belekhova and Akulina, 1970; Belekhova and Kosareva, 1971). Also, unilateral ablation of the tectum raises the threshold of rotundal units to light and movement. Restricted lesions affect responses only in the corresponding part of the visual field (Morenkov and Pivavarov, 1973, 1975).

Morenkov and Pivavarov (1973, 1975) studied the properties of 50 rotundal units in *Emys*. Less than 50% of the units showed spontaneous activity ranging from 0.8 to 6.5 Hz. The latency to light flashes was 60–100 msec. The majority (85%) of the units responded to illumination changes. These units were classified as on (9.3%), off (12.4%), on–off (37.9%), and movement sensitive (31.0%). The most effective stimuli were circles 10°–20° in diameter moving at 15°–60°/sec. A few of the units were directionally selective. The units had very large receptive fields with an unusual structure: stimuli in the lower half of the visual field produced intense responses while those in the upper field were relatively ineffective.

The relation of nucleus rotundus to ADVR was first established by Hall and Ebner (1970b) who made lesions that involved rotundus in *Pseudemys*. Degenerated axons could be traced through the lateral forebrain bundle to a terminal field in ADVR. Similar results have been obtained in *Emys orbicularis* (Kosareva, 1974). Conversely, injections of HRP into ADVR retrogradely label neurons in rotundus (*Pseudemys* and *Chrysemys:* Parent, 1976; Balaban and Ulinski, 1981a; *Emys:* Belekhova et al., 1979). The little physiological work that is available is consistent with the anatomy: lesions of nucleus rotundus suppress evoked potentials in ADVR (Belekhova, 1979).

The organization of the rotundal-ADVR projection has been studied by Balaban and Ulinski (1981b). A large lesion of nucleus rotundus produces degeneration in ADVR that is restricted precisely to zone 4 of dorsal area. A small lesion produces a band of degeneration in ADVR that extends rostrocaudally throughout the length of zone 4 of dorsal area (Fig. 4.11). Detailed examination of the degeneration indicates that rotundal axons are of coarse caliber as they run through the lateral forebrain bundle. They branch as the bundle approaches the ventromedial border of dorsal area, one branch running rostrally along the ventral border of the area and the other branch running dorsally in the transverse plane, along the area's medial border. Branches of the second type bear collaterals that have small varicosities and extend into dorsal area (Fig. 4.12). These data suggest that the axon of an individual rotundal neuron branches extensively along the borders of dorsal area and extends throughout zone 4. Results of HRP experiments are consistent with this model in that large HRP injections in dorsal area retrogradely

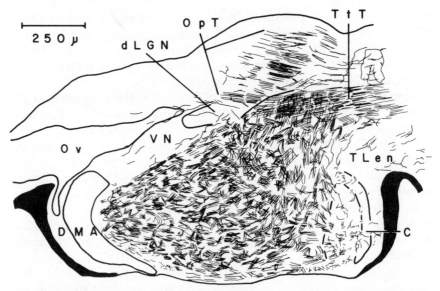

FIGURE 4.10. Tectorotundal axons in a turtle. This semischematic figure depicts the distribution of tectorotundal axons labelled after an HRP injection into the tectum in *Pseudemys*. Note the density and widespread distribution of tectorotundal axons after a subtotal tectal injection. *Abbreviations:* **C**, caudal nucleus; **dLGN**, dorsal lateral geniculate nucleus; **DMA**, dorsomedial anterior nucleus; **OpT**, optic tract; **OV**, ovalis complex; **TLen**, thalamic lentiform complex; **TtT**, tectothalamic tract; **VN**, ventral nucleus. From Rainey and Ulinski (1982b).

label a large percentage of rotundal neurons. Smaller HRP injections in dorsal area label a smaller percentage of rotundal neurons, but the labeled neurons tend to be scattered in a band that extends rostrocaudally through rotundus (Fig. 4.13).

Belekhova (1979) reports that the receptive fields of units in ADVR cover the entire visual field and respond more intensively to moving stimuli than to stationary stimuli or diffuse illumination. Dünser et al. (1981) confirmed these findings and studied the properties of units in ADVR of *Pseudemys* using extracellular recording techniques. The majority of units respond to a variety of spatial, temporal, and chromatic stimuli over most of the monocular visual field. Units respond well to slight movements anywhere in a receptive field larger than 140° in diameter, but exhibit heightened responsiveness to stimuli falling in the region of visual space corresponding to the visual streak or line of high retinal ganglion cell density (Peterson and Ulinski, 1979). Units habituate·quickly to repetitive moving and stationary stimuli. All units

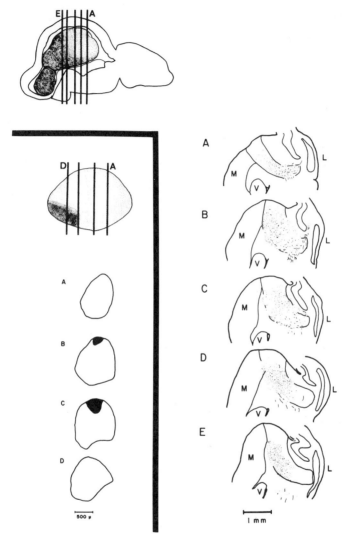

FIGURE 4.11. Rotundal-dorsal area projection in turtles. The projection of nucleus rotundus to dorsal area of ADVR is demonstrated in this experiment. The inset shows a series of sections through rotundus at the levels indicated. The extent of a rotundal lesion is shown in black. The pattern of degeneration seen in a Fink–Heimer preparation of the telencephalon is shown in the main part of the figure. A series of sections through ADVR are shown. Degenerated axons approach the ventral border of dorsal area in sections (C), (D), and (E). The full rostrocaudal extend of dorsal area is filled with particulate degeneration throughout zone 4. *Abbreviations:* **L,** lateral cortex; **M,** medial area of ADVR; **V,** ventral area of ADVR. From Balaban and Ulinski (1981b).

107

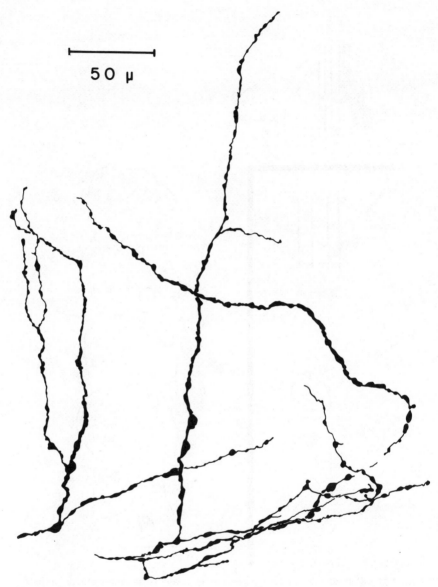

FIGURE 4.12. Rotundal axons in dorsal area. Examples of putative rotundal axons are shown from a rapid Golgi preparation of dorsal area of ADVR in *Pseudemys*. From Balaban and Ulinski (1981b).

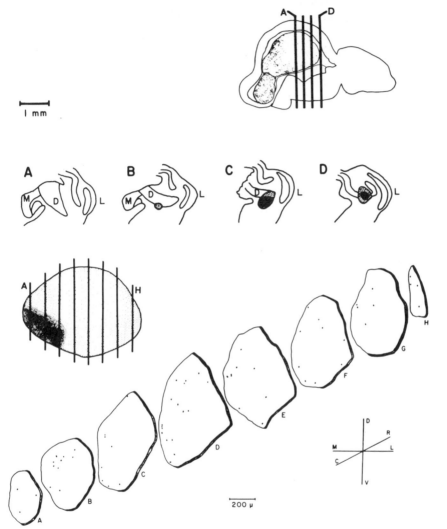

FIGURE 4.13. Rotundo-dorsal area projection in turtles. The projection of nucleus rotundus to ADVR in *Pseudemys* is demonstrated in this retrograde horseradish peroxidase experiment. The sections in the upper part of the figure show the site of an HRP injection in ADVR. Sections at the bottom of the figure show the pattern of retrogradely labeled neurons in nucleus rotundus. From Balaban and Ulinski (1981b).

respond to broad chromatic spectra in both light and dark adaptation. Although units were movement sensitive, they lacked directional sensitivity (Dünser, Maxwell, and Granda, 1981).

In summary, it appears that the projection of the retina to the optic tectum is retinotopically organized in turtles, but that the projection of tectum to nucleus rotundus is *not* retinotopically organized. Instead, the axons from a cluster of tectal neurons diverge through both rotundal nuclei. Similarly, an individual rotundal neuron has an axon that diverges widely in zone 4 of dorsal area. Thus, a given neuron in dorsal area is likely to receive convergent projections from neurons throughout rotundus and, as the physiology shows, from large regions of visual space.

5. *Crocodilians* (Figs. 4.14 and 4.15).   The tectum projects bilaterally to nucleus rotundus in *Caiman* (Braford, 1972). Nucleus rotundus is well developed in crocodilians (Huber and Crosby, 1926). Stereotaxic lesions of rotundus produce terminal degeneration in ADVR in *Caiman crocodilus* (Pritz, 1975). Efferents accumulate on the medial surface of rotundus and course rostrally in the lateral part of the lateral forebrain bundle. Degenerated axons pass through the ventrolateral area, but it could not be ascertained if synaptic contacts are made in this area. The medial border of the field is marked by a cell-free area, but the other boundaries could not be specified. The total extent of the projection area was not identified because all of the rotundal lesions were subtotal.

6. *Birds* (Fig. 4.16).   Most of the information on the tectofugal pathway in birds comes from studies of pigeons. As in the case of turtles, there is sufficient information to outline the features of the pathway from the retina, through tectum and rotundus and to ADVR.

Retinal ganglion cells in pigeons have complex receptive field properties, including motion and direction selectivity (e.g., Maturana and Frenk, 1963; Miles, 1972; Pearlman and Hughes, 1976). They project topographically (Hamdi and Whitteridge, 1954; Clarke and Whitteridge, 1976) to the superficial layers of the contralateral tectum (Acheson, Kemplay, and Webster, 1980) where they synapse on the dendrites of radial cells (Hunt and Webster, 1975).

The properties of visual units in the tectum vary as a function of depth. The receptive fields of superficial tectal units are small, usually less than 4° of visual arc (Maturana and Frenk, 1963; Jassik-Gerschenfeld, Minois, and Conde-Courtine, 1970; Jassik-Gerschenfeld and Guichard, 1972; Hughes and Pearlman, 1974). These units are movement sensitive and often directionally selective. The subjacent central gray contains some units like those in superficial tectum, but 84% of the units have receptive fields larger than 10°, with the majority ranging

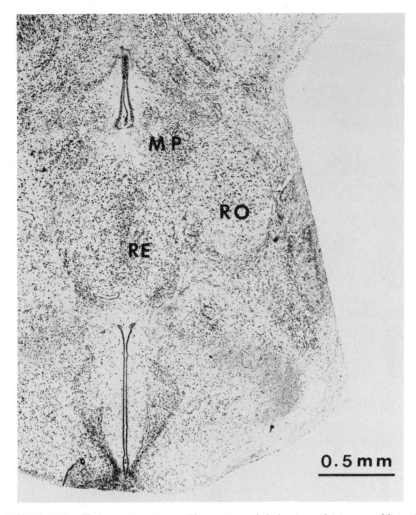

FIGURE 4.14. Thalamus in caiman. The pattern of thalamic nuclei in crocodilians is illustrated in this section through the thalamus of *Caiman sklerops*. The section passes through nucleus rotundus (RO), nucleus reuniens (RE), and nucleus medialis posterior (MP).

from 10° to 120° (Revzin, 1970). These units tend to be movement sensitive, but lack directional selectivity (Revzin, 1970; Jassik-Gerschenfeld, Guichard, and Tessier, 1975). There, therefore, seems to be a conversion of units with small receptive fields into units with very large receptive fields within the tectum, but the mechanisms underlying this transformation are not known.

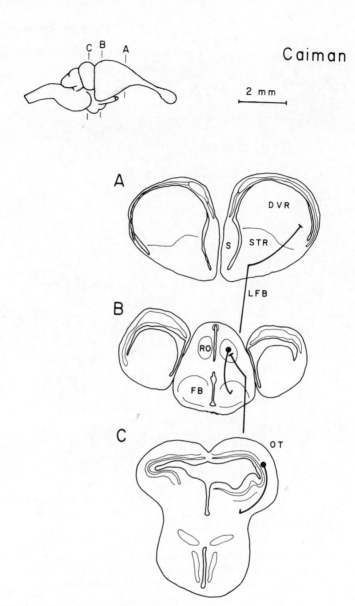

FIGURE 4.15. Tectofugal pathway in caiman. The optic tectum (OT) receives visual information from the contralateral retina. The tectum projects to nucleus rotundus (RO) in the thalamus. The projection is bilateral, but only the ipsilateral projection is shown. Neurons in rotundus project via the lateral forebrain bundle (LFB) to the lateral part of DVR (the dorsolateral area of Crosby). *Other abbreviations:* **FB,** forebrain bundles; **S,** septum; **STR,** striatum. Based on Braford (1972) and Pritz (1975).

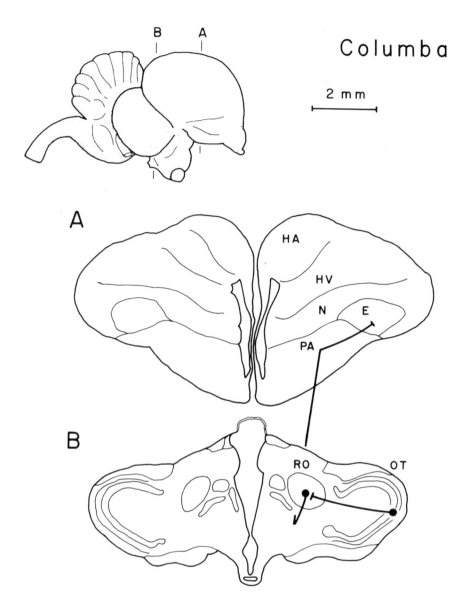

FIGURE 4.16. Tectofugal pathway in pigeon. The optic tectum (OT) receives visual information from the contralateral retina in pigeons. The tectum projects to nucleus rotundus (RO) in the thalamus. The projection in bilateral, but only the ipsilateral projection is shown. Neurons in rotundus project to the ectostriatum (E) in DVR. *Other abbreviations:* **HA**, hyperstriatum accessorium; **HV**, hyperstriatum ventrale; **N**, neostriatum; **PA**, paleostriatum augmentatum. Based on Hunt and Künzle (1976), Benowitz and Karten (1976), and Karten and Hodos (1970), and others.

Orthograde degeneration studies (Karten and Revzin, 1966) demonstrate that the optic tectum projects to nucleus rotundus and HRP experiments indicate that neurons located in the central gray of the tectum (Benowitz and Karten, 1976; Reiner and Karten, 1978) are the source of the projection (Fig. 4.17) (Karten, 1965; Hunt and Künzle, 1976). Small lesions or injections of tritiated materials anywhere in the tectum result in degeneration or radioactive label, respectively, that is scattered throughout rotundus. Conversely, small injections of HRP in rotundus label neurons in the central gray throughout the tectum (Benowitz and Karten, 1976). These experiments indicate that in pigeons, as in turtles, a given region of rotundus receives information from all points in visual space. However, Benowitz and Karten (1976) suggest that there is some organization embedded within this pattern of convergence. They divide rotundus into several cytoarchitectural areas. Injections of HRP that are restricted to a particular area of rotundus retrogradely label neurons in a particular sublayer of the central gray, but throughout the tectum. They thus suggest that the tectorotundal projection is organized according to the laminar position of neurons within the central gray.

Physiological studies have provided some information on rotundal neurons. Units in rotundus show a spontaneous discharge rate of 10 spikes per second (DeBritto et al., 1975). They are either excited or inhibited by increases in illumination (DeBritto et al., 1975). Revzin (1970) found that the majority (75%) was inhibited by increases in illumination whereas Granda and Yazulla (1971) found that the majority (66%) was excited by an increase. Rotundal units fall into two major categories when stimulated with white light. A minority are responsive to non-moving stimuli (Crossland, 1972, 22% of 68 units; Revzin, 1979). However, the majority of units in every study of rotundus (Revzin, 1979, 80% of 225; Crossland, 1972, 89% of 68; DeBritto et al., 1975, 100% of 36; Maxwell and Granda, 1979, percentage not specified) have large receptive fields, usually greater than 100° and often 180°, that are movement sensitive. They respond to small stimuli anywhere in the receptive field. Crossland (1972) found that 73% of his movement sensitive units had inhibitory surrounds. Many movement sensitive units have preferred directions (Crossland, 1972; Revzin, 1970, 1979) and, in some cases, show a null direction in which responses are inhibited by stimuli moving antiparallel to the unit's preferred direction (Revzin, 1979). Some units show responses that are dependent on stimulus size, whereas others are nonselective for size. Rotundal units are also responsive to color (Granda and Yazulla, 1971; Yazulla and Granda, 1973; Maxwell and Granda, 1979). Units may be either excited or inhibited by colored stimuli. They have spectral sensitivity curves with peaks at 500 and 600

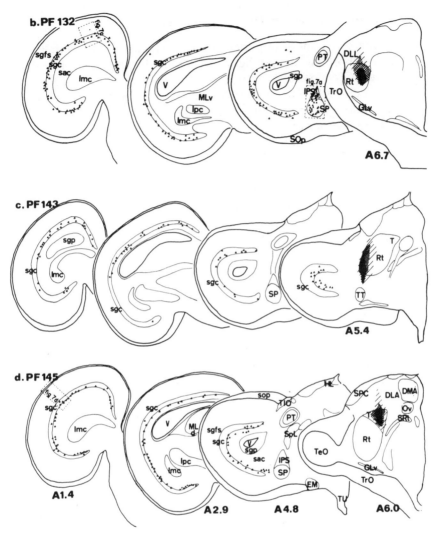

FIGURE 4.17. Tectorotundal projections in pigeon. Transverse sections through pigeon brains showing HRP injection sites in nucleus rotundus (Rt) and the resulting patterns of label in the stratum griseum centrale (SGC) of the tectum. Injections into the anteromedial rotundus (b) label cells in the superficial SGC, while injections into caudal rotundus label deeper SGC neurons only. *Abbreviations:* **DLA,** nucleus dorsalateralis anterior; **DLL,** nucleus dorsolateralis lateralis; **DMA,** nucleus dorsomedialis anterior; **HL,** lateral habenular nucleus; **Imc,** magnocellular part of nucleus isthmi; **Ipc,** parvocellular part of nucleus isthmi; **PT,** pretectum; **Ov,** nucleus ovalis; **SAC,** stratum album centrale; **SGC,** stratum griseum centrale; **SGFS,** stratum griseum et fibrosum superficiale; **SGP,** stratum griseum periventriculare; **SO,** stratum opticum; **SP,** nucleus subpretectalis; **SpL,** nucleus spiriformis lateralis; **TrO,** optic tract; **Tu,** tubercular hypothalamus; **TeO,** optic tectum. From Benowitz and Karten (1976).

nm. Some units show opponent process characteristics, either being excited by short wavelength light and inhibited by long wavelengths, or vice versa (Granda and Yazulla, 1971; Yazulla and Granda, 1973).

The study by Benowitz and Karten (1976) suggests that rotundus is divided into cytoarchitectural areas, each receiving inputs from a specific sublayer of the tectal central gray. There is also some evidence indicating that rotundus is divided into areas on physiological grounds. Yazulla and Granda (1973) and Maxwell and Granda (1979) report that color opponent units are located preferentially in ventral rotundus. Revzin (1979) found that ventral rotundus tends to contain units that were responsive to nonmoving stimuli (unlike most of the units in rotundus) and luminance related phenomena. The posterior one-third of rotundus contained units that lacked directional selectivity. The anterior part of rotundus contained directionally selective units.

It is well established that nucleus rotundus projects to the ipsilateral ectostriatum within ADVR. Lesions of the ectostriatum produce retrograde degeneration of rotundal neurons in pigeons (Karten and Hodos, 1970) and quail, *Coturnix coturnix* (Faciolli and Minelli, 1975). Degenerated axons pass radially through the paleostriatum primitivum and augmentatum on their way to ectostriatum. The projection appears topographically organized with caudolateral rotundus projecting to caudomedial ectostriatum and rostral rotundus projecting to rostrolateral ectostriatum. Lesions of the ectostriatum produce retrograde degeneration of rotundal neurons. Restricted stereotaxic injections of HRP into ectostriatum label neurons in nucleus rotundus in pigeons (Benowitz and Karten, 1976). Injections in rostral ectostriatum label neurons in dorsal anterior rotundus; lateral injections label ventral and lateral neurons; caudal injections label posterior neurons; medial injections label medial neurons. This study is consistent with the orthograde degeneration study in that they both indicate that rostral rotundus projects to rostral ectostriatum, but is inconsistent in that the degeneration study suggests a reversal of the mediolateral axis in the projection from caudal rotundus, whereas the retrograde study suggests that the projection is not reversed. Since damaged axons can transport HRP, both studies face fiber of passage problems. Revzin and Karten (1967) confirmed these projections with electrophysiological techniques by stimulating nucleus rotundus and recording evoked potentials in the ectostriatum. DeBritto et al. (1975) recorded antidromic spikes in nucleus rotundus following stimulation of the ectostriatum.

These investigations suggest that there is some organization in the rotundo-ectostriatal projection, but do not completely elucidate the nature of the organization. Notice that, although the rotundus-ectostriatal projection is topographically organized, the projection is not retinotopically organized because retinotopy is lost in the tectorotundal projection. It thus seems unlikely that the rotundal-ADVR pathway could carry detailed information about position in visual space. However, the possibility remains that the pathway conveys information about other visual parameters. A given region in the ectostriatum might receive information about stimuli with particular spectral or velocity characteristics (Revzin, 1970), say, from all points of visual space.

The involvement of ectostriatum in visual processes has been confirmed using 2-deoxyglucose (Streit et al., 1980) and physiological techniques. Evoked potentials in the forebrains of pigeons following visual stimulation were recorded in early physiological studies by Bremer, Dow, and Moruzzi (1939) and Gogan (1963), but the responsive area was not completely localized. Later studies localized visual responses to ectostriatum. Flash evoked potentials recorded from neostriatum intermedium are found to reverse as the ectostriatum is approached (Parker and Delius, 1972). Systematic exploration of the forebrain with 50-μm micropipettes localized visual responses within the ectostriatum and determined the contribution of rotundal efferents to ectostriatal evoked potentials following electrical stimulation of rotundus (Revzin and Karten, 1967). Initial, small di- or triphasic spikes were followed by larger negative–positive (N–P) waves. The amplitude of the N–P waves was reduced to about 50% when stimulus rates reached 10 per second, whereas the initial spikes were not affected by stimulus frequencies of up to 100 per second. This suggests that the spikes represent action potentials in the rotundal efferents and the N–P waves represent the envelope of summed postsynaptic activity in the ectostriatum. The latency of the initial waves was 2.5–3.5 msec. These latencies are roughly consistent with the antidromic latencies for ectostriatum to rotundus conduction times of 1.1 msec reported by DeBritto et al. (1975). The spontaneous discharge of ectostriatal units (Revzin and Karten, 1967) correlated with slow wave activity; units fired at the negative peaks of high amplitude slow waves. Only 15% of 220 ectostriatal units studied could be driven by rotundal stimulation. The lack of response of the majority of units could be due to partial suppression of activity by pentobarbital or urethane anesthesia, an inhibitory input from rotundus to ectostriatum or a dominance of ectostriatal neurons by nonrotundal (e.g., hyperstriatal) inputs.

The minimal evidence available indicates that there is little change in unit properties in the projection from rotundus to ectostriatum. Revzin (1970) studied 100 ectostriatal units. The majority (65%) responded to visual stimuli and 62% had response properties like rotundal wide field units. Kimberly, Holden, and Bambrough (1971) studied 49 ectostriatal units. The majority of these had receptive fields that covered all available visual space. The minority (16) had restricted receptive fields, but their sizes could not be determined. Movements of small ($\frac{1}{6}°$–5°) targets were the most effective stimuli and 86% of the units were directionally selective. The majority (32/44) of the units examined for this parameter had a null axis, and most preferred anterior movement.

In summary, there is excellent evidence that visual information reaches the ectostriatum in birds through nucleus rotundus. There is general agreement that the rotundal-ectostriatal system has units with large receptive fields that respond to movement of small stimuli anywhere in the receptive fields. Many of the units are directionally selective. It is not known if ectostriatal units, like those in rotundus, are color sensitive. Studies of ectostriatal physiology have not systematically studied the location of ectostriatal units. Thus, the significance of the topography of rotundal-ectostriatal projections is not known.

In addition to the well documented tecto-rotundal-ectostriatal path, Gamlin and Cohen (1982) have recently provided evidence for a second visual pathway from the tectum to ADVR in pigeons. It involves the thalamic nucleus dorsolateralis posterior (DLP). HRP injections retrogradely label neurons in the optic tectum, primarily in the stratum griseum centrale. Injections of tritiated amino acids in DLP demonstrate a projection to the neostriatum intermediale. The terminal field is located caudal and medial to the ectostriatum. The projection could be confirmed by HRP injections in the neostriatum which retrogradely labeled neurons in the posterior part of DLP. Units in DLP were responsive to visual stimuli with a latency of 30–55 msec.

(b) *Auditory Pathways*

1. *General Features of Auditory Pathways.*   The overall organization of the auditory pathways is the same in all reptiles and birds. (For a general review, see Popper and Fay, 1980.) Neurons in the acoustic ganglion project ipsilaterally to medullary nuclei, but the nature of the nuclei differs between groups (snakes: Miller, 1980; lizards: DeFina and Webster, 1974; Miller, 1975; Foster and Hall, 1978; *Caiman:* Leake, 1974; turtles: Miller and Kasahara, 1979; birds: Boord and Rasmussen, 1963). It is known that the primary acoustic nuclei are tonotopically organized at least in crocodilians (Manley, 1970) and birds (Konishi, 1970; Rubel and Parks, 1975; Sachs and Sinnett, 1978). The medullary nuclei project to a midbrain structure called nucleus mesencephalicus lateralis pars dorsalis (MLD) in birds (Boord, 1968) and the torus semicircularis in reptiles

(Foster and Hall, 1978). A tonotopic organization in the midbrain has been demonstrated with electrophysiological techniques in crocodilians (Manley, 1971) and birds (Knudsen and Konishi, 1978). The auditory midbrain projects bilaterally to a caudal thalamic nucleus in snakes (Ulinski, 1977b), lizards (Distel and Ebbesson, 1975; Foster and Hall, 1978), crocodilians (Pritz, 1974a), and birds (Karten, 1967). The subsequent projections of the auditory thalamus to DVR will now be considered for each group.

2. *Snakes.* The auditory midbrain of snakes is unusual in that it protrudes onto the surface of the brain posterior to the optic tectum (Senn, 1969). These posterior colliculi apparently receive auditory information (Hartline, 1971) and project to the most medial part of nucleus lentiformis thalami in garter snakes (Ulinski, 1977b). Lesions involving this nucleus produce terminal degeneration in ADVR (Ulinski, 1978a), but these lesions were not restricted to the lentiform nucleus and definitely damage other thalamic nuclei.

3. *Lizards* (Fig. 4.18). The torus semicircularis projects to the nucleus medialis (Fig. 4.4) in *Iguana* (Foster and Hall, 1978). Nucleus medialis projects to a terminal field in caudomedial ADVR (Foster and Hall, 1978) that corresponds to the medial projection described by Butler and Ebner (1972). Terminal debris extends to just below the ventricle. A similar situation is reported for the monitor lizard *Varanus benegalensis* (Distel and Ebbesson, 1975). HRP injections in ADVR retrogradely label neurons in a medially placed thalamic nucleus in *Tupinambis* (Lohman and van Woerden-Verkley, 1978), *Varanus exanthematicus* (ten Donkelaar and De Boer-van Huizen, 1981b) *Iguana* (Bruce, 1982) and *Gekko* (Bruce, 1982).

4. *Crocodilians* (Fig. 4.18). The torus semicircularis projects bilaterally to a midline thalamic nucleus called nucleus reuniens (Fig. 4.19) in *Caiman* (Pritz, 1974a). This is a paired structure that fuses across the midline during development (Senn, 1979). Stereotaxic lesions of the central part of nucleus reuniens demonstrate a projection to ADVR (Pritz, 1974b). Degenerated axons pass through the lateral forebrain bundle and curve radially through the ventrolateral area and ventral dorsolateral area to terminate in a region in the caudomedial dorsolateral area that seems to correspond to field G of Rose (1923) and zone 8 of Riss, Halpern, and Scalia (1969). Terminal debris reaches nearly to the ventricle. Responses to auditory stimuli have been recorded from caudomedial ADVR in *Caiman crocodilus* (Weisbach and Schwartzkopf, 1967). Single unit responses have latencies of 20–60 msec and best frequencies of 0.1–5 kHz. The structure is tonotopically organized.

5. *Birds* (Fig. 4.20). MLD projects bilaterally to nucleus ovoidalis in

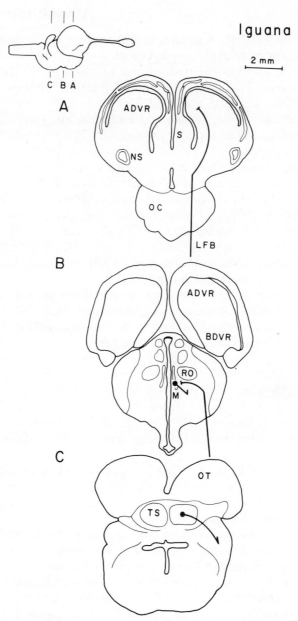

FIGURE 4.18. Auditory pathway in *Iguana*. The torus semicircularis (TS) receives projections from brainstem auditory nuclei. It projects to the nucleus medialis (M) in the caudal thalamus. Nucleus medialis projects via the lateral forebrain bundle (LFB) to the medial aspect of ADVR. *Other abbreviations:* **BDVR,** basal dorsal ventricular ridge; **NS,** nucleus sphericus; **OC,** optic chiasm; **OT,** optic tectum; **RO,** nucleus rotundus; **S,** septum. Based on Foster and Hall (1978).

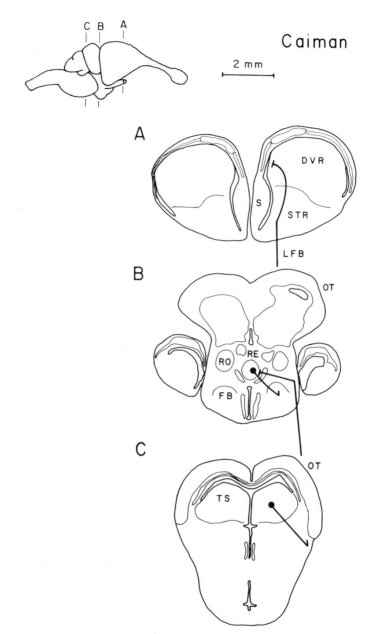

FIGURE 4.19. Auditory pathway in caiman. The torus semicircularis (TS) projects to nucleus reuniens (RE) in the caudal thalamus. This projection is bilateral, but only the ipsilateral projection is shown. Neurons in reuniens project via the lateral forebrain bundle (LFB) to the medial aspect of ADVR (the dorsolateral area of Crosby). *Other abbreviations:* **FB,** forebrain bundles; **OT,** optic tectum; **RO,** nucleus rotundus; **S,** septum; **STR,** striatum. Based on Pritz (1971a,b, 1975).

121

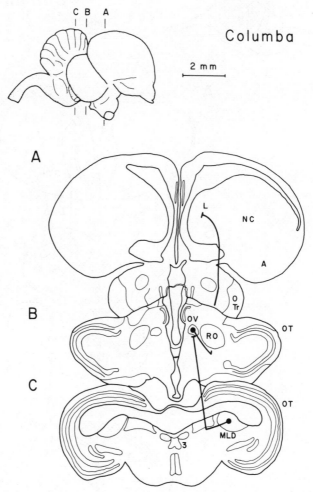

FIGURE 4.20. Auditory pathway in pigeon. The nucleus mesencephalicus lateralis pars dorsalis (MLD) receives projections from brainstem auditory nuclei. Neurons in MLD project to nucleus ovoidalis (OV) in the thalamus. This projection is bilateral, but only the ipsilateral projection is shown. Neurons in ovoidalis project via the lateral forebrain bundle to field L (L) in the caudal neostriatum (NC) of DVR. *Other abbreviations:* **A,** archistriatum; **OT,** optic tectum; **OTr,** optic tract; **RO,** nucleus rotundus; **3,** oculomotor complex. Based on Karten (1967, 1968).

the thalamus in pigeons (Karten, 1967). Stereotaxic lesions of nucleus ovoidalis demonstrate a projection to the rostral part of the caudal neostriatum in pigeons (Karten, 1968). Ovoidal efferents assemble on the lateral aspect of the nucleus and course ventrally in the medial part of the lateral forebrain bundle. The fibers turn dorsally rostral to the anterior commissure and pass through the medial paleostriatum primitivum and the paleostriatum augmentatum. Terminal degeneration is sometimes found in the paleostriatum augmentatum, but this might be due to damage of fibers ascending from the brainstem. Fibers are oriented radially as they pass through these structures. Terminal degeneration is found in field L of Rose (1914) in the neostriatum. It is situated fairly close to the ventricle caudally, but is separated from the ventricle by the hyperstriatum ventrale, rostrally. Lesions involving the caudal neostriatum produced retrograde degeneration in the nuclei ovoidalis and paraovoidalis. An essentially identical projection from nucleus ovoidalis to caudal neostriatum has been reported in the canary (*Serinus canarius*) by Nottebohm, Stokes, and Leonard (1976) and Kelly and Nottebohm (1979). The terminal field, however, does not correspond to a defined cytoarchitectonic area. The projection of ovoidalis to ADVR has been studied in some detail in the guinea fowl, *Numida meleagris*, using autoradiographic techniques (Bonke, Bonke, and Scheich, 1979). Injections in nucleus ovoidalis produce label in three zones in field L (Fig. 4.21). They are arranged concentric with the border of the hyperstriatum ventrale (HV). Zone L_1 is adjacent to HV and zones L_2 and L_3 are placed further from HV. The label is densest in L_2.

The anatomical literature, therefore, indicates that field L receives ascending auditory information from the thalamus. There have also been several physiological studies of forebrain auditory areas in birds, beginning with that of Erulkar (1955) in pigeons. Erulkar used evoked potential techniques to identify an area in the caudal neostriatum that responds to click stimuli. Subsequent studies reported similar areas in chickens (Adamo and King, 1967; Harman and Phillips, 1967), ring doves, *Streptopelia risoria* (Biederman-Thorson, 1970a), and starlings, *Sturnus vulgaris* (Leppelsack and Schwartzkopf, 1972; Leppelsack, 1974). The studies by Erulkar, Harman and Phillips, and Leppelsack employed histological verification of their recording sites. Their responsive area corresponded generally to field L, but some studies (Naumon and Iljitschow, 1964; Adamo and King, 1967) also reported areas in the hyperstriatum and basal forebrain that respond to auditory stimuli with short latencies. Similarly, Lippe and Masterton (1980) showed that exposure to white noise causes increased uptake of 2-deoxyglucose in field L. At

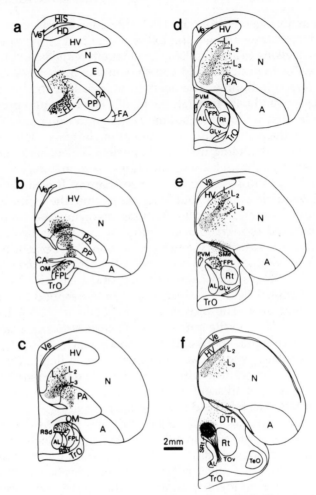

FIGURE 4.21. Auditory projections to ADVR in guinea fowl. The organization of the projection of nucleus ovoidalis (Ov) to caudal neostriatum (N) is shown in this experiment in which tritiated amino acids were injected into nucleus ovoidalis. Transported label forms three bands in the neostriatum. L_2 corresponds to the field L of Rose. L_1 and L_3 are situated on either side of L_2. *Other abbreviations:* **A,** archistriatum; **AL,** ansa lenticularis; **CA,** anterior commissure; **DTh,** dorsal thalamus; **E,** ectostriatum; **FA,** fronto-archistriatal tract; **FPL,** lateral forebrain bundle; **GLV,** ventral lateral geniculate; **HA,** hyperstriatum accesorium; **HD,** hyperstriatum dorsale; **HIS,** hyperstriatum intercalatus superior; **HV,** hyperstriatum ventrale; **OM,** occipitomesencephalic tract; **PA,** paleostriatum augmentatum; **PP,** paleostriatum primitivum; **PVM,** nucleus periventricularis magnocellularis; **RSd,** nucleus reticularis superior, pars dorsalis; **Rt,** nucleus rotundus; **Sme,** stria medullaris; **SRt,** nucleus subrotundus; **TeO,** optic tectum; **TrO,** optic tract; **Ve,** ventricle. From Bonke, Bonke, and Scheich (1979).

the present time, there is evidence for the existence of three separate auditory areas in avian ADVR.

The first area is located in the caudal neostriatum and corresponds to Rose's (1923) field L. The latency for evoked potentials in field L are surprisingly long, ranging from 12 to 25 msec in starlings (Leppelsack, 1974). Responses can always be evoked by stimuli in either ear. The latencies and amplitudes of field potentials evoked by stimuli in the contralateral ear are generally shorter and larger, respectively, than those to the ipsilateral ear. Responses to binaural stimulation are usually (Leppelsack, 1974) greater than to either ipsilateral or contralateral stimulation, but there is a substantial variation, and the responses to binaural stimulation are sometimes less than to stimulation in either ear (Biederman-Thorson, 1970a; Leppelsack, 1974). Biederman-Thorson (1970a) systematically assessed the directionality of neostriatal units by revolving a speaker around a harnessed dove. The largest response is obtained from the contralateral ear and the response falls off as the speaker crosses the bird's midline. Knudsen, Konishi, and Pettigrew (1977) found that auditory units in field L of the barn owl (*Tyto alba*) often respond to stimuli within particular regions of space. Sixty-seven percent of 213 units had spatial receptive fields, whereas only 33% responded to sounds independent of their positions. The receptive fields are vertically elongate, ranging in size from 12° azimuth by 40° elevation to 260° azimuth to 300° elevation. Units are dominated by contralateral inputs.

These physiological studies thus confirm that field L receives binaural auditory information and suggest that it may play some role in sound localization. More detailed physiological studies have pursued two lines of investigation. The first is an attempt to demonstrate a tonotopic organization within field L. Biederman-Thorson (1970a) and Leppelsack (1974) found no evidence for such an organization in field L, but the first study used stimuli at 75–85 dB, which is probably at the bases of tuning curves of field L units. Recently, Zaretsky and Konishi (1976) were successful in finding a tonotopic organization in zebra finches and Peking ducks. They reconstructed their electrode tracks and marked the positions of some units with electrolytic lesions. The best frequencies within a vertical penetration do not vary by more than 0.2 octaves. Low frequencies are found caudally and higher frequencies are represented more rostrally. A mediolateral organization was not reported. Units are recorded directly below the ventricle. Bonke, Scheich, and Langner (1979) and Bonke et al. (1981) established the existence of a tonotopic map (Fig. 4.22) in field L of the guinea fowl, *Numida meleagris*. Best frequencies of 300 Hz occur caudally in field L while frequencies of 6

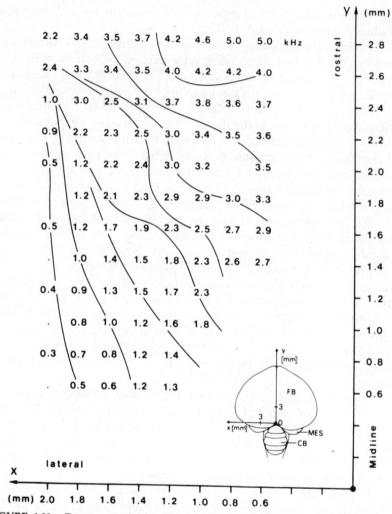

FIGURE 4.22. Tonotopy in field L. The tonotopic pattern in field L of a guinea fowl is shown projected onto an *x–y* coordinate system. The inset shows the relation of the coordinate system to the brain. The main figure shows isofrequency lines with best frequencies given in kiloHerz. *Abbreviations:* **CB,** cerebellum; **MES,** midbrain. From Bonke, Scheich, and Langner (1979).

kHz occur rostrally, in agreement with the results in ducks. Isofrequency contours run from rostral–lateral to medial–caudal. They correspond in direction to the paths taken within field L by fibers from nucleus ovoidalis (Bonke, Bonke, and Scheich, 1979). Continuous isofrequencies are also present in vertical planes perpendicular to the boundary of the hyperstriatum ventrale. The results of a 2-deoxyglucose study (Scheich et al., 1979; Scheich, Maier, and Bonke, 1980; Scheich and Maier, 1981) are consistent with this last result in that exposure of guinea fowl to pure tones produces radioactive labeling in a stripe that extends through field L perpendicular to hyperstriatum ventrale and in the correct isofrequency domain. The stripes of labeling also continued into hyperstriatum ventrale. Similarly, Zaretsky (1978) found a tonotopic organization in hyperstriatum ventrale (his area A) in the zebra finch (*Poephilla guttata*) and canary (*Serinus canarius*).

The second more detailed line of physiological investigation centers on a characterization of the auditory units in field L. The response properties of single units in field L to artificial stimuli have been characterized in ring doves (Biederman-Thorson, 1970a,b) and starlings (Leppelsack, 1974). Units in doves respond to stimulus onset. The larger sample (103 units) in starlings includes those that respond with either activation or inhibition to the stimulus onset, are tonically activated or inhibited by the stimulus, or are activated or inhibited by the termination of the stimulus. A few (2%) of the units show phase locking to rhythmic stimuli. Only 6 of 40 units responded to pure tones in doves, but a larger number of units responded to sine wave stimuli in starlings. Frequencies of 2–4 kHz and 0.5–4 kHz, respectively, were the most effective. Biederman-Thorson (1970b) reported that complex sounds such as clicks, hisses, and squeaks were effective in driving neostriatal units. Leppelsack determined tuning curves for 160 units. Of these, 75% had typical shapes with a single best frequency. However, 25% had complex tuning curves consisting of several disjunct peaks. The response patterns to the different best frequencies were often different. These units resembled those reported by Biederman-Thorson in nucleus ovoidalis (1970b) or in MLD (1967).

More recently, units in field L have been studied using species specific calls. (See Galambos and Worden, 1972, and Bullock, 1977, for general reviews of this field.) Leppelsack and Vogt (1976) studied field L units in the starling (*Sturnus vulgaris*), a species with an extensive repertoire of songs used for intraspecific communications. One hundred twenty-nine units were studied using a program of sound elements as stimuli. Units varied in their selectivity. Most responded to fewer than 10 of 80 distinct sound elements, whereas the minority responded to 61–

65 of the 80 elements. Individual units tended to respond to particular features of natural sounds rather than the song as a whole. These features included the frequency bandwidths of the stimuli and the temporal structure of the stimulus (Leppelsack, 1978). Bonke, Scheich, and Langner (1979) and Scheich, Langner, and Bonke (1979) studied field L units in the guinea fowl (*Numida meleagris*). They focused on studying the Iambus call which the hen uses to communicate with its mate or chicks when visually separated. A total of 58 of 168 auditory units could distinguish the Iambus call from other calls. Most of the energy in the Iambus call is between 1.0 and 2.3 kHz with the energy maximum at 1.8 kHz. Selective units were located preferentially in the region of field L that shows best frequencies of 1–2 kHz. They responded best to stimuli with energy concentrated at about 1.8 kHz or its harmonics (Fig. 4.23). Selective units were located preferentially in the L_1 and L_3 zones of field L whereas units that responded well to pure tones were seen in zone L_2. Langner, Bonke, and Scheich (1981a,b) investigated the responsiveness of field L neurons to spoken vowels in mynah birds. Mynah birds both imitate human speech and use vowel-like sounds in conspecific communication. One hundred thirty-two of 250 units were responsive to at least one of nine vowels from one German speaker. The mechanisms of vowel selectivity were analyzed with five synthetic vowels composed of two formants that could be presented separately. Most selective units also responded to one or both formants. Selective units were found almost exclusively in band L_1 and L_3 of field L. Finally, Leppelsack (1981) found that 11.3% of 1200 auditory units in field L of white-crowned sparrows (*Zonotrichia leucophyrs*) respond to only one of two alternate trill versions of conspecific songs. All of these studies suggest that neurons in field L are involved in the discrimination of naturally occurring sounds, but the mechanisms underlying these discriminations are not yet understood.

A particular difficulty is that some of the calls studied have much of their energy concentrated in a given bandwidth. Since call-specific units are often located preferentially in a region of field L that contains units with best frequencies close to the bandwidth, it is sometimes difficult to be certain that the call-specific units are not actually frequency specific units. However, Margoliash (1982) used electrically altered song recordings to search for song-specific units in the hyperstriatum ventrale and subjacent "shelf" of neostriatum in the white-crowned sparrow (*Zonotrichia leucophrys*). A number of units did not respond to tone and noise bursts, but could be driven by song. Phrase combinations were often necessary to elicit responses; the individual phrases of the song played backwards were ineffective. Frequency shifting one or both phrases and

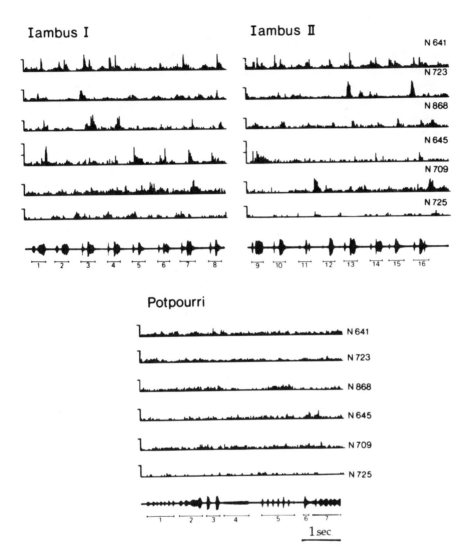

FIGURE 4.23. Neurons with selective properties for Iambus calls. Shown are the post-stimulus time histograms (PSTHs) of six neurons that responded to a large number of Iambus variations and, among the Potpourri calls, to the Iambus-like calls 5 and 6 (Rhythmic Cry and Tremolo Front). The code number of the neurons is given on the right of the PSTHs. The oscillograms of the calls and the call numbers are shown below. Scale divisions on the ordinate of the PSTHs, which represent responses to 20 repetitions of the stimuli, indicate 10 spikes/bin. From Scheich et al. (1979).

changing the interphrase interval duration could abolish the response. It was sometimes possible to model phrase combinations with simple stimuli such as consecutive tone bursts. Units would then respond only to the second tone, even when both were of identical frequency, duration and amplitude. They showed a significant degree of selectivity, responding only to the bird's own song and related songs within a large repertoire of songs.

Since field L projects to the hyperstriatum ventrale (see Section 3.6), it should also be possible to record auditory responses from hyperstriatum ventrale. Katz and Gurney (1981) have done this in zebra finches (*Poephilla guttata*). Of 59 neurons, 36 in the hyperstriatum ventrale pars caudalis responded to noise bursts. Most were excited or inhibited by the onset and/or the offset of the noise burst. Latencies to onset were 25–40 msec. Neurons located in the neostriatum immediately subjacent to the hyperstriatum ventrale are also responsive to auditory stimuli (Katz, 1982). Intracellular recordings were obtained from 32 cells in this area. The 17 cells that showed auditory responses fell into two groups. Sixty-five percent had long latencies of 100–350 msec. Thirty-five percent had short latencies of 30–40 msec. All cells had low spontaneous activities and preferred noise bursts to tones of any frequency.

The second auditory area in avian ADVR is located in the frontal neostriatum adjacent to the nucleus basalis, a structure that receives somatosensory information from the beak. This auditory area has been studied in pigeons. Iljtschow (1966) recorded auditory evoked auditory potentials dorsal to nucleus basalis. Delius, Runge, and Oeckinghaus (1979) studied the area in more detail in both chronic and acute preparations. Auditory responses had latencies of 5–8 msec to the first inflection, which are short compared to the latencies seen in field L. The best frequencies of units were between 2 and 5 kHz. Contralateral and ipsilateral stimuli were equally effective, in contrast to the contralateral dominance seen in field L. Trigeminal deafferentation did not abolish the responses, thereby ruling out the possibility that the area receives vibratory responses from the beak. On the other hand, destruction of the cochleae abolished the responses. The source of afferents to the area is not known.

The third auditory area was described in starlings and pigeons by Kirsch, Coles, and Leppelsack (1980). The area is located in the frontal neostriatum about 1.0 mm dorsal to nucleus basalis and corresponds to Rose's field G. The latencies of auditory responses in field G are 18.0 msec, as compared to latencies of about 6 msec in the short latency area adjacent to nucleus basalis. Forty-six percent (36/79) of the units showed excitatory responses; 13% showed inhibitory responses. Twenty-six percent could not be classified using pure tones or white noise. Units had classical tuning curves with best frequencies between 150 and 7.0 kHz. The majority of units had best frequencies of 600 Hz to 2.0 kHz. Response bandwidths are 0.8–2.2 octaves at 10 dB above the best frequency peak. They are, therefore, relatively broadly tuned as compared to field L units that have bandwidths of about 0.5 octaves. The sources of the afferents to field G are not known.

In summary, there appear to be three auditory areas in avian DVR. Field L receives projections from nucleus ovoidalis in the thalamus. It has long latency responses. Its units respond to pure tones and complex stimuli. They are dominated by contralateral input and may have spatial receptive fields. Units sometimes have complex tuning curves; their best frequencies extend across the species' frequency range. The area is tonotopically organized. The epibasalis area shows short latency responses. Units are equally responsive to ipsilateral and contralateral stimuli. They have best frequencies in the high end of the frequency range. Area G has long latency responses. Its units have classical tuning curves with best frequencies preferentially in the lower end of the frequency range. The sources of the afferents to the epibasalis area and field G are not known.

(c) Somatosensory Pathways

1. *General Features of Somatosensory Pathways.* Somatosensory information reaches the thalamus or telencephalon via four distinct pathways. Two carry information from the postcranial body surface and one carries information from the head. In addition, birds have a possibly unique somatosensory pathway that carries information from the trigeminal nuclei directly to ADVR.

In the spinothalamic pathway, the central processes of dorsal root ganglion cells project to the spinal gray matter (Petras, 1976; snakes: Kusuma and ten Donkelaar, 1980; lizards: Goldby and Robinson, 1962; Joseph and Whitlock, 1968; Cruce, 1979; Kusuma and ten Donkelaar, 1980; turtles: Kusuma and ten Donkelaar, 1980; birds: Leonard and Cohen, 1975; *Caiman:* Joseph and Whitlock, 1968). Spinal neurons project to the thalamus (snakes: Ebbesson, 1969; lizards: Ebbesson, 1967; Bruce, 1982; cryptodiran and pleurodiran turtles: Ebbesson, 1969; Belekhova and Kosareva, 1971; Pederson, 1973; pigeons: Karten, 1963; *Caiman:* Pritz and Northcutt, 1980; Ebbesson and Goodman, 1981). In the monitor lizard, *Varanus exanthematicus*, HRP experiments demonstrate that the spinothalamic projections originate bilaterally in laminae V–VII of the spinal cord (Hoogland, 1981).

In the dorsal column pathway, dorsal root ganglion cells project directly to the dorsal column nuclei in the caudal medulla (Jacobs and Sis, 1980, and references in previous paragraph). The size and nature of these nuclei vary with the relative development of the species' limbs. It is known that the dorsal column nuclei show a somatotopic organization in *Alligator* (Kruger and Witkovsky, 1961). They project to the thalamus in a monitor lizard, *Varanus benegalensis* (Ebbesson, 1978), and in *Caiman* (Pritz and Northcutt, 1980).

Somatosensory information from the head is carried principally by the trigeminal nerve. The central processes of neurons in the trigeminal ganglion terminate in a complex of trigeminal nuclei in the brainstem (e.g., Dubbeldam, 1980; Molenaar, 1978a). The projections have been studied using Fink–Heimer techniques in snakes (Molenaar, 1974; Schroeder and Loop, 1976; Molenaar, 1978b), pigeons (Dubbeldam and Karten, 1978), and ducks (Dubbeldam et al., 1979). It is likely that the trigeminal complex projects to the thalamus in all reptiles and birds, but this has been shown only in the python, *Python reticulatus* (Molenaar and Fizaan-Oostven, 1980). Direct projections from the principal nucleus of the trigeminal complex to nucleus basalis in DVR, bypassing the thalamus, are found in birds (see below), but it is not yet clear if a comparable pathway exists in reptiles. Molenaar and Fizaan-Oostven (1980) could not find a direct pathway to DVR in *Python*. However, ten Donkelaar and De Boer-van Huizen (1981b) were able to retrogradely label neurons in the principal trigeminal nucleus in the monitor lizard, *Varanus exanthematicus*, following forebrain injections.

The routes by which somatosensory information reaches DVR have been studied in lizards, crocodilians, and birds.

2. *Lizards.* HRP injections into the caudolateral area of ADVR in *Iguana* and *Gekko* retrogradely label neurons in the nucleus medialis posterior and posterocentralis of the thalamus (Bruce, 1982). These nuclei receive ascending somatosensory projections (Bruce, 1982).

3. *Crocodilians* (Fig. 4.24). In *Caiman*, nucleus medialis posterior (MP, Fig. 4.14) in the thalamus (Huber and Crosby, 1926) receives projections from both the spinal cord and the dorsal column nuclei (Pritz and Northcutt, 1980; Ebbesson and Goodman, 1981). This nucleus projects to a terminal field situated in central ADVR (Pritz and Northcutt, 1980). Lesions in medialis posterior produce terminal degeneration in central ADVR. Conversely, injection of HRP in the central region of ADVR retrogradely labels neurons in medialis posterior.

4. *Birds.* The thalamic nuclei that process somatosensory information have not been adequately studied in birds. However, Delius and Bennetto (1972) identified a thalamic region in pigeons which responded

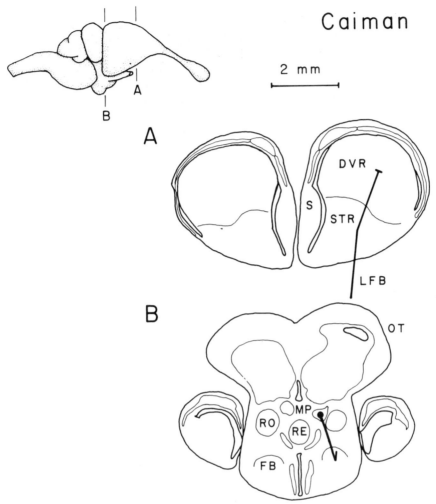

FIGURE 4.24. Somatosensory pathway in caiman. Nucleus medialis posterior (MP) receives ascending projections from the dorsal column nuclei and the spinal cord. Neurons in medialis posterior project via the lateral forebrain bundle (LFB) to the central part of DVR (the dorsolateral area of Crosby). *Other abbreviations:* **FB**, forebrain bundles; **OT**, optic tectum; **RE**, nucleus reuniens; **RO**, nucleus rotundus; **S**, septum; **STR**, striatum.

to somatosensory stimulation using bipolar electrodes. Evoked potentials and multiple unit activity centered in the nuclei superficialis parvocellularis and dorsolateralis posterior. Units responded briskly to minimal feather movements of the contralateral body surface including the head, and less well to similar movements on the ipsilateral side. Latency to a tap on the skin was 9–10 msec. The diameter of cutaneous receptive fields appeared to be on the order of 10–20 mm. Comparable results were obtained by Witkovsky, Zeigler, and Silver (1973). The ascending pathways that project to these nuclei have not been adequately studied.

Two somatosensory regions have been encountered in ADVR. The first is in the caudal neostriatum. Erulkar (1955) recorded evoked potentials in a restricted region of anterior neostriatum caudale of pigeons following light tactile stimulation of feathers on all parts of the contralateral body surface. Delius and Bennetto (1972) recorded evoked potentials and multiple unit responses from a medial region of neostriatum caudale in pigeons following tactile stimulation. Units were driven by stimuli to all parts of the contralateral body and head surface. Latencies in these studies ranged from 11 to 18 msec and it was not possible to establish a somatotopic organization. The route by which somatosensory information reaches the caudal neostriatum is not certain.

The second somatosensory region is nucleus basalis, which is situated rostrally in ADVR (Fig. 4.25). Basalis receives a bilateral projection from the principal trigeminal nucleus and processes somatosensory information from the outer surface of the bill and the oral cavity. The size of nucleus basalis varies considerably between species and is correlated with the size of the trigeminal complex and of the beak (Stingelin, 1961). Each step in this pathway has been studied in some detail and can be outlined here (Fig. 4.26).

The surface of the bill contains characteristic populations of somatosensory mechanoreceptors called Herbst and Grandry corpuscles. The Herbst corpuscles are lamellated receptors that closely resemble Pacinian corpuscles in their morphology (Munger, 1971; Gottschaldt and Lausmann, 1974). They are preferentially distributed on the rostrolateral margins of the bill in ducks (*Anas platyrhynchos*) where they are very densely packed (Berkhoudt, 1980). They are rapidly adapting mechanoreceptors that are sensitive to high frequency vibrations (e.g., Necker, 1973, 1974; Gregory, 1973; Leitner and Roumy, 1974; Gottschaldt, 1974). Grandry corpuscles are epithelial cell–neurite complexes (Munger, 1971) that are found more posteriorly on the bill (Berkhoudt, 1980). They are also rapidly adapting mechanoreceptors, but are re-

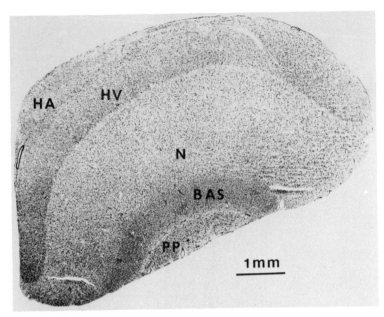

FIGURE 4.25. Nucleus basalis. The cytoarchitecture of nucleus basalis is shown in this section through the rostral telencephalon of a duck, *Anas platyrhynchos*. Nucleus basalis (BAS) forms a band of neurons situated just dorsal to the dorsal medullary laminae. *Abbreviations:* **HA,** hyperstriatum accessorium; **HV,** hyperstriatum ventrale; **N,** neostriatum; **PP,** paleostriatum primitivum.

sponsive to the velocity of moving stimuli (Gottschaldt, 1974). Both types of receptors respond best to stimuli moving tangentially over the surface of the skin. The Herbst corpuscles are also thermosensitive (Gottschaldt et al., 1982).

The bill and tongue are innervated by all three branches of the trigeminal nerve (Berkhoudt, 1980) and by the glossopharyngeal nerve. Trigeminal fibers have their somata in the trigeminal ganglion, which is somatotopically organized (Dubbeldam and Veenman, 1978). Central processes from the trigeminal ganglion project to the trigeminal complex in the brainstem (pigeon: Dubbeldam and Karten, 1978). The complex contains the principal and spinal nuclei (each of which can be subdivided into several components; see Dubbeldam, 1980). It is the principal nucleus that projects to nucleus basalis. The projections of the trigeminal (Dubbeldam, 1980; Dubbeldam and Karten, 1978; Zeigler and Witkovsky, 1968) and glossopharyngeal (Dubbeldam et al., 1979) ganglia to the principal nucleus are topographically organized. Zeigler and

Anas

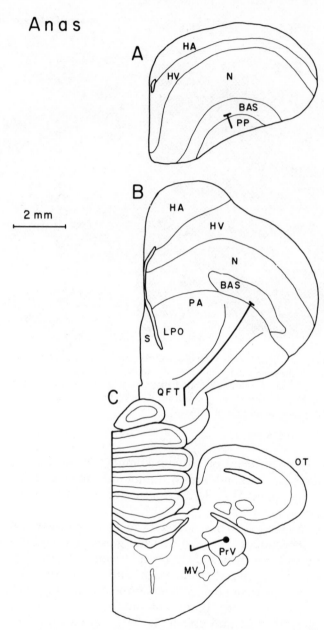

FIGURE 4.26. Quinto-frontal path. The principal trigeminal nucleus (PrV) receives projections from the trigeminal ganglion. It projects directly to nucleus basalis (BAS) in DVR via the quinto-frontal tract (QFT). *Other abbreviations:* **HA,** hyperstriatum accessorium; **HV,** hyperstriatum ventrale; **LPO,** parolfactory lobe; **MV,** motor nucleus of the trigeminal nerve; **N,** neostriatum; **OT,** optic tectum; **PA,** paleostriatum augmentatum; **PP,** paleostriatum primitivum; **S,** septum. Based on Dubbeldam, Brauch, and Don (1981).

Witkovsky (1968) studied the properties of trigeminal units in the principal sensory nucleus of pigeons. The units had small receptive fields. Seventy-two percent of 130 units were responsive to stimulation of the beak; 28% were responsive to displacement of the lower beak. A large percentage of the units responded tonically to stimulation.

Using Marchi techniques, Wallenberg (1903) showed that the trigeminal nuclei in birds project directly to nucleus basalis without a thalamic relay. Karten (Cohen and Karten, 1974), Dubbeldam and Wijsman (1975) and Dubbeldam, Brauch, and Don (1981) subsequently confirmed this projection using Fink–Heimer techniques. Trigeminal fibers ascend in the quintofrontal tract and undergo a partial decussation at the level of the trochlear nucleus. They reach the telencephalon through the lateral forebrain bundle and terminate in nucleus basalis. Karten (Cohen and Karten, 1974), working on pigeons, and Dubbeldam, Brauch, and Don (1981), working on mallard ducks, found somewhat different patterns of trigeminal terminations in basalis. In pigeons, the ipsilateral and contralateral projections terminate in alternating bands within basalis. In mallards, ipsilateral fibers terminate in the rostral two-thirds of nucleus basalis; contralateral fibers terminate in the caudal two-thirds. The intermediate part of the nucleus thus receives bilateral projections. There are also some dorsoventral differences in the terminations in that coarse caliber fibers ascend along the columns of somata in dorsal basalis.

Several lines of evidence indicate that the trigeminal projections to basalis are topographically organized. First, small lesions of the principal nucleus produce local concentrations of degeneration in basalis (Dubbeldam, Brauch, and Don, 1981). Second, restricted injections of HRP in basalis retrogradely label clusters of neurons in the principal trigeminal nucleus (Dubbeldam, Brauch, and Don, 1981). Interestingly, labeling was also seen in the nucleus superficialis parvocellularis of the thalamus, suggesting that basalis may receive convergent projections from the principal trigeminal nucleus and the somatosensory thalamus. Third, electrophysiological studies show a topographic representation of the bill and mouth in basalis. In pigeons, Witkovsky, Zeigler, and Silver (1973) found that receptive fields localized inside the mouth were grouped medially in the nucleus; receptive fields located outside the mouth were located laterally. Fifty-seven percent of the units had large receptive fields; most others were small. As the electrode advanced in the dorsoventral plane (or, because of the orientation of the nucleus in the brain, from caudal to rostral in the nucleus), receptive fields moved from proximal to distal and from the dorsal to the ventral beak. In ducks, Berkhoudt, Dubbeldam, and Zeilstra (1981) found a detailed somatotopy in basalis with the tongue represented rostrally and the tip of the bill represented caudally (Figs. 4.27 and 4.28). Contralateral fields

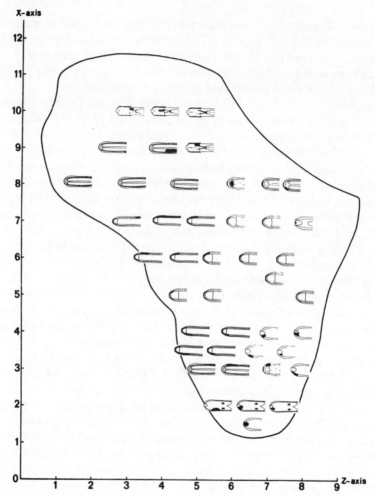

FIGURE 4.27. Receptive fields in nucleus basalis. The positions of somatosensory receptive fields are shown on a dorsal view of nucleus basalis in a duck. The small drawings show various parts of the bill. The blackened areas show the positions of receptive fields. From Berkhoudt, Dubbeldam, and Zeilstra (1981).

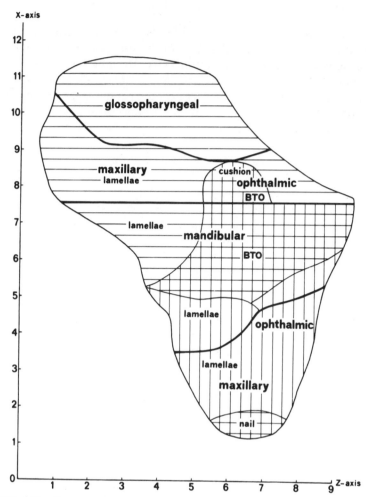

FIGURE 4.28. Somatotopy in nucleus basalis. The positions in nucleus basalis of information from various branches of the trigeminal nerve on the glossopharyngeal nerve are shown. Horizontal lines indicate contralateral representations. Vertical lines indicate ipsilateral representations. Crosshatched areas indicate bilateral representations. *Abbreviation:* **BTO,** bill-tip organ. From Berkhoudt, Dubbeldam, and Zeilstra (1981).

are represented rostrally, ipsilateral fields caudally, and bilateral fields in the central and most caudal parts of the nucleus, in agreement with the orthograde degeneration results. Densely innervated regions, like the tip of the bill, have proportionately larger representations in basalis. Receptive fields were relatively large on the caudal areas of the external bill and smaller on the tongue and bill tip. Receptive fields encountered along dorsal to ventral penetrations through basalis had similar peripheral locations.

Basalis units responded to mechanical stimulation in both pigeons (Witkovsky, Zeigler, and Silver, 1973) and ducks (Berkhoudt, Dubbeldam, and Zeilstra, 1981). The latency to stimulation was comparable (2.8 and 3.8 msec, respectively) in both cases. All of the units were rapidly adapting in ducks and showed phasic responses to vibratory stimuli. Their firing patterns also showed velocity sensitive components, suggesting that, in contrast to units in the principal trigeminal nucleus, basalis units receive information from both Herbst and Grandry corpuscles.

In summary, there is evidence for two somatosensory areas in DVR of birds. The first is in the caudal neostriatum and probably receives thalamic projections from the nuclei superficialis parvocellularis and dorsolateralis anterior. The second is nucleus basalis, which receives direct trigeminal projections bilaterally from the principal trigeminal nucleus, and possibly a thalamic projection. Nucleus basalis contains a topographic representation of the bill surface and oral cavity.

Thalamic Nuclei Involved in Diffuse Projections

The general conclusion to be drawn from the studies reported in the previous section is that thalamic nuclei that receive visual, auditory, and somatosensory information project to well-defined regions of DVR. By contrast, a second group of thalamic nuclei are involved in widespread projections to the forebrain, including DVR.

1. *Turtles.*   The perirotundal nuclei in the pond turtles *Pseudemys* and *Chrysemys* surround the rostral pole of nucleus rotundus. The largest nucleus in this group is the dorsomedial anterior nucleus (DMA). The efferent projections of DMA have been studied in *Pseudemys* and *Chrysemys* using Fink–Heimer and autoradiographic tracing techniques (Balaban and Ulinski, 1981a). DMA contributes a bilateral projection to the rostral hypothalamus, septum, dorsal and dorsomedial cortex, striatum, basal dorsal ventricular ridge, and ADVR (Fig. 4.29). The DMA

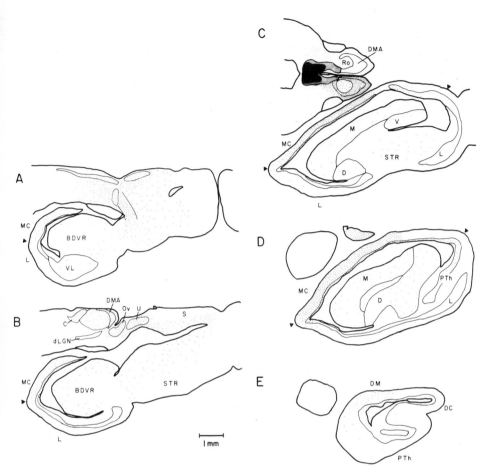

FIGURE 4.29. Projections of perirotundal nuclei in turtles. The perirotundal nuclei such as the dorsomedial anterior nucleus (DMA) give rise to a diffuse projection to the telencephalon in the red-eared turtle, *Pseudemys scripta.* This projection is demonstrated in this experiment in which tritiated amino acids were injected into caudal DMA. The sections are in the horizontal plane with rostral to the right. *Other abbreviations:* **BDVR,** basal dorsal ventricular ridge; **C,** nucleus caudalis; **D,** dorsal area of ADVR; **DC,** dorsal cortex; **dLGN,** dorsal lateral geniculate nucleus; **DM,** dorsomedial cortex; **L,** lateral cortex; **M,** medial area of ADVR; **MC,** medial cortex; **Ov,** nucleus ovalis; **PTh,** pallial thickening; **Ro,** nucleus rotundus; **S,** septum; **STR,** striatum; **U,** umbonate nucleus; **V,** ventral area. From Balaban and Ulinski (1981a).

projection to ADVR is via fine caliber, varicose axons that project sparsely to zones 2–4 of the dorsal, medial, and ventral areas. Injections of HRP in ADVR retrogradely label neurons in DMA in *Emys orbicularis* (Belekhova et al., 1979) and in *Pseudemys* and *Chrysemys* (Balaban and Ulinski, 1981a). The source of afferents to DMA in turtles is not known.

2.   *Lizards.*   HRP injections in ADVR retrogradely label neurons in DMA of lizards. Large injections in *Iguana* label neurons in DMA and the adjacent dorsolateral anterior nucleus (Bruce and Butler, 1979). Injections of HRP in tegu lizards, *Tupinambis* (Lohman and van Woerden-Verkley, 1976, 1978), and monitor lizards, *Varanus exanthematicus* (ten Donkelaar and De Boer-van Huizen, 1978, 1981b), label neurons in the dorsomedial nucleus. DMA receives projections from the septum in tegu lizards (Hoogland, ten Donkelaar, and Cruce, 1978).

3.   *Crocodilians.*   In *Caiman crocodilus*, injections of HRP in DVR retrogradely label neurons in the dorsomedial anterior nucleus and the adjacent dorsolateral anterior nucleus (Brauth and Kitt, 1980).

The Problem of Thalamostriate Projections

All of the thalamic projections to ADVR documented in the literature enter the telencephalon via the lateral forebrain bundle. Thalamic axons curve dorsally rostral to the anterior commissure and are obliged to pass through the striatum to reach ADVR. It is not yet clear whether or not these axons synapse in the striatum *en route* to ADVR because it is impossible to distinguish axons passing through the striatum from true terminal zones in either orthograde degeneration or autoradiographic experiments at the light microscopic level. Similarly, retrograde tracing techniques face a fibers of passage problem. Thus, Parent (1976) injected HRP in the lateral striatum of the turtle *Chrysemys* and reported retrograde labeling of cells in the perirotundal nuclei. However, these nuclei were also labeled by injections in ADVR, so it is not clear whether the perirotundal nuclei have projections that terminate in the striatum or whether the striatal injections merely injured axons passing through the striatum. Revzin and Karten (1967) used physiological techniques to argue that evoked potentials recorded in the paleostriatum following visual stimulation in pigeons were due to action potentials in rotundal axons. Potentials with properties similar to postsynaptic potentials were smaller than those recorded in the ectostriatum and could be due to volume conduction from the ectostriatum. This experiment suggests that rotundal fibers only pass through the paleostriatum, but the matter can be unequivocally settled only with experiments at the electron microscopic level.

4.2. CORTICAL AFFERENTS TO ADVR

Projections from cortex to ADVR have not been as completely documented as those from thalamus. However, there is evidence for cortico-ADVR projections in several groups. It is strongest in the case of projections from a visual cortical area to ADVR in turtles and birds.

Lizards

In tegu lizards, projections from the medial aspect of the cortex course laterally around the lateral recess of the ventricle and terminate in lateral ADVR (Lohman and Mentink, 1972; Lohman and van Woerden-Verkley, 1976). Also, Butler (1976) found sparse terminal degeneration in the deep parts of ADVR following lesions of dorsal cortex in the tokay gecko, *Gekko gecko*.

Turtles

Early studies (Northcutt, 1970; Gaidenko, 1978) showed that ablation of the dorsolateral region of cortex produces terminal degeneration in the ipsilateral ADVR. In a more detailed study, Balaban (1979) showed that both a lateral part of the dorsal cortex and the pallial thickening (an S-shaped specialization of the lateral edge of dorsal cortex) projects to ADVR. Pallial thickening projects to zones 2–4 of both dorsal area and medial area, rostral to the anterior commissure. The caudal part of dorsal cortex appears to project more caudally and superficially in ADVR. HRP injections in ADVR retrogradely label neurons in the second layer of the pallial thickening (Fig. 4.30; Balaban, 1978b). These neurons have dendrites that extend radially toward the pial surface (Balaban, 1979), suggesting that they intersect geniculocortical axons and thereby provide a second route by which visual information can reach ADVR.

Birds

Projections are reported from the hyperstriatum to the ectostriatum, neostriatum, and paleostriatum augmentatum in chickens, ravens, and love birds (Adamo, 1967). Karten et al. (1973) report a topographically

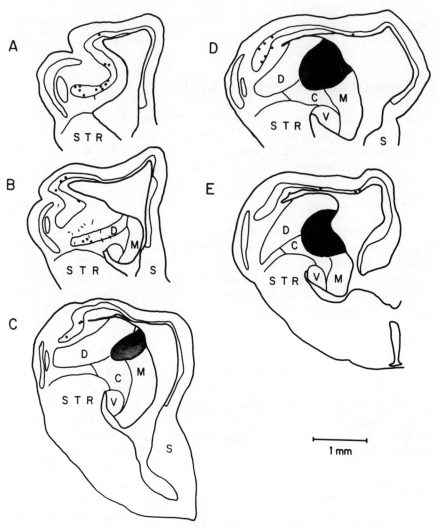

FIGURE 4.30. Projections of the pallial thickening to ADVR in a turtle. An HRP injection in ADVR (black and gray area) retrogradely labels neurons in the pallial thickening (dots) in *Pseudemys. Abbreviations:* **C,** central area of ADVR; **D,** dorsal area of ADVR; **M,** medial area of ADVR; **S,** septum; **STR,** striatum; **V,** ventral area of ADVR. From Balaban (1979).

organized projection from the visual Wulst to the periectostriatal belt in burrowing owls and pigeons.

4.3. AFFERENTS TO BDVR

The known afferents to BDVR can be divided into two groups. The first arise from cortical structures or from ADVR and are potentially a source of visual, auditory, and somatosensory projections to BDVR. The second are projections from the main or accessory olfactory bulbs, depending on the species under consideration.

Nonolfactory Afferents

These projections are discussed in detail in Section 6.1 in conjunction with the efferent projections of ADVR, but it can be noted at this point that ADVR is known to project to BDVR in snakes, lizards, and birds. These projections have not been studied in detail, so it is not known if projections from different modality specific areas within ADVR project to restricted targets in BDVR.

Olfactory Afferents

The olfactory bulb is divided into main and accessory bulbs in snakes and lizards; the situation is unclear in turtles and crocodilians; and birds have only a main olfactory bulb (Parsons, 1970; Tucker and Smith, 1976). However, the efferent projections of the olfactory bulbs include projections to BDVR in all of the reptiles studied.

(a) *Snakes and Lizards*

The accessory olfactory bulb projects to the ipsilateral nucleus sphericus in both snakes and lizards. This has been shown using degeneration techniques in garter snakes, *Thamnophis sirtalis* and *T. radix* (Fig. 4.31; Halpern, 1976), and in boa constrictors, *Constrictor constrictor*, and Florida king snakes, *Lampropeltis getulus floridanus* (Kowell, 1974). In lizards, it has been shown in *Lacerta* (Gamble, 1952), *Anolis* (Armstrong, Gamble, and Goldby, 1953), *Tupinambis* (Heimer, 1969), and *Dipsosaurus* (Ulinski and Peterson, 1981). In each case, fibers run caudally from the accessory bulb through the basal forebrain in a distinct accessory olfactory tract. They enter the rostral face of nucleus sphericus and terminate in its hilar layer. Terminal debris is present in the center of the hilar

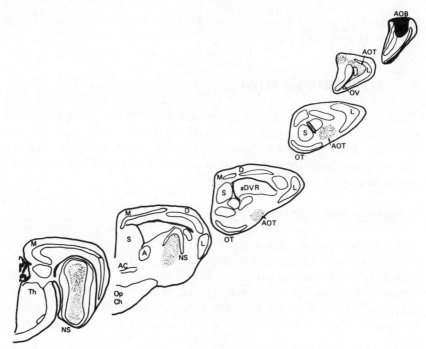

FIGURE 4.31. Projections of the accessory olfactory bulb in a snake. A lesion of the accessory olfactory bulb (AOB) in a garter snake (*Thamnophis*) produces degeneration that courses through the accessory olfactory tract (AOT) and terminates in nucleus sphericus (NS) in BDVR. *Other abbreviations:* **DVR,** anterior dorsal ventricular ridge; **A,** nucleus accumbens; **D,** dorsal cortex; **L,** lateral cortex; **M,** medial cortex; **OpCh,** optic chiasm; **OT,** olfactory tubercle; **S,** septum; **Th,** thalamus. From Halpern (1980).

layer, but is absent from the band of the layer that lies immediately internal to the mural layer.

(b) *Turtles*

Projections from the olfactory bulbs have been studied using degeneration techniques in *Testudo graeca* (Gamble, 1956) and in the pond turtles *Pseudemys* and *Chrysemys* (Northcutt, 1970; Balaban, 1977). Rolon and Skeen (1980) used the orthograde transport of HRP to study bulbar efferents in the soft-shelled turtle *Trionyx s. spinifer*. Fibers from the lateral olfactory tract extend caudally and terminate in the outer layer of ventromedial BDVR (Fig. 4.32).

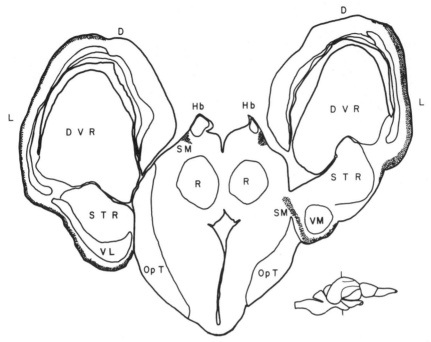

FIGURE 4.32. Projections of the olfactory bulb to BDVR in a turtle. The projections of the olfactory bulb to the caudal telencephalon in the turtle *Pseudemys* are shown as they appear in a Fink–Heimer preparation following a lesion of the olfactory bulb. The left side of the section is ipsilateral to the lesion. The inset shows the plane of the section. *Abbreviations:* **D,** dorsal cortex; **Hb,** habenula; **DVR;** anterior dorsal ventricular ridge; **L,** lateral cortex; **OpT,** optic tract; **R,** nucleus rotundus; **SM,** stria medullaris; **STR,** striatum; **VM,** ventromedial nucleus of striatum; **VL,** ventrolateral nucleus of striatum.

(c)   *Crocodilians*

Olfactory projections have been studied using degeneration techniques in *Caiman sclerops* (Scalia, Halpern, and Riss, 1969). Olfactory efferents were found to run caudally in the lateral olfactory tract and terminate in the superficial layer of BDVR (Fig. 4.33) in both the nucleus of the lateral olfactory tract and ventromedial area of Crosby (1917).

(d)   *Birds*

Rieke and Wenzel (1978) studied olfactory projections using degeneration techniques in pigeons. They did not find olfactory projections to

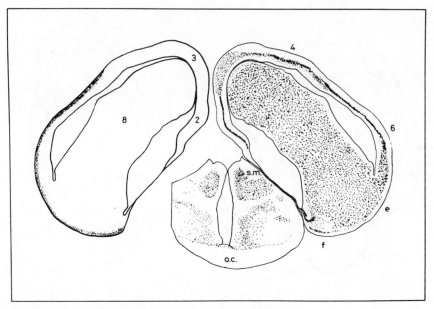

FIGURE 4.33.   Projections of the olfactory bulb to BDVR in a crocodilian. The left side of the figure shows the pattern of degeneration in a Nauta preparation of the caudal telencephalon of *Caiman* following a lesion of the olfactory bulb. The right side of the figure is a drawing of a Nissl preparation. *Abbreviations:* **o.c.,** optic chiasm; **s.m.,** stria medullaris. Numbers and letters refer to cytoarchitectonic areas defined by Riss, Halpern, and Scalia (1969). From Scalia, Halpern, and Riss (1969).

the archistriatum. It would be interesting to examine the olfactory efferents in birds with well-developed olfactory systems such as turkey vultures or petrels.

4.4.   MODALITY SPECIFIC AREAS IN DVR

The major suggestion that emerges from this chapter is that DVR includes a series of areas, each of which receives information from one of the major sensory modalities (Fig. 4.34). Visual, auditory, and somatosensory information are carried through thalamotelencephalic projections to ADVR. The pattern seems to be that visual projections terminate laterally within ADVR, somatosensory projections terminate in a central region of ADVR, and auditory projections terminate medially in ADVR. Each modality is represented at least once, but birds may have three distinct auditory areas and two visual areas within

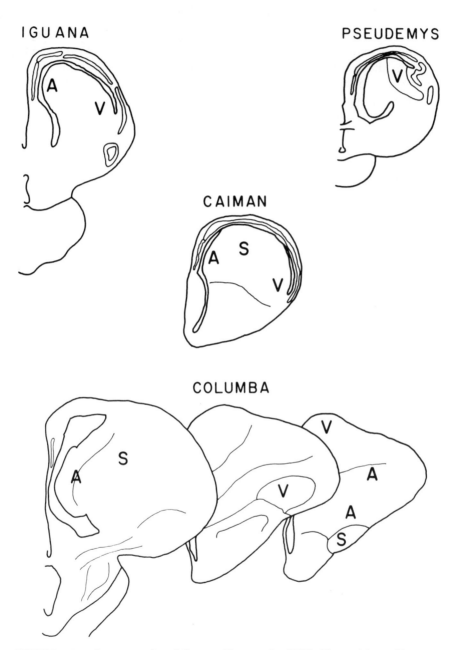

IGUANA

PSEUDEMYS

CAIMAN

COLUMBA

FIGURE 4.34. Summary of modality specific areas in ADVR. The positions of known auditory (A), somatosensory (S), and visual (V) areas in ADVR are plotted on forebrain sections of those species that have been adequately studied.

ADVR. Olfactory information is carried through either the accessory or lateral olfactory tract, depending on species, to BDVR. In snakes and lizards, the accessory olfactory bulbs terminate within BDVR in nucleus sphericus. In the other reptiles studied, olfactory efferents terminate over the ventral surface of BDVR. The situation is not well studied in birds.

In addition to these relatively direct sensory projections to DVR, there is evidence in most groups that efferents from ADVR terminate in BDVR. It is not known if information from each nonolfactory modality terminates within a specific subdivision of BDVR, in which case BDVR would contain a modality specific area for each of the major sensory modalities.

Chapter Five

BRAINSTEM AFFERENTS TO DVR

A Digression

This chapter concludes the discussion of afferents to DVR and striatum by considering the projections of brainstem neurons to the forebrain. It is something of a digression from the central argument of the treatise, but is relevant to the issue of sensory linkages in two ways. First, it is quite likely that at least some of the brainstem systems provide a general modulation of the forebrain, including a regulation of the sensory systems that reach ADVR. Second, some of the brainstem structures that project to the forebrain are also involved with the efferent pathways that link ADVR and the striatum to motor centers in the brainstem. The best-studied of the brainstem systems are those that use one of the monoamines (noradrenaline, dopamine, or serotonin) as a transmitter substance. These monoaminergic systems are treated first, followed by a brief discussion of an additional set of brainstem projections to the forebrain that apparently parallels the monoaminergic systems. The central concept of this chapter is the existence of these multiple, parallel pathways from the brainstem to the forebrain. Taken in conjunction with the available information on the distribution of transmitter substances in the telencephalon, the anatomy of the brainstem pathways reinforces the division of the dorsal telencephalon into DVR and striatum.

5.1. MONOAMINERGIC SYSTEMS

Catecholaminergic and serotonergic neurons have been localized with histofluorescent techniques in the brainstems of lizards (Baumgarten and Braak, 1968; Braak, Baumgarten, and Falck, 1968), *Caiman* (Brauth and Kitt, 1980), cryptodiran turtles (Parent, 1979), and several species of birds (Bertler et al., 1964; Fuxe and Ljungren, 1965; Tohyama et al., 1974; Ikeda and Gotoh, 1971; Yamamoto, Tohyama, and Shimizu, 1977; Dubé and Parent, 1981; Shiosaka et al., 1981). Three groups of monoaminergic neurons are potentially involved in forebrain projections. First, a group of noradrenergic neurons is present in the rostral pons in a position corresponding to the mammalian locus coeruleus. Second, dopaminergic neurons are found in the midbrain tegmentum. The more laterally placed of these correspond to the cytoarchitecturally defined substantia nigra in lizards and turtles and to the pedunculopontine nucleus in crocodilians and birds. The more medially placed dopaminergic neurons correspond to the ventral tegmental area. Third, serotonergic neurons are found throughout the raphé of the midbrain and rhombencephalon. Information relating to the projections of these nuclei in each group of reptiles and birds will now be reviewed. The general pattern is that the midbrain dopaminergic groups project to the striatum. The pontine noradrenergic group projects to DVR and possibly to the striatum. By analogy with the situation in mammals, it is likely that the serotonergic groups of the raphé also project to the forebrain, but this has not been clearly demonstrated in most cases.

Lizards

HRP injections in ADVR and striatum in the monitor lizard *Varanus exanthematicus* retrogradely label neurons in the locus coeruleus and in the substantia nigra (ten Donkelaar and De Boer-van Huizen, 1981b). Baumgarten and Braak (1968) could trace fibers from catecholaminergic neurons in the mesencephalic tegmentum (presumably the substantia nigra) through the forebrain bundles and into the striatum in *Lacerta viridis* and *L. muralis*. They are fine caliber fibers that bear small varicosities, 0.5–1.5 μm in length. Microspectrographic techniques indicate that norepinephrine is the most abundant catecholamine in this region. This finding differs from the usual report of high dopamine levels in this region in other groups of reptiles and birds. Contestabile and DiPardo (1976) examined the monoamine oxidase distribution in *L. muralis* and found weak activity in the striatum, but marked activity more ventrally in nucleus accumbens and the olfactory tubercle.

1 mm

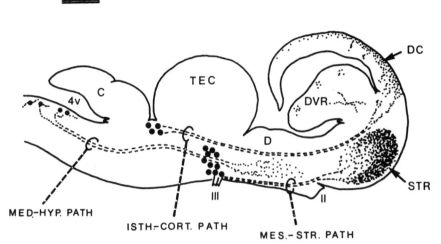

FIGURE 5.1. Catecholaminergic pathways in a turtle. The cells of origin (large dots) and axons of catecholaminergic neurons are summarized on a parasagittal section of a *Chrysemys* brain. The medullo-hypothalamic, isthmi-cortical, and mesencephalic-striated paths are indicated. *Abbreviations:* **C**, cerebellum; **D**, diencephalon; **DC**, dorsal cortex; **DVR**, anterior dorsal ventricular ridge; **TEC**, optic tectum; **STR**, striatum; **4v**, fourth ventricle; **II**, optic nerve; **III**, oculomotor nerve. From Parent (1979).

HRP injections in ADVR and striatum also retrogradely label raphé neurons in *Varanus* (ten Donkelaar and De Boer-van Huizen, 1981b). Braak, Baumgarten, and Falck (1968) followed yellow fluorescent fibers from neurons surrounding the interpeduncular nucleus of the midbrain into ADVR in *Lacerta*, where the fibers formed a diffuse plexus. This suggests the existence of a serotonergic projection to ADVR.

Turtles

Two lines of evidence indicate that dopaminergic neurons in the midbrain tegmentum project to the striatum in turtles (Fig. 5.1). First, midbrain transections rostral to this group cause an accumulation of fluorescence in the proximal axons of these cells and a depletion of fluorescence in the striatum (Parent, 1973b). Lesions caudal to the mesencephalon do not cause a decrease in striatal fluorescence, suggesting that catecholaminergic neurons present in the isthmus (Parent and Poirer, 1971; Yamamoto, Tohyama, and Shimizu, 1977) do not project to the striatum. Second, mesencephalic neurons corresponding in position to the catecholaminergic groups can be labeled retrogradely following injections of

HRP into the striatum, but not in the overlying DVR (Parent, 1976; Belekhova et al., 1978). Juorio (1969) and Parent (1979) found high dopamine concentrations in the striatum, indicating that the mesencephalic projection to the striatum is dopaminergic.

Catecholaminergic fibers encapsulate the large cell clusters in medial area of ADVR in *Chrysemys* (Parent, 1973a; Parent and Poitras, 1974). The origin of these fibers is not certain, but Balaban and Ulinski (1981a) were able to retrogradely label neurons in locus coeruleus following large injections of HRP into ADVR in *Pseudemys* and *Chrysemys*.

Crocodilians

The ventrolateral area contains a heavy concentration of catecholaminergic fibers in fluorescent preparations (Brauth and Kitt, 1980). Fluorescent fibers are most extensive in the small-celled part of ventrolateral area and only sparsely distributed in the large-celled part. HRP injections into the ventrolateral area retrogradely label neurons in the pedunculopontine nucleus of the mesencephalic tegmentum (Fig. 5.2) and in the locus coeruleus in the pontine tegmentum. These experiments show that the two brainstem groups have axons that terminate in or pass through the striatum. It is not certain which groups terminate in the striatum and which contribute to the diffuse plexus of catecholaminergic fibers seen in dorsal DVR.

Birds

There is good evidence that midbrain catecholaminergic groups in birds project to the striatum (Fig. 5.3). Bertler et al. (1964) could follow fluorescent fibers rostrad from the mesencephalon through the medial forebrain bundle in pigeons. They turn dorsally at the level of the anterior commissure and participate in a major plexus in the paleostriatum augmentatum. Fine fluorescent fibers were also found in this structure and the parolfactory lobe by Parent and Olivier (1970/1971), Karten and Dubbeldam (1973), Tohyama et al. (1974), Dubé and Parent (1981), and Lewis et al. (1981). Bertler et al. (1964) performed transections between the diencephalon and the telencephalon and found that the concentrations of dopamine and noradrenaline in the ipsilateral striatum decreased over the control side. Lewis et al. (1981) found that lesions in the pars compacta of the pedunculopontine nucleus led to a decrease in the concentration of catecholaminergic terminals in the paleostriatum augmentatum, but not in the parolfactory lobe. By contrast, lesions in the ventral tegmental area depleted catecholamine terminals in the parolfac-

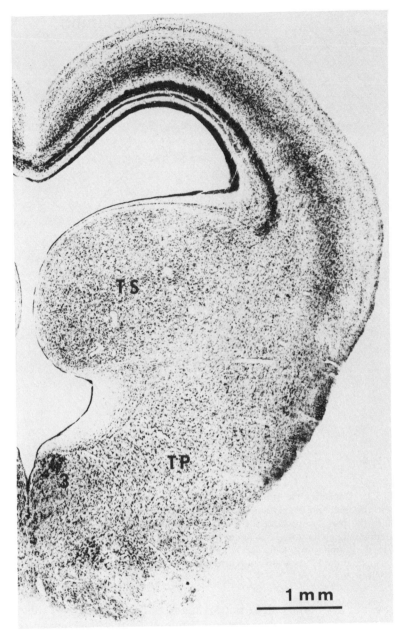

FIGURE 5.2. Midbrain tegmentum in a crocodilian. A cross section through the mid-brain of *Alligator mississippiensis* shows the pedunculopontine nucleus (TP). *Other abbreviations:* **TS**, torus semicircularis; **3**, oculomotor nucleus.

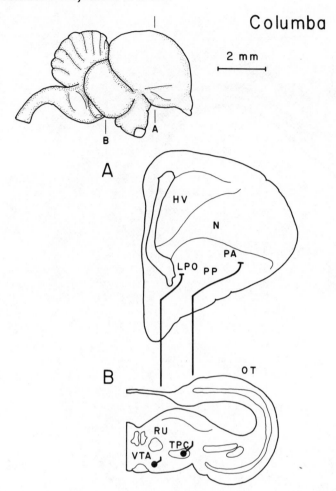

FIGURE 5.3. Dopaminergic projections to the striatum in pigeons. Dopaminergic neurons in the midbrain tegmentum project topographically to the striatum in pigeons. Neurons in the pars compacta of the pedunculopontine nucleus (TPC) project to the paleostriatum augmentatum (PP). Neurons in the ventral tegmental area (VTA) project to the parolfactory lobe (LPO). *Other abbreviations:* **HV,** hyperstriatum ventrale; **N,** neostriatum; **PP,** paleostriatum primitivum; **RU,** red nucleus. Based on Kitt and Brauth (1981a), and others.

tory lobe, but not in the paleostriatum augmentatum. Similarly, Kitt and Brauth (1980) used autoradiographic techniques to trace the connections of the pedunculopontine nucleus in pigeons and found that this nucleus projects heavily to the rostral and lateral regions of the paleostriatum augmentatum and lightly to the parolfactory lobe and intrapeduncular nucleus. The ventral tegmental area projects primarily to the parolfactory lobe and nucleus accumbens. The projections from midbrain cate-cholaminergic groups to the striatum are thus topographically orga-nized.

In addition to the catecholaminergic projections of the striatum, fluorescent fibers are seen in ADVR, particularly in the hyperstriatum ventrale. These fibers probably originate at least in part in the locus coeruleus. Lesions of pontine catecholaminergic groups lead to de-creases in the concentration of fluorescent fibers in the hyperstriatum (Tohyama et al., 1974), and Kitt and Brauth (1980) could show with autoradiographic techniques that the locus coeruleus in pigeons has a light projection to the hyperstriatum ventrale and neostriatum. Injec-tions of HRP in the hyperstriatum of chicks retrogradely label neurons in the locus coeruleus (Miceli et al., 1980).

These studies demonstrating monoaminergic projections to DVR and striatum are consistent with the distribution of monoamines and their degratory enzymes in the forebrain. Juorio and Vogt (1967) found that the anterior part of the paleostriatum augmentatum has high concentra-tions of dopamine (3.00 ± 0.24 μg/g), norepinephrine (0.40 ± 0.05 μg/g), and epinephrine (0.11 ± 0.02 μg/g) in pigeons, chickens, ducks, and spice finches (*Lonchura punctulata*). Lewis et al. (1981) adduced phar-macological data suggesting that the fluorescence present in the paleo-striatum augmentatum and parolfactory lobe is due principally to dopamine. Pretreatment of zebra finches with a monoamine depletor (tetrabenazine), or an inhibitor of catecholamine biosynthesis (α-methyl-p-tyrosine) led to a decrease of fluorescence in the striatum, whereas treatment with an inhibitor of norepinephrine synthesis (disulfiram) led to no change in striatal fluorescence. In addition to these catechol-amines, the paleostriatum augmentatum has a high concentration (1.39 ± 0.05 μg/g) of serotonin (Juorio and Vogt, 1967). Positive reactions for the enzyme monoamine oxidase have been reported in the paleostri-atum augmentatum, parolfactory lobe (Kusunoki, 1969; Minelli, 1970), and hyperstriatum accessoriuim (Kusunoki, 1969).

5.2. THICK CALIBER SYSTEMS

The axons of the monoaminergic systems characteristically have wide-spread projections within the telencephalon and thin, highly varicose axons. In addition, there is evidence for the existence of a projection from the brainstem to ADVR that also has widespread projections. However, its axons are of a thick caliber. The projections to ADVR appear to be only part of a more extensive projection system (Ulinski, 1981).

Snakes

Projections from the brainstem to ADVR have been studied with Fink–Heimer techniques in garter and water snakes following unilateral transections of the midbrain (Ulinski, 1978a). A system of thick caliber fibers could be followed into the telencephalon via the forebrain bundles (Fig. 5.4). Some of the fibers decussate over the anterior commissure. A contingent enters caudal ADVR bilaterally. Other fibers turn dorsally into rostral ADVR from the lateral forebrain bundle. The thick parent fibers are confined primarily to zones C + D, but bear thin collaterals with small varicosities that extend radially into zone B. The remaining thick caliber fibers project to septum and cortex. The organization of the cortical projections has been studied in some detail (Ulinski, 1981). In particular, HRP injections in cortex retrogradely label neurons situated dorsolateral to the oculomotor rootlets in the midbrain tegmentum.

Lizards

Thick caliber projections to ADVR have been described in the green iguana, *Iguana iguana* (Butler, 1980), the tokay gecko, *Gekko gecko* (Butler, 1980), and the tegu lizard, *Tupinambis* (ten Donkelaar and De Boer-van Huizen, 1981b) following midbrain transections. The projections are bilateral. HRP injections in ADVR retrogradely label neurons in the lateral mesencephalic tegmentum in *Iguana* (Bruce and Butler, 1979), tegu lizards (Lohman and van Woerden-Verkley, 1978), and *Varanus* (ten Donkelaar and De Boer-van Huizen, 1981b).

Turtles

Hall and Ebner (1970b) could not trace degeneration into ADVR following midbrain transections in *Pseudemys*. However, Balaban and Ulinski (1981a) report a few retrogradely labeled neurons in the nucleus profundus mesencephali of *Pseudemys* following large HRP injections in ADVR.

5.3.   PARALLEL PATHWAYS FROM THE BRAINSTEM

The complete pattern of brainstem projections to the telencephalon has not been adequately worked out for any one given species. However, the overall similarity in the bits and pieces of information that are available makes it possible to outline the nature of the pattern with some confidence. Three monoaminergic systems apparently project from the

NATRIX

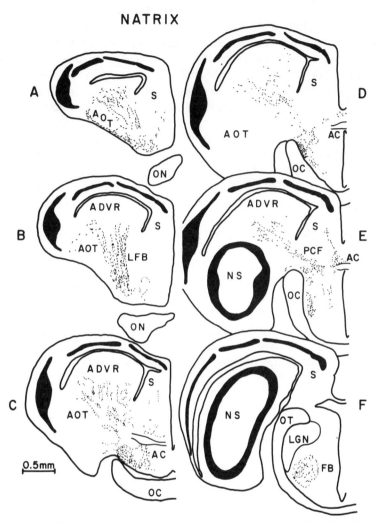

FIGURE 5.4. Thick caliber projections to ADVR. The pattern of thick caliber degeneration seen in a Fink–Heimer preparation of the water snake, *Natrix sipedon,* is shown plotted on a series of forebrain sections. *Abbreviations:* **AC,** anterior commissure; **ADVR,** anterior dorsal ventricular ridge; **AOT,** accessory olfactory tract; **FB,** forebrain bundles; **LFB,** lateral forebrain bundle; **LGN,** lateral geniculate nucleus; **OC,** optic chiasm; **ON,** optic nerve; **OT,** optic tract; **NS,** nucleus sphericus; **PCF,** postcommissural fascicle; **S,** septum. From Ulinski (1978a).

brainstem to the telencephalon, terminating differentially in the striatum and ADVR. The striatum receives a topographically organized, dopaminergic projection from the midbrain tegmentum. Data considered in the next chapter indicate that this projection is one limb of a set of reciprocal projections that interconnect the striatum and the mesencephalic tegmentum. ADVR receives serotonergic projections from the raphé nuclei and noradrenergic projections from the locus coeruleus. There is no evidence for a topography to these projections. The precise terminal zones of these projections is not yet known, but they may be restricted preferentially to periventricular regions of ADVR. There is an additional thick caliber projection from the midbrain tegmentum to the telencephalon; the transmitter substance associated with this system of fibers is not known.

Because of the mesencephalic projection to the striatum, this region of the telencephalon has a characteristically high concentration of dopamine. It also has relatively high concentrations of several other substances related to transmitter metabolism, such as acetylcholinesterase, suggesting that it contains a relatively large number of cholinergic neurons or terminals. The striatum also demonstrates strong enkephalin-like and substance P-like immunoreactivity, indicating the presence of systems that may use the enkephalins and substance P as transmitter substances. The nature of these systems is not yet known.

Chapter Six

EFFERENT CONNECTIONS

Last Steps in the Linkages

The preceding chapters discussed the principal afferent systems that carry information to DVR and striatum, and therefore include a characterization of the sensory linkages to DVR. The ultimate task in the characterization of the linkages is to consider those efferent systems that carry information away from DVR, and therefore form the last steps in the linkages. Figure 6.1 displays the overall pattern of these projections. ADVR projects to the underlying striatum and to BDVR or archistriatum. These structures, receiving projections from ADVR, in turn issue three major pathways. First, predominantly striatal projections reach the brainstem reticular formation through the optic tectum, and thereby place ADVR in contact with major descending motor pathways. Second, there are striatal projections that engage ADVR in a series of feedback loops through a variety of thalamic and brainstem structures. Finally, there are projections from BDVR to the hypothalamus.

6.1. EFFERENTS FROM ADVR

Most investigations of ADVR's efferents show two major projections. The first is a projection of ADVR onto the subjacent striatum. The second is a projection to the basal dorsal ventricular ridge or archistriatum. These projections will now be considered for each of the groups of reptiles and birds.

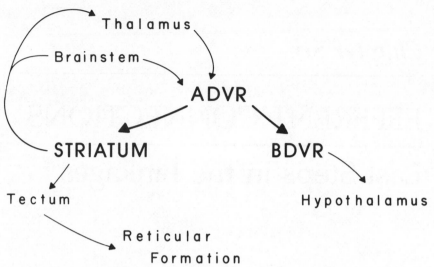

FIGURE 6.1.   Overview of sensory–motor linkages. The basic pattern of efferent projections from ADVR is summarized.

Snakes

Neurons in zones A, B, and C in garter and water snake ADVR have axons that are confined to ADVR, and superficial lesions of ADVR produce degeneration only within this structure (Ulinski, 1978a). However, neurons in zone D have axons that course ventrally out of ADVR, and lesions that encroach deeply into ADVR demonstrate efferent projections to the striatum (Fig. 6.2). Axons coursing ventromedially terminate in the medial striatal nucleus. A second contingent of fibers courses ventrally and terminates in the intrapeduncular nucleus. Fibers coursing ventrolaterally terminate in the perifascicular complex. The most laterally situated of these continues caudally to terminate in the ventral two-thirds of the posterior dorsal ventricular ridge within BDVR. ADVR efferents in snakes thus seem to be topographically organized, with medial ADVR projecting to medial striatum and lateral ADVR projecting to lateral striatum and BDVR.

Lizards

Stereotaxic lesions demonstrate a pattern of ADVR efferents in tegu lizards (Hoogland, 1977) resembling that seen in snakes (Fig. 6.3). Lesions in rostral ADVR produce degeneration in the small-celled and

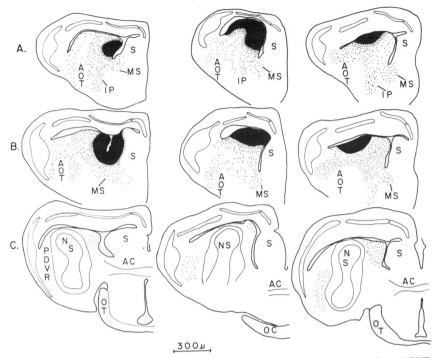

FIGURE 6.2.   ADVR efferents in snakes. The pattern of efferent projections from ADVR is shown in three experiments on **garter** snakes, *Thamnophis sirtalis*. Three sections from Fink–Heimer preparations of each case are shown. *Abbreviations:* **AC,** anterior commissure; **ADVR,** anterior dorsal ventricular ridge; **AOT,** accessory olfactory tract; **IP,** intrapeduncular nucleus; **MS,** medial striatal nucleus; **NS,** nucleus sphericus; **OC,** optic chiasm; **OT,** optic tract; **PDVR,** posterior dorsal ventricular ridge; **S,** septum. From Ulinski (1978a).

large-celled ventral striatum and lateral amygdaloid nucleus (Hoogland, 1977) within BDVR. Lesions in caudal ADVR produce degeneration in the contralateral ventral striatum. ADVR efferents have also been studied in tegu lizards using autoradiographic tracing techniques (Voneida and Sligar, 1979). Labeled material was transported ventromedially through the stria terminalis to the hypothalamus, to the striatum and to the nucleus accumbens, olfactory tubercle and posterior dorsal ventricular ridge.

Efferent projections of ADVR in the Type I lizard, the tokay gecko (*Gekko gecko*), have been described following suction aspiration of the dorsal cortex and ADVR (Butler, 1976). Lesions of ADVR produced degeneration throughout ipsilateral ADVR. Degeneration was also present

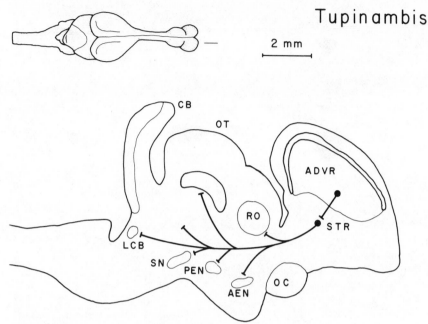

FIGURE 6.3. ADVR efferents in tegu lizards. ADVR projects to the striatum (STR) in *Tupinambis*. Neurons in the striatum project to nucleus rotundus (RO) in the dorsal thalamus, the anterior (AEN) and posterior (PEN) entopeduncular nuclei, the substantia nigra (SN), and the lateral cerebellar nucleus (LCB). It is not known if these projections are effected by collaterals from the same neurons. *Other abbreviations:* **CB,** cerebellum; **OT,** optic tectum. Based on Hoogland (1977) and Voneida and Sligar (1979).

in the striatum, but its distribution was not described in relation to specific nuclear groups. Terminal degeneration was reported, however, to be particularly dense around the medial recess of the lateral ventricle. As in tegu lizards, fibers decussate over the anterior commissure and terminate around the medial recess of the contralateral lateral ventricle.

Injections of HRP in ADVR of *Iguana* label neurons in the lateral forebrain bundle (the nucleus intrapeduncularis) and in the posterior dorsal ventricular ridge (Bruce and Butler, 1979), indicating that the projections between ADVR and striatum are reciprocal.

Turtles

Efferent projections of ADVR in *Chrysemys* have been studied following suction lesions (Northcutt, 1970). Degeneration attributed to damage of ADVR was found throughout ipsilateral ADVR and striatum (Fig. 6.4).

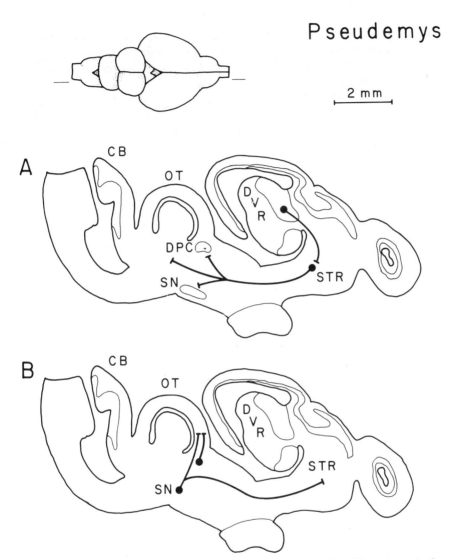

FIGURE 6.4. DVR efferents in turtles. The connections of ADVR and the striatum in the red-eared turtle, *Pseudemys scripta,* and the painted turtle, *Chrysemys picta,* are shown in two diagrams drawn on the same parasagittal section. (A) ADVR projects to the striatum (STR). Neurons in the striatum project to the dorsal nucleus of the posterior commissure (DPC) in the pretectum, the substantia nigra (SN), and the nucleus profundus mesencephali (shown but not labeled). (B) Reciprocal projections reach the striatum from the substantia nigra (SN). Both the substantia nigra and the dorsal nucleus of the posterior commissure (not labeled) project to the optic tectum. *Other abbreviation:* **CB,** cerebellum. Based on Northcutt (1970), Reiner et al. (1980), and others.

The degeneration in the striatum was not related to specific nuclear groups. Degeneration could also be traced through the anterior commissure to the contralateral ADVR and through the lateral forebrain bundle to nucleus rotundus and the mesencephalon.

Following injections of HRP in ADVR, labeled neurons were present in the small-celled striatum, the large-celled striatum, and embedded in the lateral forebrain bundle (Belekhova et al., 1979; Balaban and Ulinski, 1981a).

Crocodilians

Schapiro (1964) made stereotaxic lesions in DVR in *Caiman* and traced its efferent pathways using Nauta–Gygax techniques. Degeneration could be followed from the dorsolateral area, through the intermediolateral area of ADVR and into the ventrolateral area of the striatum (Fig. 6.5A). Degeneration could also be traced into the ipsilateral lateral forebrain bundle. A few fibers decussate at the anterior commissure.

Birds

The efferents of lateral ADVR, field L and neighboring neostriatum, the hyperstriatum ventrale and nucleus basalis have been studied with experimental techniques (Fig. 6.6).

Karten and Dubbeldam (1973) made initial observations on the efferent projections from the lateral part of ADVR in pigeons by making horizontal knife cuts through the ectostriatum. These lesions could have damaged efferents from the ectostriatum (Fig. 6.6E), from areas of ADVR situated dorsolateral to the ectostriatum, or both. Dense terminal degeneration was present in the subjacent paleostriatum augmentatum (PA); sparse degeneration was also seen in the paleostriatum primitivum (PP) and intrapeduncular nucleus. Kitt and Brauth (1978) made injections of tritiated amino acids into the temporo-parieto-occipital area (not labeled in Fig. 6.6), which is situated dorsolateral to the ectostriatum. Projections could be traced to the paleostriatum augmentatum (PA) and ventromedial parolfactory lobe (LPO). In addition to these projections to the striatum, Zeier and Karten (1971) report that the lateral regions of ADVR project to the archistriatum through the dorsal archistriatal pathway. The projections terminate in the intermediate part of the archistriatum (A). HRP injections in the archistriatum of parakeets retrogradely label neurons in an area that appears topographically equivalent to the temporo-parieto-occipital area (Paton, Manogue, and Nottebohm, 1981). (The authors, however, label this area as the hyper-

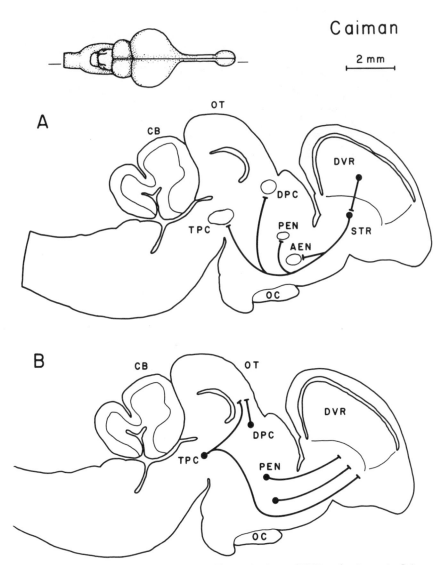

Caiman

2 mm

FIGURE 6.5. ADVR efferents in caiman. The projections of DVR and striatum in *Caiman* are shown on two diagrams of the same parasagittal section. (A) DVR projects to the striatum (STR). Neurons in the striatum project to the anterior (AEN) and posterior (PEN) entopeduncular nuclei, the dorsal nucleus of the posterior commissure (DPC) in the pretectum, and the pars compacta of the pedunculopontine nucleus (TPC). (B) Reciprocal projections to the striatum are effected by the posterior entopeduncular nucleus (PEN), anterior entopeduncular nucleus (not labeled) and the pedunculopontine nucleus (TPC). The pedunculopontine nucleus and the dorsal nucleus of the posterior commissure (DPC) project to the optic tectum (OT). *Other abbreviations:* **CB,** cerebellum; **OT,** optic chiasm. Based on Schapiro (1964), Brauth and Kitt (1980), and Reiner et al. (1980).

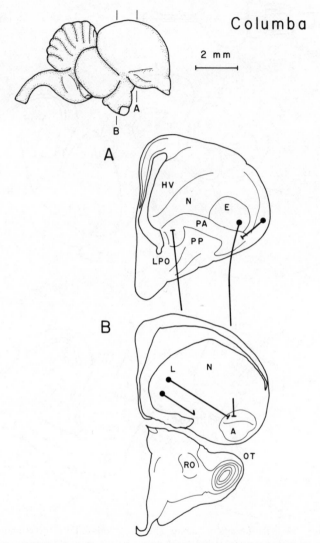

FIGURE 6.6. ADVR efferents in pigeon. DVR in pigeon projects to the striatum and archistriatum. Neurons in field L (L) project ventromedially to the medial paleostriatum augmentatum (PA) and ventrolaterally to the intermediate archistriatum (A). Neurons in the ectostriatum (E) project to the intermediate archistriatum. The temporo-parieto-occipital area (not labeled) also projects to the paleostriatum augmentatum. Notice that the overall pattern of DVR projections to the paleostriatum augmentatum is topographically organized. *Other abbreviations:* **HV**, hyperstriatum ventrale; **LPO**, parolfactory lobe; **N**, neostriatum; **OT**, optic tectum; **PP**, paleostriatum primitivum; **RO**, nucleus rotundus. Based on Karten and Dubbeldam (1973), Kitt and Brauth (1978), and Zeier and Karten (1971).

striatum.) It is therefore likely that the temporo-parieto-occipital area projects to the striatum.

A comparable set of projections have been demonstrated for field L and neighboring regions of the caudal neostriatum. First, injections of tritiated amino acids into field L demonstrate a projection to the medial part of the paleostriatum augmentatum in canaries (Kelly and Nottebohm, 1979) and in guinea fowl, *Numida meleagris* (Bonke, Bonke, and Scheich, 1979). Second, projections from field L course ventrolaterally and terminate in the archistriatum. Knife cuts that damage the neostriatum caudale in pigeons produce dense degeneration that proceeds ventrolaterally through the dorsal archistriatal tract to the intermediate part of the archistriatum (Zeier and Karten, 1971). A comparable projection to the nucleus robustus of the archistriatum is present in canaries (Nottebohm, Stokes, and Leonard, 1976).

The projections of the hyperstriatum ventrale have been studied in songbirds (Fig. 6.7) and guinea fowl. Lesions or injections of tritiated amino acids or HRP into the hyperstriatum ventrale pars caudalis (HVc) of canaries demonstrate two projections (Nottebohm and Kelly, 1979; Nottebohm, Kelly and Paton, 1982). The first is to nucleus robustus (RA). The fibers pass through the neostriatum via the dorsal archistriatal path and terminate in the center of nucleus robustus, thus complementing the field L projection which terminates at its borders. The second projection is to a tear-shaped region within the parolfactory lobe that is called area X. These projections have also been demonstrated in zebra finches in that injections of HRP in the parolfactory lobe, including area X, and in nucleus robustus (Gurney, 1981) retrogradely label neurons in the hyperstriatum ventrale pars caudalis. Comparable projections are present in guinea fowl (Bonke, Bonke, and Scheich, 1979). Autoradiographic studies show that the hyperstriatum ventrale projects to the medial paleostriatum augmentatum and to the intermediate archistriatum.

The frontoarchistriatal path can be followed from nucleus basalis into the anterior and intermediate parts of the archistriatum (Wallenberg, 1903). Zeier and Karten (1971) studied this projection using degeneration techniques in pigeons. They indicate that the dorsoarchistriatal path originates in nucleus basalis and terminates in the archistriatum intermedium and overlying neostriatum. Similarly, injections of tritiated proline in nucleus basalis label a terminal field in the neostriatum caudale just dorsal to the archistriatum (Wild and Zeigler, 1982). In the same set of experiments, injections of HRP in the terminal field retrogradely label neurons in nucleus basalis. Both orthograde and retrograde HRP experiments indicate that this region of the neostriatum projects to the archi-

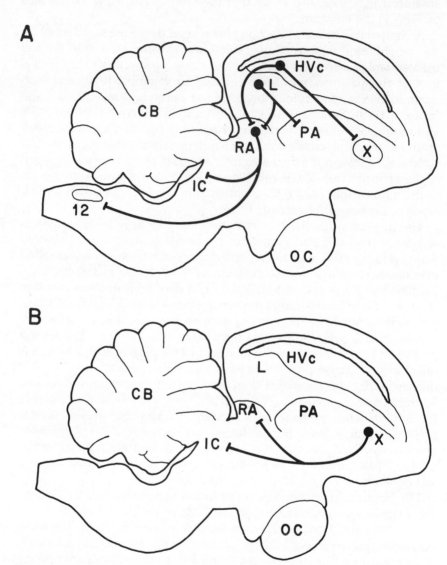

FIGURE 6.7. Efferent projections of ADVR and striatum in canary. The descending projections from DVR in the canary, *Serinus canarius,* are shown on two diagrams of the same parasagittal section. (A) The caudal part of the hyperstriatum ventrale (HVc) receives projections from field L (L) and projects to area X in the parolfactory lobe and nucleus robustus (RA) in the archistriatum. Field L projects additionally to RA and the paleostriatum augmentatum (PA). Nucleus robustus projects to the intercollicular area (IC) of the midbrain and the hypoglossal nucleus (12). (B) Area X projects to the nucleus robustus (RA) and the intercollicular area (IC). *Other abbreviations:* **CB,** cerebellum; **OC,** optic chiasm. Based on Nottebohm, Stokes, and Leonard (1976) and Stokes, Leonard, and Nottebohm (1974).

striatum. The projections from nucleus basalis to the archistriatum thus appear to involve a synapse in the caudal neostriatum.

6.2.   EFFERENTS FROM THE STRIATUM

The efferent projections of the striatum have been studied in lizards, turtles, *Caiman*, and birds.

Lizards

Efferent projections of the striatum have been studied in tegu lizards using Fink–Heimer techniques (Hoogland, 1977). Efferents leave the striatum and terminate in the diencephalon, mesencephalon, and metencephalon (Fig. 6.3B). Lesions of the mediobasal striatum produce degeneration in the lateral hypothalamus, but this may be due to the interruption of fibers from the olfactory tubercle. Lesions anywhere in the striatum produce degeneration in two structures that are associated with the ventral peduncle of the lateral forebrain bundle. These are the anterior entopeduncular nucleus (AEN), in the diencephalon, and the posterior entopeduncular nucleus (PEN), in the mesencephalon just rostral to the substantia nigra (SN). In addition, the striatum projects to the substantia nigra, the prerubral field, and the central gray of the mesencephalon. Finally, there are projections to the lateral cerebellar nucleus (LCB). This general pattern of projections has been confirmed in *Tupinambis* using autoradiographic techniques (Voneida and Sligar, 1979). Striatal projections have also been studied in the monitor lizard *Varanus exanthematicus* by ten Donkelaar and De Boer-van Huizen (1981a). They showed that HRP injections in the vicinity of the substantia nigra retrogradely label neurons in the striatum. Their experiments also demonstrate the existence of more extensive striatal projections in that HRP injections in the rhombencephalic reticular formation also label striatal neurons. By injecting HRP in the optic tectum, it was shown that both the dorsal nucleus of the posterior commissure and the substantia nigra, in turn, project to the optic tectum. The substantia nigra, ventral tegmental area, and the anterior entopeduncular nucleus project to the striatum in *Varanus* (ten Donkelaar and De Boer-van Huizen, 1981b).

Turtles

The striatal projections in *Chrysemys* generally resemble those in *Caiman* (Reiner et al., 1980). Striatal efferents (Fig. 6.4A) have been traced, using both the orthograde transport of tritiated materials and HRP, through the ventral peduncle of the lateral forebrain bundle to the dorsal nucleus of the posterior commissure (DPC), the nucleus profundus mesencephali, and the substantia nigra (SN). The nucleus of the posterior commissure (Fig. 6.4B) projects to the optic tectum (Reiner et al., 1980). Finally, the substantia nigra projects both to the striatum and to the optic tectum. Thus, the nucleus profundus mesencephali, the nucleus of the posterior commissure, and the substantia nigra all involve ADVR in projections to the optic tectum (Fig. 6.4B).

Crocodilians

Projections of the striatum have been studied in *Caiman* using both orthograde and retrograde tracing techniques (Brauth and Kitt, 1980; Reiner et al., 1980). Injections of tritiated amino acids in the large-celled ventrolateral area (VLA) demonstrate projections to the diencephalon and mesencephalon (Fig. 6.5A). Targets in the diencephalon are limited to the anterior entopeduncular nucleus (AEN) and the ventrolateral and ventromedial areas of the thalamus (not shown in Fig. 6.5). The mesencephalic targets are the posterior entopeduncular nucleus (PEN), the dorsal nucleus of the posterior commissure (DPC), and the pedunculopontine nucleus (TPC). Injections of tritiated amino acids into the small-celled VLA show clear projections only to the pedunculopontine nucleus. It is possible in some cases, to confirm these projections using the retrograde transport of HRP. Thus, injections of HRP into the pedunculopontine nucleus retrogradely labeled neurons in the ventral parts of both the small-celled and large-celled ventrolateral area. HRP injections in the ventrolateral thalamus retrogradely label cells in the ventrocaudal large-celled ventrolateral area. Although no cells are labeled in the small-celled ventrolateral area, those labeled cells in large-celled ventrolateral area occupy the same position as cells projecting to the pedunculopontine nucleus.

The structures in the brainstem and thalamus that receive striatal input can be divided into three groups (Fig. 6.5B). First, the anterior entopeduncular nucleus and the ventrolateral area of the thalamus have reciprocal projections back to the striatum and ADVR, respectively (Brauth and Kitt, 1980). They, thus, involve ADVR in a set of feedback loops through the brainstem and thalamus. Second, the dorsal nucleus of the posterior commissure involves ADVR in projections to the optic tectum. It receives striatal afferents and projects in turn to the optic tectum. Thus, injections of HRP into the optic tectum retrogradely label neurons in the dorsal nucleus of the posterior commissure. Third, the pedunculopontine nucleus is involved in both feedback projections to the striatum and in projections to the optic tectum (Reiner et al., 1980).

Birds

Three groups of structures receive projections from ADVR in birds: (1) the paleostriatum augmentatum and parolfactory lobe, (2) the paleostriatum primitivum and intrapeduncular nucleus, and (3) the archistriatum. The subsequent efferent projections of each of these structures will be considered in turn (Fig. 6.8).

Efferents from the paleostriatum augmentatum (PA) terminate in the underlying paleostriatum primitivum (PP) and intrapeduncular nucleus (Fig. 6.8A). This point has been demonstrated in two ways. First, small lesions of the paleostriatum augmentatum produce degeneration in the augmentatum and intrapeduncular nucleus (Karten and Dubbeldam, 1973). Second, HRP injections in the paleostriatum primitivum retrogradely label neurons in the overlying paleostriatum augmentatum (Brauth, Ferguson, and Kitt, 1978). The projections of the augmentatum onto the primitivum may be topographically organized. Kitt and Brauth (1981a) have used autoradiographic tracing techniques to demonstrate a projection from the paleostriatum augmentatum to a restricted region of the pedunculopontine nucleus of the midbrain projection. This projection terminates in both the pars compacta, which contains catecholaminergic neurons, and a field of neurons dorsomedial to the pars compacta which does not contain catecholaminergic neurons. They confirmed the projection by showing that HRP injections in the pedunculopontine nucleus retrogradely label small neurons in the dorsomedial paleostriatum augmentatum.

The parolfactory lobe lies medial to the paleostriatum. Lesions of the parolfactory lobe in pigeons (Karten and Dubbeldam, 1973) demonstrated projections via the medial forebrain bundle to the lateral preoptic area and anterior hypothalamus. However, Kitt and Brauth (1981a) were unable to confirm this projection using autoradiographic techniques. They found instead that the parolfactory lobe in pigeons projects caudally via the medial forebrain bundle into the lateral habenular nucleus, the dorsomedial anterior and posterior nuclei in the thalamus, both the pedunculopontine nucleus and ventral tegmental area, and the locus coeruleus. The projections to the habenula, midbrain tegmentum, and locus coeruleus were confirmed by retrograde HRP experiments. Lesions of area X within the parolfactory lobe of canaries (Nottebohm, Stokes, and Leonard, 1976) showed projections to a thalamic nucleus (dorsolateralis anterior pars medialis) that is situated immediately dorsal

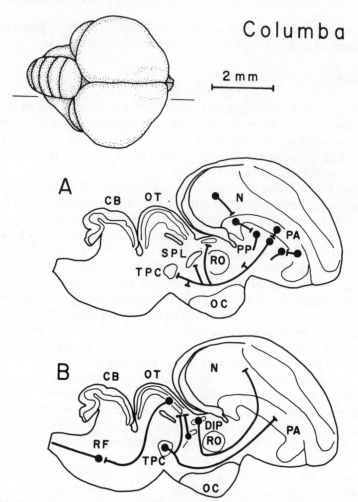

Columba

2 mm

FIGURE 6.8. Striatal connections in pigeons. Connections of the striatum in pigeons are shown on two diagrams of the same parasagittal section. (A) The paleostriatum augmentatum (PA) receives projections from the overlying ADVR, such as the neostriatum (N). Neurons in PA project to the underlying paleostriatum primitivum (PP). Neurons in PP project to the nucleus dorsalis-intermedius posterior of the thalamus (shown but not labeled), the nucleus spiriformis lateralis (SPL) in the pretectum, the pars compacta of the pedunculopontine nucleus (TPC), and the anterior and posterior nuclei of the ansa lenticularis (shown but not labeled). (B) The nucleus dorsalis-intermedius posterior (DIP) of the thalamus projects to the neostriatum. The pedunculopontine nucleus (TPC) projects to the paleostriatum augmentatum. Finally, the nucleus spiriformis lateralis (SPL) and pedunculopontine nucleus (TPC) project to the optic tectum (OT). *Other abbreviations:* **CB,** cerebellum; **OC,** optic chiasm; **RF,** reticular formation; **RO,** nucleus rotundus.

and caudal to nucleus ovoidalis and to the nucleus robustus within the archistriatum (Stokes, Leonard, and Nottebohm, 1974). The projection of the parolfactory lobe to the dorsomedial pedunculopontine nucleus apparently uses substance P as a transmitter substance (Reiner, Karten, and Korte, 1980).

The efferents from the paleostriatum augmentatum and intrapeduncular nucleus are of thick caliber and pass to the brainstem via the ventromedial part of the lateral forebrain bundle. They have been studied with degeneration techniques in pigeons by Karten and Dubbeldam (1973) and with autoradiographic techniques in guinea fowl by Bonke, Bonke, and Scheich (1979). Karten and Dubbeldam (1973) refer to this fiber bundle as the ansa lenticularis. The system terminates (Fig. 6.8B), first, in two nuclei embedded within the forebrain bundle: the anterior and posterior nuclei of the ansa lenticularis. They correspond in position to the entopeduncular nuclei in reptiles. Second, it terminates in the nucleus dorsalis-intermedius posterior (DIP), a thalamic nucleus. Third, it terminates in the nucleus spiriformis lateralis (SPL), a group of cells situated in the vicinity of the caudal thalamus and pretectum. Finally, the efferents from the paleostriatum primitivum and intrapeduncular nucleus terminate in the pars compacta of the pedunculopontine nucleus (TPC). This projection has also been confirmed in pigeons by Kitt and Brauth (1981a) who showed that injections of HRP in the pedunculopontine nucleus retrogradely label neurons in the paleostriatum augmentatum and intrapeduncular nucleus.

Details of the component of this system that involves the nucleus spiriformis lateralis have been recently examined by Reiner, Brecha, and Karten (1982). This is a crescent-shaped nucleus situated at the mesodiencephalic junction anterolateral to the descending fibers of the posterior commissure. Neurons in its dorsal part are more densely packed than are those in its ventral part. The source of striatal projections to the spiriform nucleus was first examined by placing HRP injections in the nucleus. Large neurons were labeled in the paleostriatum primitivum, but not in the intrapeduncular nucleus. These neurons are then the source of the thick caliber ansa lenticularis fibers that terminate in the spiriform nucleus. The spiriform injections also label neurons in the pars compacta of the pedunculopontine nucleus. Since this nucleus also receives projections from the ansa, it forms an indirect route by which striatal afferents can reach the spiriform nucleus. These projections to the spiriform nucleus were confirmed using autoradiographic tracing techniques.

As in reptiles, the striatal efferents fall into three groups (Fig. 6.8B).

The nucleus dorsalis-intermedius posterior receives striatal projections and projects to ADVR, thereby involving it in a feedback loop. Injections of HRP in dorsalis-intermedius posterior retrogradely label neurons in the paleostriatum primitivum and lobus parolfactorius (Kitt and Brauth, 1981b). They also demonstrate a projection from the lateral cerebellar nucleus to dorsalis-intermedius posterior. Autoradiographic studies demonstrate that dorsalis-intermedius posterior projects to the rostromedial neostriatum intermediale via the lateral forebrain bundle (Kitt and Brauth, 1981b). The nucleus spiriformis lateralis receives striatal projections and projects to the tectum (pigeons: Brecha, Hunt, and Karten, 1976; Reiner, Brecha, and Karten, 1982; quail: Minelli, Faccioli, and DeLiberali, 1979), thereby involving ADVR in projections to the optic tectum. This projection appears to be roughly topographic, but highly collateralized in pigeons (Reiner, Brecha, and Karten, 1982). Spiriform neurons contain the peptide enkephalin and terminate in enkephalinergic bands in layers 8–13 of the ipsilateral tectum (Reiner, Karten, and Brecha, 1982). Finally, the pedunculopontine nucleus receives striatal projections and projects to both the striatum and optic tectum (pigeons: Brecha, Hunt, and Karten, 1976; quail: Minelli, Faccioli, and DeLiberali, 1979).

6.3.   EFFERENTS FROM BDVR

Efferent projections from BDVR have been studied only in snakes and in birds.

Snakes

The efferent projections of nucleus sphericus have been studied in garter snakes, *Thamnophis sirtalis* and *T. radix*, using Fink–Heimer techniques (Halpern and Silfen, 1974; Halpern, 1980). Degenerated fibers from lesions in nucleus sphericus pass medially and enter the diencephalon just caudal to the anterior commissure. They pass into the preoptic area and hypothalamus and terminate in the ventromedial hypothalamus. Other fibers course medially, enter the anterior commissure, and terminate in the marginal and mural layers of the contralateral nucleus sphericus. Finally, some fibers travel rostrally from nucleus sphericus to terminate in the granular and internal plexiform layers of the ipsilateral accessory olfactory bulb.

Birds

Efferents from the archistriatum have been studied in both pigeons, ducks, and canaries. In pigeons (Fig. 6.9), lesions of the intermediate part of the archistriatum produce degeneration in a major descending path, the occipitomesencephalic tract, that terminates throughout the brainstem (Zeier and Karten, 1971). In the thalamus, degeneration is seen in the nucleus dorsolateralis posterior, several small nuclei, and the nucleus dorsalis-intermedius posterior. The latter nucleus also receives projections from the paleostriatum primitivum and intrapeduncular nucleus. In the midbrain, degeneration is seen in the intercollicular nucleus and optic tectum. In the pons and medulla, degeneration is seen in the locus coeruleus, lateral pontine nucleus, parvocellular reticular formation, trigeminal nuclei, and cuneate and gracile nuclei. Comparable projections are present in mallard ducks (Arends and Dubbeldam, 1982).

The projections of the nucleus robustus of the archistriatum in canaries (Nottebohm, Stokes, and Leonard, 1976) generally resemble the projections of the intermediate archistriatum in pigeons (Fig. 6.10). Lesions in nucleus robustus show that its major projections are to the nucleus intercollicularis in the midbrain and, particularly, to the hypoglossal nucleus. The latter projection makes sense in that the nucleus robustus seems to be involved in the control of song (see Section 7.2), and the hypoglossal motoneurons innervate the muscles of the syrinx. Comparable projections have been demonstrated with autoradiographic techniques in zebra finches (Gurney, 1981). Projections from nucleus robustus to the hypoglossal nucleus are not unique to songbirds. Paton, Manogue, and Nottebohm (1980, 1981) used orthograde tracing techniques to demonstrate that nucleus robustus of parakeets, *Melopsittacus undulatus*, projects bilaterally to the tracheosyringeal part of the hypoglossal nucleus. Conversely, injections of HRP unilaterally in the hypoglossal nucleus retrogradely label neurons bilaterally in the nucleus intercollicularis and in nucleus robustus.

In addition to these brainstem projections, the archistriatum gives rise to major projections to the hypothalamus (Zeier and Karten, 1971). These projections arise from the medial and posterior components of the archistriatum. They course medially in the occipitomesencephalic tract and run just caudal to the anterior commissure. At this point, a fascicle of fine caliber fibers turns ventrally as the pars hypothalami of the occipitomesencephalic tract. They terminate predominantly in the posterior, medial hypothalamus. Commissural connections interconnect the anterior components of the archistriatum via the anterior commissure (Zeier and Karten, 1973).

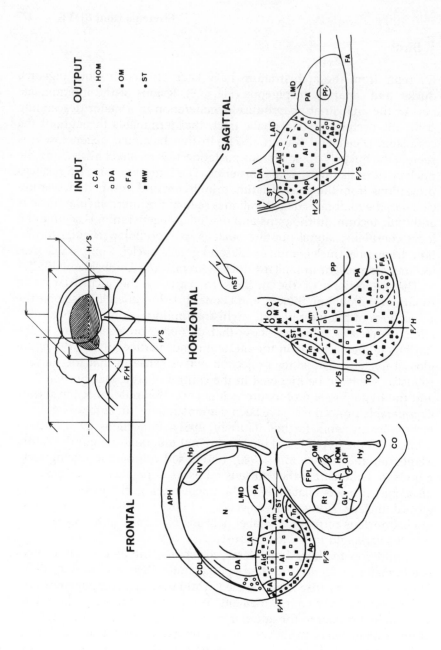

6.4. SENSORY–MOTOR AND SENSORY–HYPOTHALAMIC LINKAGES

The overall implication of the rather formidable set of connections that issue from ADVR is that sensory information that reaches ADVR can be distributed to two major regions of the brain (Fig. 6.11A). Several pathways carry information to the brainstem reticular formation, which is a premotor structure in the sense that it projects to the motoneuron pools of both the spinal cord and brainstem. First, the striatum projects to a pretectal nucleus that is called either the dorsal nucleus of the posterior commissure or the nucleus spiriformis lateralis. This nucleus projects in turn to the deeper layers of the optic tectum. Tectal neurons are known to give rise to a complex set of projections to the brainstem reticular formation. Second, the striatum projects to a dopaminergic cell group in the midbrain tegmentum. It is called the substantia nigra or the pedunculopontine nucleus. This nucleus also projects to the optic tectum. Finally, BDVR gives rise to direct projections to the reticular formation, at least in birds. The reticular formation then projects to motoneurons, including those in the facial and trigeminal motor nuclei (Arends and Dubbeldam, 1982). These projections thus constitute sensory–motor linkages. Efferents from BDVR also project medially to the hypothalamus to form sensory–hypothalamic linkages.

In addition to these projections, which carry information away from ADVR, several structures engage ADVR in feedback loops (Fig. 6.11B).

FIGURE 6.9. Schematic diagram of the major subdivisions of the archistriatum, and loci of major afferent and efferent connections. The upper diagram shows a view of the gross brain with three intersecting planes. Representative outlines through each of these planes is shown in the three lower diagrams. Each diagram also shows a key to the planes illustrated in the two accompanying figures. Thus in the frontal plane, F/S represents the sagittal plane and F/H the horizontal plane in the diagrams to the right. *Abbreviations:* **Aa,** archistriatum anterior; **Ai,** archistriatum intermedium; **Aid,** archistriatum intermedium dorsalis; **AL,** ansa lenticularis; **Am,** archistriatum medialis; **Ap,** archistriatum posterior; **APH,** area parahippocampalis; **CA,** anterior commissure; **CDL,** area corticoidea dorsolateralis; **CO,** optic chiasm; **GLv,** ventral lateral geniculate; **DA,** dorsal archistriatal tract; **FA,** fronto archistriatal tract; **FPL,** lateral forebrain bundle; **HOM,** occipito-mesencephalic tract, pars hypothalamicus; **Hp,** hippocampus; **HV,** hyperstriatum ventrale; **Hy,** hypothalamus; **LAD,** lamina archistriatalis dorsalis; **LMD,** dorsal medullary lamina; **MW,** medial wall; **N,** neostriatum; **nST,** bed nucleus of the stria terminalis; **OM,** occipito-mesencephalic tract; **PA,** paleostriatum augmentatum; **PP,** paleostriatum primitivum; **QF,** quintofrontal tract; **RT,** nucleus rotundus; **ST,** stria terminalis; **Tn,** nucleus taeniae; **V,** ventricle. From Zeier and Karten (1973).

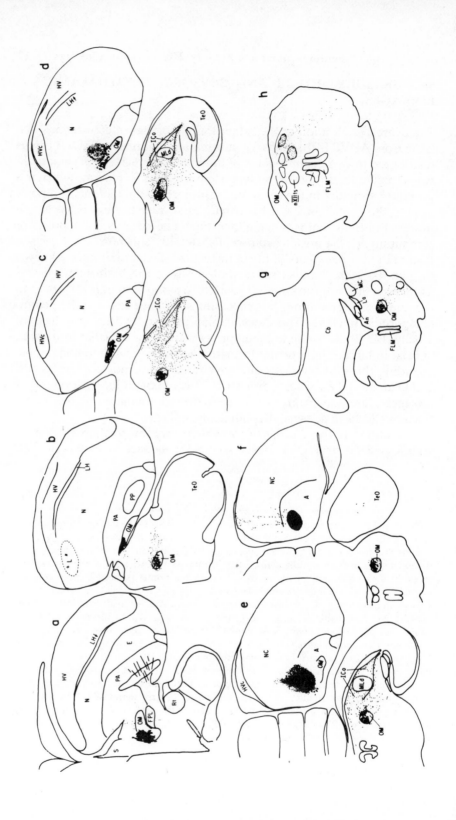

A.

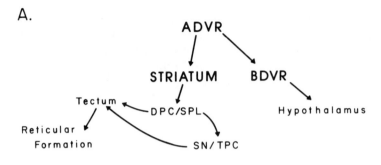

B.

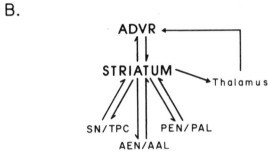

FIGURE 6.11. Summary of the efferent projections of DVR. (A) Efferent projections involved in sensory–motor linkages from ADVR and BDVR to the tectum and to the hypothalamus. (B) Efferent projections involving ADVR in feedback loops.

FIGURE 6.10. Archistriatal projections in song birds. Fink–Heimer degeneration charted from a lesion of the nucleus robustus archistriatalis (RA) (d, e, f). Fibers from the destroyed area join the occipitomesencephalic tract (OM) and travel rostrally (c, b, a) to enter the brainstem. Extensive degeneration is seen in the mesencephalon, particularly nucleus intercollicularis. No degenerating fibers entered the auditory relay nucleus (MLd). Fibers continued caudally in OM giving off projections occasionally to the reticular formation and probably to the facial nucleus. In the caudal medulla a massive projection left OM and entered the nucleus hypoglossi, pars tracheosyringealis (nXIIts), with many fibers ramifying directly around the cell bodies. *Abbreviations:* **A,** archistriatum; **An,** nucleus angularis; **Cb,** cerebellum; **E,** ectostriatum; **FLM,** medial longitudinal fasciculus; **FPL,** lateral forebrain bundle; **HV,** hyperstriatum ventrale; **HVc,** hyperstriatum ventrale, pars caudalis; **ICo,** nucleus intercollicularis; **L,** field L; **La,** nucleus laminaris; **LH,** lamina hyperstriatica; **MC,** nucleus magnocellularis; **MLd,** nucleus mesencephalicus lateralis pars dorsalis; **N,** neostriatum; **Nc,** neostriatum caudale; **nXIIts,** tracheosyringeal part of the hypoglossal nucleus; **OM,** occipitomesencephalic tract; **Rt,** nucleus rotundus; **S,** septum; **TeO,** optic tectum; **PA,** paleostriatum augmentatum; **PP,** paleostriatum primitivum. From Nottebohm, Stokes, and Leonard (1976).

181

The striatum itself has reciprocal connections with ADVR. A dopaminergic cell group in the midbrain tegmentum (the substantia nigra or pedunculopontine nucleus) has reciprocal connections with the striatum, as do nuclei scattered within the tegmentum (the entopeduncular nuclei or nuclei of the ansa lenticularis). Thalamic nuclei can receive projections from the striatum and project back to ADVR.

Chapter Seven

TELENCEPHALIC PATTERN AND FUNCTION

Strategies of Comparison

The first chapter pointed out that telencephalic anatomy varies significantly between vertebrates such that each major group has a distinct pattern of telencephalic organization, DVR being the elaboration of the telencephalon that is characteristic of reptiles and birds. The previous five chapters have reviewed the information currently available on various aspects of DVR organization with the intention of identifying its structural features. This chapter uses the results of the preceding chapters to summarize some of the DVR's structural features and then addresses two general problems. First is the problem of what roles DVR plays in the behavior of reptiles and birds. The central idea is that ADVR forms a linkage between sensory projections to the telencephalon and particular brainstem structures that are involved in the modulation of behavior. Efferents that connect the striatum with the brainstem reticular formation place ADVR in a position to modulate the activity of motoneurons. Efferents that connect BDVR with the hypothalamus and nuclei in the autonomic nervous system place ADVR in a position to modulate effector systems more concerned with the internal milieu. The second general problem concerns the relation of DVR to other patterns of telencephalic organization. It would be ideally appropriate to discuss each of the major variants of telencephalic organization. However, almost nothing is known of telencephalic organization in any of the other vertebrate groups except mammals. This chapter, therefore, concludes with a comparison of the organization of DVR and of equivalent regions of mammalian forebrains.

7.1. STRUCTURAL FEATURES OF DVR

This section returns to the question "What is DVR?" that was posed in Chapter 1 and provides a more satisfactory answer by discussing some features that appear characteristic of DVR. DVR as a whole is divisible into an ADVR and BDVR in all reptiles and birds. There have been very few studies of the structure of BDVR, so almost nothing can be said about its organization. There is by contrast an extensive literature on ADVR and several aspects of its organization probably apply to ADVR in all of the groups of reptiles and birds. This section summarizes these design features and then discusses the two major variations that occur in ADVR organization.

Neuronal Structure

Two types of neurons can usually be distinguished in ADVR. The minority are juxtaependymal cells that have discoidal dendritic fields and are situated near the ventricle. Juxtaependymal cells are present in all of the reptiles that have been investigated, but have not been described in birds. The majority of ADVR neurons are stellate cells and are situated farther from the ventricle. There are variations between species in the number of dendrites on stellate cells, the details of their branching patterns, and the number of dendritic spines that they bear. Most species have a large population of stellate cells with very spiny dendrites and a smaller population with spine-poor or aspiny dendrites. The dendritic field sizes of ADVR neurons are approximately constant across species in spite of the interspecific size variation seen in ADVR. Stellate cells in snakes (Ulinski, 1978a), turtles (Balaban, 1978a), and chickens (Palacios, 1976) all have dendritic field diameters of about 300 μm, and a consequence of ADVR size variation is a variation in the size of ADVR neurons relative to ADVR's overall size. Thus, the ratio of ADVR diameter to stellate cell dendritic field diameter is about 3:1 for garter snakes, 6:1 for turtles, and greater than 10:1 for chickens.

There is a strong tendency for neurons in ADVR to form clusters of touching neurons. Electron microscopy indicates that the plasma membranes of somata in these clusters are directly apposed and sometimes bear specialized junctions. These clusters vary in distribution. Clusters occur preferentially near ADVR's ventricular surface in snakes, lizards,

Sphenodon, and turtles. They are found frequently throughout DVR in crocodilians and birds. The clusters also vary in the number of constituent neurons. They contain only a few neurons in most forms, but the zone 2 clusters of turtles contain large numbers of neurons. All of the neurons in a given cluster are usually the same size, but clusters in some lizards contain a single large neuron surrounded by several smaller neurons, and there are less dramatic differences in the sizes of neurons within a given cluster in birds. The significance of ADVR clusters is not known, but they may be groups of electrotonically coupled neurons in some species that could serve as a substrate for rather complex neuronal computations (see Berry and Pentreath, 1977). The variations in the sizes of neurons in a cluster and the numbers of neurons in a cluster would have functional significance because these variables would alter electrical properties of the cluster (Getting, 1974; Getting and Willows, 1974).

Thalamic Afferents

Thalamotelencephalic fibers form a large proportion of the afferents to ADVR in all groups of reptiles and birds. However, the relation of the thalamic fibers to ADVR varies between species and between different regions within ADVR in a given species. In snakes, thalamic fibers extend into all four zones. They are, therefore, positioned to synapse on both the juxtaependymal cells that lie in the periventricular zones as well as the stellate cells that lie in the deeper zones. In tegu lizards, degeneration following thalamic lesions extends up to, but not into, the periventricular zone. By contrast, the cell cluster zone in turtles is separated from deeper zones by a cell-poor region. Thalamic fibers from nuclei with restricted projections tend to terminate exclusively in the deepest zone. They, therefore, probably do not reach either the stellate cells in the cell cluster zone or the juxtaependymal cells of the periventricular zone. The relation of thalamic afferents to zones varies somewhat between the different areas of ADVR as discussed by Balaban and Ulinski (1981a). Thalamic afferents in birds tend to terminate quite deep in ADVR. Thus, ectostriatum receives fibers from nucleus rotundus and is situated near ADVR's ventral border. Field L receives fibers from nucleus ovoidalis and is separated from the ventricle by the hyperstriatum ventrale. Similarly, nucleus basalis receives trigeminal afferents and is distant from the ventricle.

Balaban and Ulinski (1981a) divided thalamotelencephalic pathways in turtles into two groups. Although direct evidence for a comparable division in other groups of reptiles and birds is limited to lizards, it is likely that both types of projections are present in all species. The first type of thalamic projections are diffuse projections that involve a sparse termination in several telencephalic targets. They are typically effected by fine caliber axons that reach the telencephalon via both the lateral forebrain bundle system and a medial pathway that proceeds through the medial forebrain bundle and dorsally up the medial wall of the telencephalon. Diffuse projections originate from perirotundal nuclei such as the dorsomedial anterior and dorsolateral anterior nuclei. These nuclei project bilaterally to ADVR as well as to several other telencephalic targets such as the septum, cortex, and striatum. Within ADVR the projections are diffusely distributed to all regions of ADVR. The functional significance of such diffuse thalamic projections is unknown.

The second type of thalamic projections are restricted projections that involve a dense termination in a single telencephalic target. These include the projections of thalamic sensory nuclei to ADVR. Thus, discrete thalamic nuclei that receive visual information from the optic tectum, auditory information from the torus semicircularis, and somatosensory information from the spinal cord and dorsal column nuclei have been identified in most groups of reptiles and birds. Each of these nuclei has a restricted projection to ADVR. The consequence of this arrangement is that there are modality specific areas in ADVR.

Modality Specific Areas

There is reasonably good evidence that the pattern of restricted thalamic projections to ADVR results in a set of areas in ADVR, each of which receives a significant input from a specific sensory modality. These areas appear to be situated in topologically equivalent regions of ADVR in the various groups. Nucleus rotundus universally receives visual projections from the tectum and, in those cases where its efferents have been studied, projects to a terminal field situated laterally in ADVR. Radially oriented intrinsic connections link this region with overlying regions, thus forming a radial sector of ADVR that receives visual information from the tectum. An auditory thalamic nucleus projects to a caudomedial terminal field in ADVR in all species examined, so that an auditory area is probably generally present in medial ADVR. Additional auditory areas may be present in rostral ADVR, but these have not been adequately studied. A somatosensory nucleus projects to a central area of ADVR in *Caiman* and probably birds. There is too little information on ascending somatosensory paths to know if this is a general pattern. The principal trigeminal nucleus projects to nucleus basalis in at least birds.

It is often the case in neural systems that a restricted afferent system terminates in a cytoarchitecturally distinct region of its target. It might be expected, then, that the modality specific areas would correspond to cytoarchitecturally distinct areas in ADVR. A pattern of this type is present in the cryptodiran turtles in which areas can be defined on cytoarchitectonic grounds. Each area displays a variant of the basic pattern of three zones and receives projections from a particular thalamic nucleus. However, there are significant variations in the degree to which such areas are segregated from each other. In snakes, it is difficult to recognize cytoarchitectonic areas within ADVR. Golgi studies indicate that an individual thalamic axon initially runs vertically into ADVR, but eventually curves and can extend throughout much of ADVR's mediolateral extent. There is some variation in the cytoarchitecture of lizard ADVR in Nissl preparations, and it is possible to recognize fairly discrete patches in material prepared to demonstrate the enzyme succinic dehydrogenase (SDH). These patches may correspond to the terminal fields of specific thalamic nuclei. Similarly, cytoarchitectonic subdivisions of ADVR are not sharply defined in crocodilians, but discrete patches that correspond to the terminal fields of thalamic nuclei are visible in SDH material. Cytoarchitectonic subdivisions are somewhat clearer in birds. The ectostriatum, in particular, has sharp anatomical boundaries and is the target of the rotundo-DVR projection. Thus, the concept of areas in ADVR is a reflection of the pattern of ADVR's afferent and intrinsic connections that does not always correspond to cytoarchitecturally distinct entities.

The sensory information that reaches the modality specific areas seems to be highly processed. That is, the receptive field properties of units in ADVR tend to differ significantly from those of the corresponding primary sensory neurons. Retinal ganglion cells in turtles and pigeons have small receptive fields, but the receptive fields of units in the rotundal target within ADVR of both species are very large. This difference in receptive field properties presumably reflects intratectal transformations as well as the convergences seen in the tectorotundal and, possibly, rotundal-DVR projections. Similarly, acoustic nerve fibers in birds have relatively sharp tuning curves and respond well to pure tone stimuli. However, units in field L have broader tuning curves, often with multiple peaks, and may respond preferentially to complex stimuli such as species-specific calls or position in visual space. The nature of receptive fields in nucleus basalis is not yet entirely clear: very large fields have been reported in basalis in pigeons, whereas relatively small fields have been reported in ducks. These may be technical differences in the conduct of the experiments rather than real interspecific variations (Berkhoudt, Dubbeldam, and Zeilstra, 1981).

Two different variations in the topographic organization of the modality specific areas can be recognized. On the one hand, the projections to the medial auditory area in at least birds and crocodilians and to nucleus basalis in birds are receptotopically organized. A series of isofrequency contours can be defined in both field L and its adjacent zones and a somatotopic map can be defined in both the dorsal and ventral parts of nucleus basalis in ducks. There is some evidence for a differential magnification of parts of the receptor surface in basalis, and the overall size of the nucleus does vary with the size and degree of innervation of the bill.

On the other hand, the laterally placed visual area apparently lacks a topographic representation of visual space. This lack of retinotopy is presumably a result of the nontopographic organization of both the tectorotundal projection and the rotundal-DVR projection. The functional significance of such nontopographic projections is not known, but Dacey and Ulinski (1983) have recently reviewed some hypotheses. First, it is conceivable that the rotundal-DVR pathway encodes information about position in visual space in spite of the extensive convergence seen in its projections. This hypothesis is consistent with behavioral data implicating nucleus rotundus in pattern vision and acuity discriminations in pigeons (Macko and Hodos, 1979; Mulvanny, 1979). One mechanism that would preserve information about position in visual space involves coding spatial position in discharge frequency. In turtles, for example, tectal neurons are distributed nonhomogeneously within the tectum (Ulinski, 1978b). There is an increase in the density of tectal neurons within the tectal representation of the retinal visual streak, a linear area of increased ganglion cell density (Peterson and Ulinski, 1979). A given rotundal neuron could receive a sample of information from all regions of visual space, but with a greater number of neurons from within the streak representation synapsing on each rotundal neuron than from the representation of the peripheral retina. Rotundal neurons would then be stimulated by visual stimuli anywhere in visual space, but with a greater synaptic strength by stimuli within the visual streak. Consistent with this model, there is some evidence that rotundal units with large receptive fields in turtles respond preferentially to stimuli within certain regions of visual space (Morenkov and Pivavarov, 1975). Visual units in ADVR also have large receptive fields that respond preferentially to stimuli within the visual streak (Dünser et al., 1981). A similar model has been suggested for the spatial to frequency transformation in the projection from the superior colliculus to the paramedian pontine reticular formation in primates (Wurtz and Albano, 1980).

A second hypothesis is that spatial information is not encoded in the rotundal-DVR pathway, but that rotundal neurons encode information about some other parameters of visual stimuli. Evidence from physiological studies of avian rotundus suggests that large field units with different stimulus preferences are differently distributed within rotundus (Revzin, 1979; Maxwell and Granda, 1979). Rotundus would then resemble other sensory structures that lack a receptotopic organization but contain neurons that encode other features of sensory stimuli. The space mapped component of the torus semicircularis of owls is an auditory structure that lacks a tonotopic organization, but contains neurons that code position in auditory space (Knudsen and Konishi, 1978). Similarly, the FM-FM region of auditory cortex in the mustache bat is not tonotopically organized, but contains neurons that are tuned to particular delays between the bat's high frequency pulse and its echo (O'Neill and Suga, 1982).

A third hypothesis is that the rotundal-DVR pathway contains a distributed representation of a spatiotemporal pattern of activity in the tectum in which information is coded in the patterned activity of an entire population of cells. (See Anderson and Hinton, 1981, for a discussion of distributed representations.) No individual unit would uniquely specify a particular position in space or be selective for a single feature, but would respond instead to many input patterns with information being coded as a variation in the strength and temporal position of the unit's output relative to the output of others. This hypothesis would also be compatible with the proposed role for rotundus in pattern discrimination and is consistent with the finding that many rotundal cells respond to any change in the visual image (Revzin, 1979). It suggests that physiological analysis of rotundus should involve recording from several units simultaneously, so that the relative activities of single units can be correlated with changes in the visual stimulus.

These hypotheses may not be mutually exclusive, and there are certainly other hypotheses that are equally plausible. The limited evidence that can be cited in support of each hypothesis emphasizes that it is much too early to argue strongly for any one model of nontopographic projections.

Radial Organization

There is a tendency for connections within ADVR to be radially organized. This is seen in Golgi preparations by the predominance of neurons with radially oriented collaterals and in axonal tracing experiments by the presence of projections that either ascend or descend within ADVR along its radii. The consequence of such radial connections is that the information that is transmitted to a patch within ADVR will be secondarily relayed to neurons lying above and below the patch within a radial sector. Thus, information from a specific thalamic nucleus can reach all of the zones in a particular area of ADVR in all reptiles and birds. However, the degree to which direct thalamic information reaches periventricular neurons varies, so that thalamic information can gain access to periventricular neurons in turtles and birds only via vertical interconnections within ADVR.

One implication is that neurons situated along a given radius in ADVR may share common physiological properties due to the combined tendencies of thalamic afferents to pursue a radial course into ADVR and of neurons within ADVR to have axons that ascend and descend along radii. This property has been demonstrated by physiological experiments in some cases. An electrode that is advanced radially through the auditory area of ADVR in crocodilians and birds tends to encounter units with the same best frequencies. Electrodes advanced radially in nucleus basalis in ducks encounters units with similarly placed receptive fields. Comparable results have not been obtained in the visual areas of ADVR, but the properties of the rotundal-DVR projection make it difficult to know which stimulus parameters might be relevant.

At the same time, there should be some variation in the detailed physiology of neurons situated in different positions within a given radial sector due to variations in the properties of neurons, particularly those involved in clusters, and to differences in the placement and effect of afferent systems within the sector. Limited physiological studies on field L and nucleus basalis provide some evidence for such differences. The properties of auditory units in bands L_1, L_2, and L_3 in field L are slightly different, and receptive fields are smaller in the dorsal part of nucleus basalis than they are in the ventral part.

Nonthalamic Afferents

Although the thalamic projections to ADVR have been the most intensively studied, HRP injections into ADVR reveal that a large number of ascending projections reach ADVR. The best studied of these form a series of parallel pathways from the brainstem reticular formation to ADVR and the striatum. Serotonergic projections from the raphé nuclei to ADVR and noradrenergic projections from the locus coeruleus to ADVR have now been demonstrated in most of the groups of reptiles and birds. However, their termination patterns have not been studied in enough detail to identify what the fundamental pattern might be. It does seem clear though that dopaminergic neurons in the midbrain tegmentum project to the striatum in all groups. There is also evidence that thick caliber projections originate from neurons in the midbrain tegmentum and project to ADVR in at least reptiles.

Efferent Projections

The final structural feature that is characteristic of ADVR is an overall similarity between groups of reptiles and birds in the pattern of efferent connections that issue from ADVR. Degeneration and autoradiographic tracing experiments and Golgi preparations all indicate that neurons in ADVR project ventrally to the striatum and to BDVR. The efferents seem to originate from the spiny stellate cells that are predominant in ADVR, but very little is known about the organization of these efferent projections. Golgi preparations in snakes indicate that the most ventrally situated neurons in ADVR project to the striatum. However, neurons situated near the ventricular surface in the hyperstriatum ventrale are known to project to both the striatum and archistriatum in birds. Thus, it is not yet clear how the efferent projections from ADVR are related to its neuronal organization.

There is some indication that the efferent projections as a whole are topographically organized with neurons situated most medially in ADVR projecting to the medial aspects of the striatum and neurons situated most laterally projecting to BDVR, but this pattern may not hold universally. Also, the branching patterns of ADVR axons within the striatum or BDVR have not been studied, so the nature of the transformation that occurs as information leaves the modality specific sensory areas of ADVR is a complete unknown.

The subsequent connections of the striatum and BDVR form a complex network that links ADVR to many structures in the brainstem. Three major pathways can be identified within these connections. The first are projections that carry information from the forebrain to the optic tectum either directly or indirectly. The striatum typically projects to a pretectal nucleus (called variously the dorsal nucleus of the posterior commissure or the nucleus spiriformis lateralis) and to a catecholaminergic group in the midbrain tegmentum (called either the substantia nigra or the pedunculopontine nucleus). Both of these structures project to the optic tectum. The significance of these projections is that they establish a potential contact between the striatal efferents and the massive, bilateral tectoreticular projections. These pathways originate in the optic tectum of both reptiles and birds (Ulinski, 1977a) as they apparently do in all vertebrates. The reticular formation in turn projects bilaterally to the spinal cord in snakes (ten Donkelaar, 1976a,b), lizards (Robinson, 1969; Cruce, 1975; ten Donkelaar, 1976a,b; ten Donkelaar and de Boer-van Huizen, 1978; Cruce and Newman, 1981), turtles (ten Donkelaar, 1976a,b), and birds. The tectum, thus, serves to link ADVR and the striatum with major descending motor pathways.

Additional descending projections originate in the rostral parts of the archistriatum in birds and travel through the occipitomesencephalic tract to a variety of brainstem structures that include the midbrain and pontine reticular formations. In songbirds, there are also direct projections to hypoglossal motoneurons involved in the control of song. These projections would thereby serve to establish a second, relatively direct link between ADVR and the reticulospinal pathways. It is not known if comparable projections originate from the BDVR of reptiles.

A third group of afferent projections participate in feedback loops with the forebrain. First, injections of HRP into ADVR provide evidence that the striatum projects back to ADVR in at least some species. Second, nuclei in the lateral forebrain bundle often have reciprocal relations with the striatum. These are the entopeduncular nuclei or the nuclei of the ansa lenticularis. Third, a catecholaminergic group of nuclei in the midbrain tegmentum has reciprocal relations with the striatum. These are the substantia nigra, pedunculopontine nuclei, and ventral tegmental area. Each of these receives projections from the striatum and projects to the striatum. Fourth, the striatum participates in some longer feedback loops involving thalamic nuclei. In tegu lizards, there is evidence for striatal projections to nucleus rotundus, which projects back to ADVR. In *Caiman*, the ventrolateral area of the thalamus receives both striatal and cerebellar inputs and projects to ADVR. In canaries, nucleus ovoidalis receives projections from area X of the parolfactory lobe and projects to field L in ADVR. The functions of loops of this type are not well understood, except that they conceivably serve as control loops that regulate ongoing movements (see Evarts, 1970).

Two Patterns of DVR Organization

The features discussed in the preceding sections are those that seem generally characteristic of ADVR in all groups of reptiles and birds. However, in spite of these similarities, there are significant variations in the neuronal structure of ADVR between species. The suggestion being made here is that two basic patterns of ADVR organization can be recognized and that the variations that do occur are variations on these two basic themes.

The first pattern is one of three zones and is found in the majority of reptiles. A zone immediately deep to the ventricular surface contains juxtaependymal cells with discoidal dendritic fields. A second zone contains a large number of clusters of stellate cells. A third zone contains fewer clusters and a larger proportion of isolated stellate cells. The major variation within this pattern is in the degree of development of the second or cell cluster zone. In snakes and Type II lizards, the cell cluster zone is relatively indistinct. In Type I lizards, *Sphenodon* and turtles, the cell cluster zone is more distinct and is separated from the underlying zone by a cell-poor zone. In all of these forms, information that reaches a restricted patch of DVR will be relayed to neurons above and below the patch within a radial sector by radially oriented connections, but the number of relays needed for information to reach the full extent of the sector will depend in part on the size of ADVR.

The second organizational pattern involves the presence of clusters scattered throughout ADVR and is found in crocodilians and birds. As in the first pattern, radially oriented connections seem to spread information throughout a radial sector within ADVR, but there is no single structural feature comparable to the cell cluster zone that defines zones in the second pattern. There tend to be instead relatively subtle differences in cell size, packing density, or dendritic field properties such as those found in the central and peripheral parts of the auditory area of the neostriatum, in the dorsal and ventral parts of nucleus basalis, or in the ectostriatum and periectostriatal belt. There tend to be horizontally aligned fibrous layers in ADVR such as the lamina hyperstriatica in birds or the cell-poor areas in crocodilian ADVR.

The existence of these two major organizational patterns clearly reflects the phylogenetic relationships within reptiles. The snakes, lizards, and rhynchocephalians, which share the first organizational pattern, are all lepidosaurian reptiles (Romer, 1956), so that the similarities seen in their ADVRs is not surprising. However, the relationship of the turtles to other reptiles is not clear (e.g., Caroll, 1969) and the overall similarity of ADVR organization seen between turtles and lepidosaurs is somewhat unexpected. Northcutt (1978a) has suggested that the presence of a distinct cell cluster zone is a primitive character because it is found in three phylogenetic lineages (turtles, rhynchocephalians, and Type I lizards). The implication is that the common ancestors of the lineages had distinct cell cluster zones that became less distinct during the evolution of snakes and Type II lizards. (See Switzer, Kirsch and Johnson, 1980, for the rationale behind this type of argument.) However, there is a relatively small number of surviving lineages within the reptilian radiation, so it is difficult to know how widespread any one pattern of ADVR organization may have been. Also, no other group of tetrapods have DVRs, so it is not possible to effect comparisons with members of other, closely related radiations. Thus, it is possible that a distinct cell cluster zone evolved in parallel in the three lineages. Similarly, it is possible that ADVR organization within both Type I and Type II lizards represents some degree of parallel evolution.

The living crocodilians and birds, which share the second pattern of ADVR organization, are both derived from archosaurian reptiles (e.g., Caroll, 1969; Ostrom, 1976). Since archosaurs have been an extremely large and diverse radiation, and since crocodilians and birds are probably only distantly related within the archosaurs, it is difficult to assess the degree to which the DVRs of crocodilians and birds represent an organizational pattern common to stem archosaurs, on the one hand, versus parallel elaborations of a common pattern, on the other.

The almost complete absence of detailed physiological studies on snakes, lizards, or turtles makes it difficult to compare the functional properties of neurons in ADVRs with the first organizational pattern to those of neurons in ADVRs with the second organizational pattern in the better studied forebrains of birds. However, there are overall similarities across species in both the afferent pathways that carry sensory information to ADVR and the efferent pathways that carry transformed information away from ADVR. The organizational differences seen within ADVR may then be a major factor in determining interspecific differences that occur in the overall sequence of transformations to and from ADVR. Appropriate investigations on the intrinsic organization of ADVR in several species are potentially very useful in clarifying the role that ADVR plays in modulating behavior.

7.2. SENSORY–MOTOR AND SENSORY–HYPOTHALAMIC LINKAGES

Given these structural features, what can be said about DVR's functional significance? The central theme in this treatise is that DVR forms a set of linkages between the principal sources of sensory information to the brain and some of the structures that modulate behavior. Its afferents arise largely from nuclei involved in carrying visual, auditory, somatosensory, and olfactory information to the forebrain. The sole targets of its efferent projections are structures in the base of the forebrain that engage it in a series of feedback loops and place it in contact with descending pathways to the reticular formation and to the hypothalamus. The possible roles of these linkages can now be evaluated.

Both its position relative to descending motor pathways and its involvement in a series of feedback loops hint that ADVR plays some role in the genesis or control of movement, but the persistence of basic movement sequences after bilateral hemispherectomies in reptiles (Peterson, 1980) and birds (Pearson, 1972; Benowitz, 1980) indicates that neither ADVR nor the striatum is essential for the generation of movement per se. Studies in which large lesions were made in ADVR, or in which ADVR was electrically stimulated in chronic preparations, have produced results that are consistent with the idea that ADVR has some involvement in the control of movement without yielding much insight into its specific role. (For a summary of this literature, see the reviews by Benowitz, 1980; Pearson, 1972; and Peterson, 1980.) However, some promising results have been obtained in recent years by assessing the effects of restricted lesions on the performance of natural behaviors in reptiles and birds.

For example, ADVR's role in processing visual information has been studied using visually guided pecking in pigeons (Bugbee and Hodos, 1979). Birds were trained to perform a series of visual discriminations, including several that involved following moving stimuli. Lesions of the nucleus spiriformis lateralis, one of the nuclei that link the striatum to the tectum, did not impair postoperative ability to perform color, intensity, or pattern discriminations. However, they did impair the ability to perform on two tasks that involved following moving stimuli. Normal pigeons could be trained to rapidly peck a sequence of response keys illuminated in random order, but following lesions of nucleus spiriformis lateralis this task took much longer than it did preoperatively. Normal pigeons could be trained to track a target that continuously changes position (a piece of grain on a revolving drum), but lesioned birds were totally incapable of pecking moving grain, even when it was revolving as slowly as 8 cm/sec. Control lesions of nucleus rotundus did not produce these deficits (Hodos, 1976). These experiments suggest that striatal efferent pathways provide information to the tectum that is critical in responding to objects that are changing position in visual space.

A second line of inquiry into ADVR's role in processing visual information has used visual displays in anoline lizards (Greenberg, 1977, 1978; Greenberg, MacLean, and Ferguson, 1979). Like many lizards, those in the genus *Anolis* have a repertoire of visual displays that are used in social communication. Displays in male *Anolis carolinensis* include a signature display that consists of three to five vertical movements of the forebody with a brief extension of the dewlap (or throat pouch) and the challenge display that involves similar vertical somatic movements and dewlap extension, but includes a sagittal expansion of the body profile. The signature display typically precedes the challenge display in territorial confrontations and occurs in confrontations between males. The roles of ADVR and striatum in controlling visual displays were investigated by exposing single male lizards to displaying conspecifics in an adjacent tank. The lizard received a unilateral forebrain lesion and was tested with an eyepatch over one eye. Each lizard could thus serve as its own control by moving the patch to the eye contralateral to the lesion. Lesions restricted to ADVR had no clear effect on displays in *Anolis*. However, lesions involving the striatum produced complete or near-complete failure to perform the challenge display. Control procedures indicated that visual cues were involved. The experiments thus point to the involvement of ADVR's efferent pathways in rather selective visually guided behaviors.

ADVR's role in processing auditory information has been studied by examining the neural control of song production in songbirds such as canaries, chaffinches, white-crowned sparrows, or zebra finches (Nottebohm, 1980a). Birdsong is produced by the syrinx, which lies in the bird's chest where the two bronchi join the trachea. The syrinx contains two independent vibrating membranes; each is innervated by a tracheosyringeal branch of the hypoglossal nerve (e.g., Manogue and Nottebohm, 1982). Only male birds produce song and they first sing as they approach sexual maturity. The ability to produce song is under hormonal control. The control of song is lateralized, with the left syringeal half normally producing 90% or more of the song. The song itself is highly individualized and consists of stereotyped units called "syllables" that are repeated several times in succession to form "phrases." The acquisition of normal song in some species is known to depend on the bird being able to hear.

The neural control of song has been investigated by determining the effects of lesions of ADVR and its efferent pathways in adult male canaries (Nottebohm, Stokes, and Leonard, 1976). Lesions of field L produce a partial loss in song variety leaving song structure basically intact, but lesions of components of the efferent pathways originating in the auditory area of ADVR produce major deficits. Ipsilateral destruction of the left hyperstriatum ventrale pars caudalis (HVc) is followed by a marked loss of phrase structure. Ipsilateral destruction of the right HVc results in a reduction of song frequency. Bilateral destruction of HVc results in silent song. Electrical stimulation of HVc in parakeets, canaries and zebra finches elicits electrical activity in the tracheosyringeal nerves (Manogue, Paton and Nottebohm, 1982; Paton and Manogue, 1982). Similarly, destruction of nucleus robustus of the archistriatum results in major loss in song structure, with lesions of the left nucleus having a greater effect. These findings are generally consistent with earlier electrical stimulation studies of parrots (Kalischer, 1905) and a variety of other birds (Brown, 1971, 1973, 1974; Delius, 1971) that implicated the archistriatum or neighboring structures in the control of vocalization. The mechanisms underlying the interruption of song structure are unknown, but the fact that bilateral deafening in canaries produces only a partial and progressive deterioration of song (Nottebohm, Stokes, and Leonard, 1976) indicates that something more than a simple relay of auditory information to motor centers is involved.

Finally, ADVR's role in processing somatosensory information has been studied using feeding in pigeons (Zeigler, 1974, 1976). The act of feeding in pigeons can be divided into a series of components that altogether last about 300 msec (Zeigler, Levitt, and Levine, 1980). The feeding cycle begins with pecking, which consists of a downward movement of the head. Contact with the grain terminates the downward movement and initiates mandibulation, which involves an upward movement of the head synchronized with a series of tongue movements that propel the grain from the beak tip to the rear of the buccal cavity. Swallowing terminates the cycle. Bilateral lesions of the quintofrontal tract or nucleus basalis produce an aphagia as well as interfering with the neural control of movement patterns involved in eating (Zeigler and Karten, 1973a,b). Birds with such deficits can peck normally and will swallow food if placed manually at the back of the mouth, but have difficulty grasping and mandibulating kernels of grain. Lesions in the occipitomesencephalic tract also lead to deficits in feeding behavior (Zeigler, 1974; Levine and Zeigler, 1981). The pecking movements are hesitant and frequently incomplete. In many cases the oral cavity fails to open sufficiently to permit grasping and mandibulation of grain kernels, even when the peck is completed.

These four examples involve different behaviors in different organisms, but have several factors in common. All of the behaviors involve a naturally occurring sequence of movements. In each case, the sequence is more complex than a simple rhythmical or oscillatory set of movements. Lesions of ADVR or its efferent pathways do not produce paralysis or inability to move, and they do not generally lead to an alteration in arousal state or motivation. (Lesions involving nucleus basalis are an exception, but it is not known if the motivational changes are due to involvement of basalis or of other structures.) In each case, however, the lesions lead to a significant alteration of the movement sequence. In each case, the successful execution of the movement sequence is dependent on one or more sensory cues. It would appear that there is some breakdown at the interface between the reception of the appropriate sensory cues and the genesis of movement. The nature of this interface is not known and, in fact, is likely to be different in the various sensory systems. In the case of song production, it seems that there is a difficulty somewhere between the "auditory template" and the "motor tape." The concept of an auditory template derives from the fact that birds deafened after they have learned to sing can produce fairly normal song: they must have an internal template to which songs can be compared (e.g., Galambos and Worden, 1972). The concept of a "motor tape" or "schema" is a general one in theories dealing with the organization of movement (e.g., Gallistel, 1980). It is generally agreed that there must be a central representation of the entire movement because the nervous system could not adequately control the movements of each individual muscle in a way that could lead to movement patterns that are constant regardless of environmental circumstance or perturbation. Lesions in the hyperstriatum ventrale or archistriatum seem to interfere with the reading of the "song tapes." Comparable formalizations have not been derived for the other behaviors discussed in this section. However, the best hypothesis at this point is that ADVR and the striatum in reptiles and birds play a role in supplying the sensory information that is prerequisite to the correct reading out of the schemata or motor tapes involved in a variety of behaviors.

The same strategy of using analyses of naturally occurring behaviors to study the sensory modulation of movement have also proved valuable in analyzing the sensory modulation of hypothalamic and autonomic activity. A first example comes from studies of the role of the accessory olfactory system in snakes. There have been no direct investigations involving lesions of nucleus sphericus, but the direct connections that exist between the vomeronasal organ, accessory olfactory bulb, and nucleus sphericus indicate that manipulations of the peripheral components of the vomeronasal system are having significant effects on the activity of BDVR neurons. Snakes use their slender, bifid tongues to transfer odorants from the substrate to their vomeronasal organs (Halpern and Kubie, 1980). Experimental manipulations implicate tongue flicking in several behaviors related to reproduction and prey acquisition. Tongue flicking is known to be involved in the response of both newborn (Burghardt and Pruitt, 1975) and adult (Kubie and Halpern, 1978) garter snakes to prey odors. It can be used to follow trails of substrate bound prey odors (Kubie and Halpern, 1978). Interruption of the vomeronasal, but not the main olfactory system, abolishes prey tracking behaviors (Kubie and Halpern, 1979). Tongue flicking also appears to be important in the mating behaviors of male garter snakes. During the courtship sequence, male garter snakes tongue flick the dorsal body surface of female snakes, presumably sensing pheromones (Kubie, 1977). Interruption of the vomeronasal system leads to a disruption of male mating behaviors (Kubie, Vagvolgyi, and Halpern, 1978). Thus, the projections from the accessory olfactory bulb, through nucleus sphericus in BDVR, and to the hypothalamus appear to provide sensory information that is essential to the organization of specific behavior in snakes.

A second example of a sensory linkage provided by BDVR comes from studies on the role of the archistriatum in agonistic behaviors in birds. Wild birds typically show a variety of fear responses in captivity, frequently refusing to eat, struggling, and attempting to escape. It has been known for some time (Pearson, 1972) that total telencephalic extirpations abolish this "wildness." Phillips (1964) studied the neural bases for this taming effect in mallard ducks and showed that lesions involving the medial archistriatum or the occipitomesencephalic tract produced taming. Such lesions also had effects on ovarian development. Captivity has an inhibiting effect on reproductive capabilities in mallard ducks that is believed to be mediated by a lowered level of hypophyseal gonadotropic hormones (Phillips and Tienhoven, 1960). Medial archistriatal lesions blocked the inhibitory effect of captivity on ovarian development (Phillips, 1964). Conversely, electrical stimulation of the medial archistriatum produced crouching, sneaking, or running movements (Phillips, 1964). Phillips suggested that these effects are mediated via the projections of the medial archistriatum to the hypothalamus.

Phillips (1964) also observed that electrical stimulation of the archistriatum produced cardiovascular changes, possibly representing an autonomic component of general fear reactions. Cohen and his colleagues have examined the neural substrates for these reactions (Cohen and Trauner, 1969; MacDonald and Cohen, 1973; Cohen, 1980). Cohen (1975) showed that normal pigeons establish a strong conditioned aversive reaction to a light flash associated with foot shock within 20 pairings. Conditioned animals show an increase in heart rate above base line in response to whole-field retinal illumination. Control lesions, including damage to the anterior and intermediate parts of the archistriatum, produce no deficits in the conditioned response. However, damage to the medial and posterior components of the archistriatum shows a very severe deficit in the conditioned response. The interpretation is that the lesions interrupt pathways from the medial/posterior archistriatum to the hypothalamus and then to parasympathetic and sympathetic centers modulating cardiac function. Consistent with this hypothesis, electrical stimulation of these regions of the archistriatum produce marked changes in heart rate. The afferent limb of the linkage is not entirely certain because projections from the ectostriatum to the archistriatum are preferentially to the anterior and intermediate parts of the archistriatum, but it is possible that intra-archistriatal projections are involved (Benowitz, 1980).

All of these studies lend support to the idea that the sensory linkages that can be traced through ADVR to the brainstem recticular formation and the hypothalamus by anatomical or physiological techniques have real, functional roles in the modulation of behavior. The behaviors are in each case relatively complex and naturally occurring. The analyses completed so far have been sufficient only to implicate sensory linkages through ADVR in the modulation of the behaviors. However, it is likely that continued efforts can begin to determine the precise mechanisms underlying these modulations.

7.3.   COMPARISONS WITH THE FOREBRAIN OF MAMMALS

It remains now to place what is known about the organization of DVR into the larger context of vertebrate forebrain organization. Because of the absence of information on the forebrains of other groups of non-mammalian vertebrates, the task is to compare the organization of DVR to the organization of equivalent structures in the forebrains of mammals. The problem that arises immediately is exactly what the word "equivalent" means in this case. It is of course a fundamental problem in comparative biology, and it has long been recognized that two bases of comparison are possible when assessing the structures of different organisms.

Comparisons Based on Homology

The approach that has been traditional in comparative neurology is to search for brain regions in reptiles and birds that are equivalent to specific components of the forebrains of mammals in the sense of being homologues. The question usually posed has been: "What regions of the forebrains of reptiles and birds are equivalent to (that is homologous to) the isocortex of mammals?" This approach has been plagued by several deep-seated misconceptions and confusions.

One area of confusion has to do with the definition of homology itself. It occurs in large part because evolutionary biologists have over the years employed several, at least partially contradictory definitions of homology (see Ghiselin, 1976). A complete account of the pros and cons of various definitions is well beyond the purview of this book and it is sufficient to point out that virtually all modern discussions of forebrain homologies have used a definition suggested by Simpson (1961) that holds two structures in different organisms to be homologous if they are derived from the same structure in the common ancestor of the two organisms. The thrust of the homology concept is then a statement about the evolutionary history of a set of organisms and their anatomical parts.

However, even accepting this definition, there is often confusion about the relation of *homology* to *similarity*. Comparative analyses usually begin by listing similarities that exist between the different species or groups of species under consideration. Two different, evolutionary explanations can always be offered for whatever similarities are demonstrated. The first is that similarities are present because two structures in different species are derived from a single structure in a common ancestor of the two species. The similarities then reflect a relative lack of morphological change in two related, but parallel evolutionary lineages. The structures are similar in structure because they are homologous. The other explanation is that the similarities are present because two nonhomologous structures have become structurally similar due to similar, but independent responses to common functional demands. The structures are then said to be homoplastic. The important point is that *a demonstration that two structures are similar in a particular set of ways is not a demonstration that the structure are homologous*. There must also be an explicit demonstration that the similarities are not due to homoplasy.

The other side of the coin is that dissimilar structures in different organisms can be homologous. The best-known example of this is that of the malleus and incus in the inner ears of mammals, which are homologous to specific jaw bones in reptiles even though the two sets of bones are morphologically quite different. The homology in this case can be demonstrated with embryological and paleontological data (e.g., Crompton and Parker, 1978). The morphological differences reflect different functions. Similarity, thus, has no necessary relation to homology.

The need to eliminate the possibility of similarity due to homoplasy makes it difficult in many cases to prove that similar structures in different organisms are indeed homologous. This is particularly true in the case of the nervous system because most of the neural features that are studied by neurobiologists are likely to be functionally important. Consequently, most of the features or characters that have been used in discussing forebrain homologies are poor choices because it is difficult to evaluate the extent to which functional factors have resulted in similarities. The best characters are those that lack functional significance. For example, Switzer, Kirsch, and Johnson (1980) use the relation of lateral olfactory tract fibers to the accessory olfactory formation in a phylogenetic analysis of mammals because this character has no known functional significance.

The approach that has been used most often in attempting to establish homologies in the central nervous system is to use as many characters as is possible and argue that an overall similarity in a large number of independent characters (e.g., Campbell and Hodos, 1970) is unlikely to have evolved two or more times in separate evolutionary lineages. A common difficulty in using this approach is that the nervous system tends to be highly interconnected, so it is difficult to find characters that are unequivocally independent of each other. The approach is valid if the conditions are met, but it ultimately results only in a statement that two structures are *probably* homologous.

A final area of frequent confusion has to do with the ancestral relationships between groups of living vertebrates. The nature of these relationships is important to the kinds of comparisons being discussed here because the definition of homology presumes some knowledge of the ancestral relationships of the organisms being compared. An overwhelming misconception is that living animals can be validly arranged into a linear scale that reflects an evolutionary progression, a so called "phylogenetic tree" or *scala naturae*. In fact, the major reason for a burgeoning interest in the forebrain anatomy of reptiles in the late 1800s and early decades of this century was the idea that reptiles are situated "below" mammals on the phylogenetic tree. The hope was that it would then be possible to trace the evolutionary history of the mammalian (and ultimately the human) brain from a reptilian condition.

This idea of a *scala naturae* is one that has a long history in Western philosophy (Lovejoy, 1960), but has never had any scientific basis. Hodos and Campbell (1969) and Hodos (1970) have reviewed the nature of the fallacy and its impact on ideas of brain evolution. In particular, there is good paleontological data that mammals evolved from a specific group of Mesozoic reptiles, the therapsids (e.g., Hopson, 1969; Crompton and Jenkins, 1979); so the notion that mammals evolved from reptiles is an accurate one. However, the fossil record also indicates that therapsids were only distantly related to the direct ancestors of the various groups of modern reptiles. The radiation of reptiles that dominated the fauna of the Mesozoic era divided into two major lineages shortly after the first or stem reptiles evolved from their amphibian ancestors. The lineage leading to mammals proceeded through two major stages. The first stage was the evolution of the pelycosaurs, a large assemblage of reptiles that included carnivorous, herbivorous, and fish-eating forms. Some of the carnivorous pelycosaurs are believed to be the ancestors of the therapsids. Therapsids are the second stage and were in themselves a large group of reptiles, many of which gradually attained some of the morphological features characteristic of mammals. Mesozoic mammals probably evolved from cynodont therapsids. The second major lineage of reptiles led to the archosaurs or "ruling reptiles" and the lepidosaurs or "slender lizards." The archosaurs included the dinosaurs and crocodilians. A currently favored thesis is that birds were derived from dinosaurs (Ostrom, 1976). The lepidosaurs include the lizards, snakes, and rhynchocephalians. The ancestral relations of turtles remain a puzzle (e.g., Caroll, 1969), but there is no real evidence that modern turtles are more closly related to mammals than are the other groups of living reptiles, as is sometimes asserted (e.g., see Northcutt, 1970).

Putting the problem of comparing forebrain organization in reptiles, birds, and mammals into this phylogenetic framework, it is important to realize that the analysis must proceed in two steps. The first step is to determine if the structures that have been identified as DVR in the major groups of reptiles, on the one hand, and in the birds, on the other hand, are homologous. It is not possible to do this directly because the common ancestor of the turtles, lepidosaurs, and archosaurs is not known. Similarly, the common ancestor of birds and crocodilians is presumably close to the base of the archosaurian radiation and it is not possible to directly determine if it had anything like DVR. An alternative approach is to argue indirectly that the similarities in the neuronal structure and connections of DVR that have been reviewed here make it unlikely that DVR-like structures evolved independently two or three times. The basic similarity in the pattern of DVR development that was used in Chapter 2 to establish a definition of DVR in both reptiles and birds is also consistent with the idea that DVR is homologous in both groups. However, the fact that the two major patterns of DVR organization discussed in Section 7.1 correspond roughly to the lepidosaurian and archosaurian lineages suggests that DVR evolved prior to the separation of the lepidosaurs and archosaurs and was then modified in somewhat different ways in the two lineages.

Accepting for the sake of discussion the idea that the DVRs of reptiles and birds are homologous, the second step of the analysis is to determine if there are structures in the brains of modern mammals that are homologous to DVR. The requirement is a demonstration that the precursor of DVR in the brains of the common ancestor of the turtles, lepidosaurs, and archosaurs was derived from the same structure in the brain of a stem reptile as was some particular component of the forebrain of mammals.

Some data that bear on the issue are available in the fossil record because the brain morphology of fossil animals is often preserved in the form of endocasts (see Hopson, 1979). Thus, the fossil record provides a sketch of the changes that took place in the shape of the brain from the stem reptiles and, through the evolution of the major lineages (Fig. 7.1).

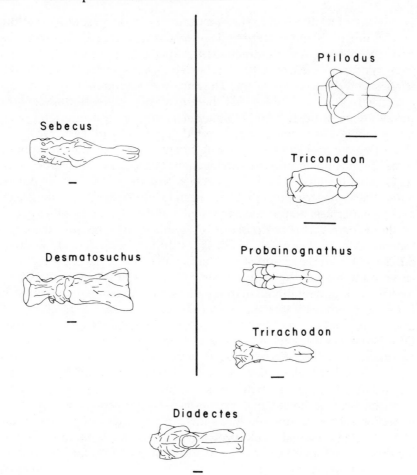

FIGURE 7.1. Endocasts of fossil reptiles and mammals. The endocast at the bottom of the figure is of *Diadectes*, a form believed to lie close to the stem reptiles. Endocasts to the left of the line are of archosaurs. Those to the right of the line are of mammal-like reptiles (*Trirachodon, Probainognathus*) and prototherian mammals (*Triconodon, Ptilodus*). Based primarily on Hopson (1979) and Quiroga (1979a, 1980a).

The endocast of *Diadectes*, a genus close to the stem reptiles, shows a very narrow midbrain and forebrain (Hopson, 1979). If this condition held generally, members of the basal reptilian stock may have had tubular forebrains that anatomically resembled the forebrains of Recent lungfishes and amphibians. Unfortunately, it may be dangerous to use amphibian forebrains as a model for the functional organization of the forebrains of stem reptiles because of the real possibility that the central nervous system of Recent amphibians shows substantial secondary simplifications, comparable to those that occurred within their skeletal system. In any case, there is no sign of the forebrain shapes characteristic of either Recent reptiles or Recent mammals in the stem reptiles.

In the archosaurian reptiles, it appears that pseudosuchians of the middle Triassic may have had narrow midbrains and forebrains, whereas the aetosaurid *Desmatosuchus* of the late Triassic shows forebrain proportions comparable to those of Recent crocodilians (Hopson, 1979). There was a clear expansion of the forebrain in several lines of archosaurs by the middle Jurassic (Hopson, 1979). The situation is basically not known in the lepidosaurs. The turtles show an expansion of their forebrain by the late Cretaceous (Hopson, 1979). It seems likely, then, that reptiles in each of the evolutionary lines leading to the Recent groups showed an expansion of the forebrain throughout the Jurassic and Cretaceous.

All of the available endocasts from pelycosaurs show narrow midbrains and forebrains (Case, 1897; Hopson, 1979). Similarly, all the available therapsid endocasts including those of the cynodonts *Probainognathus, Massetognathus,* and *Probelesodon* (Quiroga, 1979a, 1980a,b) show a telencephalon consisting of a pair of elongate tubes (Hopson, 1979). By contrast, the endocasts of Mesozoic mammals typically show an expansion or widening of the forebrain. The expansion is slight in the triconodont, *Tricondon,* but more extensive in the multituberculate, *Ptilodus,* and in later mammals (Simpson, 1927, 1937; Edinger, 1956, 1964; Jerison, 1973; Hopson, 1979; Quiroga, 1979a, 1980a,b). Endocasts from placental mammals show large cerebral hemispheres (Jerison, 1973). It is possible in some cases to trace the progressive development of the sulcal patterns that are characteristic of the various orders of placental mammals (e.g., Radinsky, 1975a,b, 1977).

The endocasts of therapsids and early mammals also suggest that there was a gradual increase in the relative size of the brain along the therapsid–mammal sequence. It has been known for some time that there is an orderly relation between brain weights and body weights across the range of vertebrates. Jerison (1973) has shown that brain weights and body weights for each class of vertebrates fall within a circumscribed area, called a minimum convex polygon, on double logarithmic plots of brain weight versus body weight. The polygon for reptiles lies slightly below the polygon for mammals (Platel, 1979). The brain weight–body weight values for therapsids lie at the upper edge of, or perhaps slightly above, the reptile polygon (Hopson, 1980; Quiroga, 1979a, 1980a,b).

To summarize, the data available from the fossil record suggest that the stem reptiles, pelycosaurs, and at least most of the therapsids had narrow forebrains. However, there was an independent, parallel expansion of the forebrain in the archosaurs and turtles and with the evolution of the Mesozoic mammals. The interpretation would be that forebrain expansion in the lineages leading to Recent reptiles is a reflection of the gradual evolution of DVR, whereas forebrain expansion in the lineages leading to mammals is a reflection of the evolution of the mammalian pattern of isocortex and basal ganglia.

The limitation of the endocast data is, of course, that they give no information on what is happening to neuronal masses inside of the forebrain as animals are evolving. The only avenue open for further, more detailed investigation is to analyze similarities in the organization of the brains of Recent reptiles, birds, and mammals. This enterprise occupied much of the time of classical neuroanatomists and produced a rather complex and confusing literature which is summarized by Ariëns Kappers, Huber, and Crosby (1936). Instead of attempting a complete historical account of this literature, it is perhaps most useful to identify three related issues that have figured in attempts to work out the relationships between forebrain components in vertebrates.

The first issue concerns which regions of the adult forebrain are derived from the pallial and basal sectors of the embryonic forebrain. It was prompted by the substantial successes of the early comparative anatomists and embryologists in dealing with the rhombencephalon (Nieuwenhuys, 1974). They had argued that the dorsal walls of the rhombencephalon (derived from the alar plates) subserve sensory functions, whereas the ventral rhombencephalic walls (derived from the basal plates) subserve motor functions. The pallium or dorsal component of the telencephalon was seen as a rostral continuation of the alar plates and assigned functions that were mediated in mammals via the ascending projections from specific sensory nuclei of the thalamus. The striatum was seen as a continuation of the basal plates and assigned motor functions.

In mammals, the basal ganglia were regarded as derivatives of the basal plate, whereas the various cortical areas of the hippocampal formation, isocortex, and pyriform lobe were seen as pallial derivative (e.g., His, 1888). The first impression gained when looking at sections through the forebrains of reptiles and birds is that DVR occupies a position, protruding into the lateral ventricle, that is comparable to that occupied by the basal ganglia in mammals. The classical viewpoint was, then, that the structures that have been termed the striatum here and DVR were both derived from the basal plate, whereas the cortex in reptiles was of pallial origin. This view is expressed in the nomenclature suggested by Ariens Kappers (e.g., 1921) which refers to an archistriatum, paleostriatum, and neostriatum. The archistriatum and neostriatum of reptiles and birds included much of what has been called DVR here. The archistriatum and neostriatum of mammals included the amygdala and caudatoputamen, respectively. The paleostriatum of reptiles and birds corresponded roughly to the globus pallidus in mammals.

This viewpoint suffered a gradual erosion in the early decades of this century. Some investigators began to point out a close, topographic association between DVR and the overlying cortical areas, suggesting that DVR was of pallial rather than basal origin. In his 1916 study of turtle forebrain morphology, Johnston noted that DVR arises by a thickening of the lateral border of the pallium. Its continued growth causes it to project into the ventricle and produces the middle and dorsal ventricular grooves. Crosby (1917) argued in her analysis of the forebrain in *Alligator* that the rostral part of DVR is pallial in origin and is primarily "neopallial" in function. Elliot Smith (1919) used the position of the lateral striate artery to argue that DVR is closely related to the pallium and referred to it as the lower part of the pallium or "hypopallium." Somewhat later, Källén (e.g., 1951, 1953, 1956, 1962) conducted an extensive series of studies on forebrain embryology in reptiles and birds and concluded that DVR is derived from the pallium on the basis of its relation to the ventricular sulci present in embryonic forebrains. The crux of this argument is to use the middle ventricular sulcus as the dividing line between the pallium and basal forebrain. Most recently, the unequivocal demonstrations of thalamic projections to ADVR have been used to argue that DVR should be regarded as a derivative of the pallium (e.g., Karten, 1969).

The consensus at this time is that there is at least an overall similarity in the basic organization of the forebrain of reptiles, birds, and mammals, if not amphibians and sarcopterygian fishes as well (see Northcutt, 1981). This similarity is partially obscured in adult forebrains, but is quite clear in the forebrains of embryonic forms. There is in each case a septum that forms the medial wall of the hemisphere. The septum is continuous under the lateral ventricle with the striatum, which makes up the ventrolateral wall of the hemisphere. The striatum is typically separated by a ventricular sulcus from the pallium, which forms the dorsolateral wall of the hemisphere. Each of these components is elaborated somewhat differently in each major group of vertebrates, but can be identified with some confidence in each case. Whether or not these similarities reflect homologies is difficult to prove unequivocally. However, the similarities are striking enough, particularly in embryos, to make it probable that they reflect homologies rather than independent derivations in two or more of the lineages. In Simpson's (1961) nomenclature, most workers would currently agree that there is a "field homology" between the pallium in the various groups of tetrapod vertebrates.

The second issue that arises in pursuing comparisons between the forebrains of reptiles, birds, and mammals is whether or not it is possible to go further and establish homologies between particular components of the pallium in the three groups. This issue also has a long history, with most of the classical workers attempting to establish homologies between the mammalian basal ganglia and isocortex and specific components of DVR and striatum in reptiles and birds. Essentially all of these arguments were based on superficial similarities between structures and made no effort to exclude similarity due to homoplasy. They will not be discussed further and the interested reader is referred to Ariëns Kappers, Huber, and Crosby (1936).

The same issue has been raised in the more recent literature by several authors who argue that DVR is homologous to various regions of mammalian isocortex. This literature can be adequately treated by restricting the discussion to comparisons of the visual components of the forebrain in reptiles, birds, and mammals. Prior to the 1960s, the literature on visual systems in nonmammals maintained that there were few if any direct retinal projections to the dorsal thalamus and that the optic tectum was the major recipient of retinal information in nonmammals. By contrast, direct retinal projections to the dorsal lateral geniculate complex of mammals were well documented and it was known that the lateral geniculate complex projected to the primary visual cortex. The dominant view of the evolution of mammalian visual systems was that of a progressive invasion of the dorsal thalamus by retinal fibers in parallel with the development of thalamotelencephalic projections during the transition from reptiles to mammals (e.g., Herrick, 1926, 1948).

This view changed in two ways during the 1960s. There was first a demonstration (Altmann and Carpenter, 1961) that the superior colliculus projects to the lateral posterior–pulvinar complex in the dorsal thalamus of cats. Since these thalamic regions were already known to project to cortex, this indicated the existence of a second route by which visual information could reach the isocortex and led to the suggestion of "two visual systems" in mammals, each of which subserves a different function (Schneider, 1969). The introduction of modern axonal tracing techniques confirmed and expanded this view (e.g., Rodieck, 1979) and it is now well documented that retinal information can reach a complex array of isocortical visual areas via a network of subcortical pathways (e.g., Graybiel and Berson, 1980).

The 1960s also saw a demonstration that the retina projects directly to the dorsal thalamus in a wide range of vertebrates, including reptiles and birds, and that the dorsal thalamus projects in turn to the pallium. In the case of reptiles and birds, Karten (1965), Karten and Hodos (1970), and Hall and Ebner (1970a,b) demonstrated pathways by which retinal information can reach the pallium in pigeons and turtles. The thalamofugal pathway involved direct retinal projections to a dorsal thalamic target and then thalamic projections to the Wulst in pigeons or the dorsal cortex in turtles. The tectofugal pathway involved projections from the retina to the optic tectum, from the tectum to nucleus rotundus in the dorsal thalamus, and from rotundus to ADVR. On the basis of these similarities in afferent pathways, it was suggested that the pallial component of the thalamofugal path (Wulst or dorsal cortex) is homologous to the primary visual cortex of mammals, whereas the pallial component of the tectofugal path (the visual area of ADVR) is homologous to peristriate cortex of mammals (e.g., Karten, 1969).

A difficulty with the suggestion is that, in spite of the similarity in visual input, there are a number of differences between the visual components of the pallium within the reptiles, between reptiles and birds, and between either reptiles or birds and mammals. There are, for example, significant differences in the nature of thalamic visual projections to the cortical part of the pallium in reptiles. In turtles, the dorsal lateral geniculate nucleus projects to the outer layer of the dorsal cortex (Hall and Ebner, 1970b; Ebner and Colonnier, 1975), whereas the visual input in lizards appears instead to be to the dorsomedial cortex (Distel and Ebbesson, 1975). There are also differences in the neuronal organization of the Wulst in birds and the dorsal cortex in turtles. The Wulst is a multilayered structure that contains exclusively stellate neurons (Pettigrew, 1979). Dorsal cortex, on the other hand, contains a single layer of densely packed neurons whose dendrites extend radially toward the pial surface. Axons from the dorsal lateral geniculate nucleus synapse on the distal dendrites of the cortical neurons (Ebner and Colonnier, 1975). Finally, the neuronal organization of both the Wulst and dorsal cortex is substantially different from that of six layered isocortex with its characteristic pyramidal cells.

These and other differences make it necessary to simultaneously entertain the alternate hypothesis that similarities in visual components of the pallium between reptiles and birds, on the one hand, and mammals, on the other, are instances of homoplasy rather than homology. Pettigrew (1979) has argued for the homoplasy hypothesis. He examined the physiology of the Wulst of owls and noted several similarities with the striate cortex of cat, including the receptive field properties of neurons, the existence of ocular dominance columns, orientation columns, and the orientation of the visual field representation. However, he felt that differences in the neuronal cytology of the Wulst and striate cortex, the placement of efferent neurons that project to the tectum in the two structures, and, most importantly, differences in the subcortical pathways that carry binocular information supported the hypothesis that similarities between the Wulst and visual cortex were due to parallel evolution or homoplasy. Similar difficulties hold for the relation between DVR and components of mammalian isocortex, so that there is at this time no compelling assignments of homologies between individual pallial components in reptiles, birds, and mammals.

The last issue that merits discussion in attempts to compare the forebrains of reptiles, birds, and mammals on the basis of homology is an attempt to deal with the differences that often exist between pallial components that share similar inputs. A particular difficulty in all attempts to homologize components of DVR with components of mammalian isocortex is that DVR is a subcortical structure with a basically nuclear organization, whereas isocortex is a laminated structure situated above the lateral ventricle. However, Karten (1969) and Nauta and Karten (1970) have suggested a homologous neuron hypothesis postulating that populations of neurons, rather than cytoarchitecturally defined nuclei, are the appropriate focus for homology arguments. Thus, neuronal populations in the ectostriatum (which receive thalamic input from nucleus rotundus) might be homologous to stellate neurons in peristriate cortex (which receive thalamic input from the lateral posterior–pulvinar complex). To deal with the difference in position, Nauta and Karten suggest that this population of neurons migrates from a subcortical position into the fourth layer of peristriate cortex during the embryonic development of mammals. This is a specific and entirely acceptable hypothesis that makes a testable prediction. It is known that migrations of this type do occur in the case of the migration of telencephalic neurons into the pulvinar during the development of fetal human brains (Rakic and Sidman, 1969), and in the case of the migration of field L neurons from a subpallial position into ADVR in chickens (Jones and Levi-Montalcini, 1958; Tsai, 1977). However, autoradiographic tracing experiments in mammals (e.g., Angevine and Sidman, 1961) have failed to demonstrate the migration of subcortical neurons into the fourth layer of the cortex. The specific suggestion made by Nauta and Karten thus lacks current experimental support.

A second homologous neuron hypothesis was suggested by Zeier and Karten (1971) in their study of the efferent connections of the archistriatum. They noted that the projections from the medial and posterior parts of the archistriatum in pigeons to the hypothalamus resemble the classically established connections of the amygdala to the hypothalamus in mammals. By contrast, the projections from the anterior and intermediate parts of the archistriatum to the brainstem lacked obvious counterparts to the amygdalar efferents known at that time. Similar projections from the central nucleus of the amygdala have been subsequently reported (Hopkins, 1975; Hopkins and Holstege, 1978; Price and Amaral, 1981). They suggested instead that the projections of the occipitomesencephalic tract to the brainstem correspond to components of the mammalian pyramidal tract that project to the brainstem (Haartsen and Verhaart, 1967). These similarities led to the idea that the medial and posterior parts of the archistriatum are homologous to the mammalian amygdaloid complex, whereas neurons in the anterior and intermediate parts of the archistriatum are homologous to layer five pyramidal neurons in the motor cortex of mammals. There would then be a similarity in the course and targets of efferent projections from the population of neurons in both birds and mammals, but the neurons would differ in their morphology and position in the telencephalon. An implication of the suggestion is that either embryonic neurons migrate from the primordium of the amygdala into the isocortex during the embryological development of mammals, or that embryonic neurons migrate from a pallial equivalent of isocortex in birds into the archistriatum. Neither alternative is supported by studies in which the paths of migrating neurons are traced using tritiated thymidine techniques.

Whether or not hypotheses of this sort have a general heuristic value is open to discussion. Webster (1979) has discussed some specific difficulties in applying the concept of homologous neuronal populations. However, it can be said generally that the same difficulties in deciding which similarities in the properties of nuclear groups are due to common ancestry and which are due to homoplasy also plague attempts at establishing homologies between populations of neurons. This point can be made by considering a specific and ostensibly clear-cut example. The basic organization of the retina is identical in all of the vertebrates so that the retinas of vertebrates are homologous by any reasonable criteria. There is also an overall similarity in the morphology of each major population of retinal neurons. Thus, the retinal ganglion cells in fishes, for example, may be reasonably considered homologous to the retinal ganglion cells of birds. What this implies is that the ultimate common ancestors of bony fishes and birds had identifiable retinal ganglion cells, as did all of the vertebrates intervening in the evolutionary lineages leading to both groups. It is difficult to see how the idea can be demonstrated explicitly, but the universal distribution of retinal ganglion cells in all of the extant vertebrate lineages is consistent with the hypothesis.

Similarly, rods in the retinas of lizards, say, might be reasonably considered homologous to rods in the retinas of turtles. However, the distribution of rods in members of the various lineages of reptiles suggests that this may not be the case (e.g., Underwood, 1970). Lizards are generally diurnal animals and typically have pure cone retinas. Rods are found only in the retinas of certain nocturnal groups such as some geckoes, but the chemistry of rod photopigments in geckoes more closely resembles that of the cone pigments of other lizards than it does of rod pigments. Thus, Walls (1942) has suggested that the "rods" of geckoes are actually transmuted cones derived during the evolution of geckoes from an ancestral group of lizards with pure cone retinas. The "rods" of geckoes would then not be homologous to the rods of turtles. It is not important here whether or not this idea is true. The point is that it can be quite difficult, even at the cellular level, to sort out which similarities are due to homology and which are due to homoplasy.

To summarize, attempts at comparisons among the forebrains of reptiles, birds, and mammals have led to a general clarification of forebrain structure in tetrapod vertebrates. A septum, striatum, and pallium can be recognized in each case and a field homology between the pallium of all three groups seems probable. DVR is most likely a pallial derivative in both reptiles and birds. However, attempts at assigning homologies between components of the pallium in reptiles, birds, and mammals have not been conclusive. A major difficulty is that of excluding the possibility that similarities in the properties of various components of the pallium are due to homoplasy rather than inheritance from a common ancestor. Although some progress has been made in establishing homologies between components of the pallium in reptiles and birds, it is more difficult to relate components of the forebrain in either of these groups to those in mammals.

Comparisons Based on Design

A classical alternative to comparisons based on homology is to compare and contrast structures that have apparently similar functions. The difficulty here is usually one of achieving a precise definition of "function." In the case of DVR, Section 7.2 has already pointed out that little is known about what roles DVR might play in the generation of naturally occurring behaviors. However, the premise of this treatise is that the information currently available is sufficient to indicate that the overall position of DVR in the organization of the brain is to effect a series of *linkages* between ascending sensory pathways and other regions of the brain known to modulate either movements or behaviors controlled by the hypothalamus. A reasonable basis for comparison between the forebrains of birds and reptiles, on the one hand, and mammals, on the other, is to compare and contrast DVR to structures that occupy similar positions in the forebrains of mammals. The question is whether or not there are components of the pallium in mammals that establish sensory linkages with the brainstem and with the hypothalamus comparable to those that DVR establishes in reptiles and birds. The answer to be explored in this section is that the isocortex of mammals occupies a functional position in the brain that is equivalent to the role played by ADVR in the brains of reptiles and birds. Thus, both ADVR and the isocortex receive ascending sensory information from specific nuclei in the thalamus. Both ADVR and the isocortex project to the striatum and to a structure (BDVR or the amygdala) in the caudal telencephalon. The projections to the striatum establish linkages between ADVR or isocortex and the brainstem reticular formation via the optic tectum. The projections to the caudal telencephalon establish linkages between ADVR or isocortex and the hypothalamus and brainstem.

It should be stressed that this comparison sets aside all considerations of the evolutionary history of the structures. ADVR may or may not be homologous to the isocortex; BDVR may or may not be homologous to the amygdala. The point is that they occupy similar positions in the organization of the forebrain and could play the same general roles in the generation of behavior. It is also important to notice that the approach requires only an overall similarity in the properties of the structures being compared. It is virtually certain that there will be significant differences due both to the evolutionary histories of reptiles, birds, and mammals and to more detailed differences in the ways in which members of the various groups use sensory information in the modulation of behavior.

It is nevertheless likely that an analysis based on similarity in design will provide useful information. Thus, the eyes of insects, molluscs, and vertebrates are not clearly homologous. However, it is useful to compare and contrast the design features of the three types of eyes because they play similar roles in the processing of visual information, and the exercise will generally lend insights into factors that are important in the design of eyes as optical devices. The question then becomes one of attempting to determine aspects of design that are important in forebrain structures that serve as linkages between sensory information and the modulation of behavior. Is it possible to discern general features or rules? Also, what is the functional and behavioral significance of the more detailed differences in design that can always be demonstrated when comparing structures between organisms? An analysis of this type will be pursued in this section by discussing each feature of DVR organization identified in Section 7.1 and then speculating on the functional implications of similarities and differences of design that are seen between reptiles and birds and mammals in Section 7.3.

(a) *Neuronal Structure*

Because of the lack of detailed information about BDVR, this section is limited to a comparison of the neuronal structure of ADVR to isocortex. An overall similarity is the presence of neurons with stellate-shaped dendritic fields in both structures. It is also possible to divide these into subclasses containing relatively spine-laden and relatively aspiny neurons in both cases. It is known that the spiny stellate cells are a major postsynaptic target for thalamic afferents to the isocortex (e.g., White, 1979). Appropriate studies have not been done for ADVR, but it is likely that spiny stellate neurons are also a major target for thalamic afferents. An initial design feature that holds for both ADVR and isocortex is then the role that stellate neurons play in receiving ascending sensory projections from the thalamus. The significance of differences in spine density is not clear, but there is some initial data that aspiny neurons in isocortex may be involved in intrinsic inhibitory interactions, whereas spiny neurons are involved in intrinsic excitatory interactions (Lund, 1978; Peters and Regidor, 1981). It is conceivable that the same distinction holds in ADVR. This idea could be evaluated by using electron microscopic techniques to examine neurons identified by either Golgi or HRP procedures.

One difference between the neuronal structure of ADVR and isocortex is that the latter structure contains a greater range of neuronal cell types. Most obvious is the lack of true pyramidal neurons in ADVR, whereas isocortex has pyramidal neurons in layers six, five, three, and two. They vary in size with the largest ones being found in layers six and five. The general rule is the pyramidal neurons have axons with collaterals that leave the confines of a particular isocortical area. Pyramidal neurons are stratified according to the destination of their axons. Those in layer two generally effect association projections to other cortical areas (e.g., Jones, Coulter, and Hendry, 1978; Fitzpatrick and Imig, 1982), those in layer three are involved primarily in commissural projections (e.g., Gilbert and Kelly, 1975; Jones, Coulter, and Wise, 1979; Imig and Brugge, 1978), those in layer five project to subcortical targets such as the spinal cord, basal ganglia, and superior colliculus, whereas those in layer six give rise to reciprocal projections to thalamic sensory nuclei (e.g., Gilbert and Kelly, 1975; Jones and Wise, 1977; Kelly and Wong, 1981) and to the claustrum (LeVay and Sherk, 1981).

The relative roles of stellate and pyramidal neurons in isocortex have been a subject of conjecture for some time. The model of information flow in visual cortex suggested by Hubel and Wiesel (1962) posited that the stellate neurons were the initial postsynaptic target for thalamic inputs and that pyramidal neurons received thalamic inputs secondarily from the stellate cells. More recent anatomical (e.g., White, 1979) and physiological (e.g., Stone, Dreher, and Leventhal, 1979) studies indicate that both stellate and pyramidal neurons receive direct thalamic inputs and the relative contributions of thalamic and intrinsic cortical inputs in shaping the receptive field properties of cortical neurons are areas of major concern. One thing that is clear, however, is that the dendrites of pyramidal neurons often extend radially across several cortical layers so that a pyramidal neuron in layer five or six, for example, is in potential receipt of inputs that are restricted to each of the various cortical layers. The output from the pyramidal neurons can therefore be modulated by a sample of all of the major cortical inputs, whereas the output from stellate cells is more likely to be dominated by inputs to the particular layer in which it is situated.

Thus, one initial impression of the neuronal structure of ADVR and isocortex is that there is a fairly sharp division into intrinsic and extrinsically projecting neurons according to their morphology in isocortex that is not seen in ADVR. The significance of this difference is not yet clear because almost nothing is known about the organization of efferent projections from ADVR. Most efferents must arise from stellate neurons, but it is not known what proportion of the stellate neurons participate in extrinsic projections and whether or not there is anything like a laminar or zonal organization.

The presence of clusters of neurons with apposed somata in ADVR is a major difference with isocortex. Although isocortical neurons may occasionally have touching somata and interactions between their dendrites are common (e.g., Roney, Scheibel, and Shaw, 1979), nothing like the massive occurrence of cell clusters that characterizes ADVR is seen in isocortex. The significance of this difference is unknown because of the lack of physiological information on cell clusters. However, it hints that there may be interesting differences in the neuronal mechanisms that underlie information processing in the two structures.

(b) *Thalamic Afferents*

Afferents from thalamic nuclei are a major source of inputs to both ADVR and isocortex. Lorente de Nó (1938) provided a classification of thalamic afferents in isocortex by recognizing specific and nonspecific afferents. Specific afferents were believed to arise from thalamic sensory nuclei such as the dorsal lateral geniculate, medial geniculate, and ventrobasal complex. Their axons coursed without much branching through the deeper layers of the cortex and arborized into a restricted tuft of collaterals in the fourth layer. Nonspecific afferents have been usually attributed to the intralaminar nuclei without definitive evidence. Their axons extended throughout the depth of the cortex, giving off collaterals in many of the layers and ultimately branching into rather widespread but diffuse arbors in the upper two layers.

Recent studies in which the morphology of thalamic afferents has been visualized by intracellular HRP injections confirmed the idea that some of the afferents from thalamic sensory nuclei resemble Lorente de Nó's specific afferents (Ferster and LeVay, 1978; Landry and Deschenes, 1981). However, they also indicate that other sensory thalamic afferents, such as those from the C laminae of cat lateral geniculate, resemble the nonspecific afferents in having widespread branches in the upper cortical layers. The morphology of afferents from other thalamic nuclei has not been established, but degeneration and autoradiographic studies show that the variety of thalamic projections is greater than suspected by Lorente de Nó (see Frost and Caviness, 1980). Thalamic projections range from restricted projections to specific isocortical areas that correspond to Lorente de Nó's specific afferents, to axons that branch and terminate as specific afferents in two or more isocortical areas, to axons that appear to project widely within isocortex, to axons that collateralize extensively and project to several different regions of the telencephalon (e.g., Caviness and Frost, 1980).

Balaban and Ulinski (1981a) described two types of thalamic projections to ADVR. Restricted projections are confined to specific areas of ADVR in turtles and, like Lorente de Nó's specific afferents, arise from thalamic sensory nuclei. However, the information available on the morphology of rotundal axons within the dorsal area of turtle ADVR (Balaban and Ulinski, 1981b) suggests that they differ considerably from mammalian specific afferents. Each individual rotundal axon apparently branches widely throughout much of dorsal area. The morphology of axons from other sensory thalamic nuclei is not known, but it does seem clear at this point that sensory thalamic nuclei do not necessarily give rise to specific-type afferents. The second type of projections to ADVR are diffuse projections that terminate in several regions of the forebrain. They seem to have characteristically thin caliber, varicose axons, but little more is known about their morphology.

The varieties of thalamic afferents to isocortex and ADVR thus greatly exceed the variety recognized by Lorente de Nó, but it will be necessary to achieve complete morphological descriptions of a larger number of afferent types before it is even possible to attempt a classification of thalamic afferents.

(c) Modality Specific Areas

Both ADVR and isocortex contain modality specific areas. Physiological techniques indicate that these areas receive projections from a particular sensory modality; anatomical techniques indicate that they receive projections from corresponding thalamic sensory nuclei.

Central to the literature on isocortex is the idea that modality specific areas correspond to particular regions of the isocortex identified on the basis of cytoarchitectonic criteria such as those described by Brodmann, O. and C. Vogt, and Bailey and von Bonin (e.g., Brazier, 1978). The significance of cytoarchitectonic areas was challenged in the 1930s, principally by Lashley and his collaborators (Lashley and Clark, 1946). However, subsequent physiological and anatomical studies have usually validated the idea of cytoarchitectonic areas in isocortex, so that cytoarchitecturally distinct regions of the isocortex usually receive projections from a particular set of thalamic nuclei and have particular physiological properties. By contrast, cytoarchitectonic areas in ADVR are much less distinct. Relatively clear areas have been recognized in ADVR of turtles by Balaban (1978a). However, unequivocal areas have not been generally recognized in other groups. Thus, the correspondence between restricted thalamic inputs and cytoarchitectonic areas seems to be a particular feature of thalamic receiving structures in some groups rather than a general feature.

The number of areas that receive information from a given sensory modality varies widely. Single visual, auditory, and somatosensory areas seem to be present in at least some reptiles (such as *Caiman*) and in the monotreme mammals (Lende, 1964; Bohringer and Rowe, 1977). However, a second visual area is present in the more medial components of the pallium in at least turtles and birds. Birds seem to have at least three auditory areas in ADVR and probably have two somatosensory areas, one caudally placed area receives information from the entire body and head and a second rostrally placed area receives information only from the head. Many marsupial and placental mammals have duplicate visual, auditory, and somatosensory areas, whereas others have multiple modality specific areas (Woolsey, 1981a,b, 1982). Cats, for example, have as many as a dozen visual areas in isocortex and some monkeys may have as many as four somatosensory areas (e.g., Van Essen, 1979). When multiple modality specific areas occur, each area seems to receive its own set of thalamic afferents and to have its own physiological properties. A common working hypothesis is that each area is a distinct functional unit, but it has proved difficult to produce clear behavioral data in support of this hypothesis in many cases (e.g., Cowey, 1981; Carlson and Welt, 1981).

Modality specific areas in both ADVR and isocortex often contain topologically organized representations of the various receptor sheets. Adjacent regions of the receptor surface are represented by adjacent regions of the modality specific area in many cases. There may be discontinuities in the maps in other instances or the maps may be broken up into a series of blocks, each of which is continuous. These discontinuities appear to be related to the geometrical constraints posed by the need to represent a two-dimensional map on a curved surface (e.g., Allman, 1977; Kaas et al., 1981a,b). However, the discontinuities occur in an orderly pattern so that the overall topological nature of the representations is not destroyed. Although each part of the receptor sheet is represented in many of the modality specific areas, there is commonly a differential representation or relative magnification of particular regions of the receptor sheet. The extent of the magnification may vary roughly with the density of receptors or ganglion cells in particular regions of the receptor sheets, or with the behavioral importance of particular regions of the periphery (e.g., Tusa, Palmer, and Rosenquist, 1978; Sur, Merzenich, and Kaas, 1980).

Other modality specific areas of both ADVR and isocortex apparently lack topographic representations of the receptor sheets. This appears to be the case in the visual area of ADVR, in some of the visual areas of primates (e.g., Gross et al., 1981) and in some of the auditory areas of bats (Suga, 1982). The significance of the apparent lack of topography in the visual representations is not clear and some hypotheses have been discussed in Section 7.1 above. In the case of the auditory cortex of bats, there is evidence for orderly representations of variables that are behaviorally important in echolocation (Suga, 1982). It may be, then, that the modality specific areas generally contain orderly representations of variables that are behaviorally important or that are needed for various neural computations; these variables may correspond to positions on the receptor surface in some cases but not in others.

A difference between the modality specific representations in ADVR and isocortex is the apparent lack of commissural connections in ADVR. Although the cerebral hemispheres are richly interconnected by commissural projections originating principally from layer three pyramidal cells in mammals, there is no clear evidence for commissural connections in ADVR. The general rule in mammals seems to be that commissural connections link together portions of the hemispheres involved in bilateral interactions. Thus, commissural connections in the somatosensory areas are present principally between representations of the proximal parts of the body, whereas the representations of the distal parts of the limbs generally lack commissural connections (e.g., Ebner and Myers, 1975). Commissural connections in the visual areas are involved principally in connecting together representations of the vertical meridian of the visual field, which falls in the center of the binocular field (e.g., Van Essen, Newsome, and Bixby, 1982). Commissural connections in the auditory areas appear to be effected between binaural columns involved in facilitatory interactions between the two ears (Imig and Brugge, 1978). It is perhaps not surprising then that modality specific areas of ADVR that lack topological representations of the periphery lack commissural connections. However, it seems likely that a detailed study of the efferents of nucleus basalis would show commissural connections because this structure both has a topological representation of the bill and is apparently involved in behaviors requiring bilateral coordination.

An unresolved issue is whether or not ADVR contains regions that receive polysensory inputs. Such regions are present in isocortex, generally positioned between two areas that receive specific inputs from different modalities (e.g., Irvine and Phillips, 1982). The boundaries of modality specific areas in ADVR are not sufficiently well mapped out to know if areas of overlap occur, and there are essentially no relevant physiological data. The course of axons from the thalamus to ADVR in snakes suggest that zones B, C, and D may receive modality specific inputs, whereas zone A receives polysensory input because the thalamic axons curve and run concentric to the ventricle for considerable distances in this zone (Ulinski, 1978a). There are physiological data that neurons in the cortex of *Alligator* are polysensory (Moore and Tschirigi, 1962).

Much less information is available on the nature of modality specific areas in BDVR and the amygdala. What is clear is that a specific region of BDVR and the amygdala receives direct projections from the accessory olfactory bulb, when this structure is present. Nucleus sphericus in snakes and lizards is a circumscribed area of BDVR that receives direct information from the vomeronasal system, and the posterior corticomedial amygdala plays the same role in many mammals (e.g., Scalia and Winans, 1975). There is thus generally a chemosensory area in both BDVR and the amygdala. Some evidence for the existence of additional modality specific areas in the amygdala has recently become available. In primates (Turner, Mishkin, and Knapp, 1980), isocortical sensory areas project to restricted regions of the basolateral complex of the amygdala. These projections can conceivably serve as an anatomical substrate for modality specific visual, auditory, and somatosensory areas in the amygdala, but nothing is known of the organization of such areas. There appear to be comparable projections from modality specific areas in ADVR to the posterior dorsal ventricular ridge (PDVR) in reptiles and the intermediate archistriatum in birds. However, it is not known if the efferents from modality specific areas in ADVR terminate in restricted parts of BDVR.

(d) *Radial Organization*

Both ADVR and isocortex demonstrate a radial organization in that an electrode passing radially through a modality specific area tends to encounter units with similar physiological properties, such as receptive field location or submodality coding properties. This is reasonably well established for the auditory area of ADVR in birds and is firmly established for several of the isocortical sensory areas.

The idea of a radial organization in isocortex received its contemporary formulation in the work of Mountcastle and Powell (Powell and Mountcastle, 1959) who recorded from the somatosensory areas of monkey cortex and found that units along a given, radially oriented electrode penetration usually had similarly placed receptive fields sharing the same submodality (deep versus cutaneous sensation, for example). They coined the word "column" for radially oriented units of the isocortex that share stimulus properties. Hubel and Wiesel (1963, 1974) extended the concept to the visual isocortex of cats and monkeys by demonstrating columns containing units that were driven preferentially by either the right or the left eye (ocular dominance columns) or by stimuli consisting of lines with particular orientations (orientation columns). The nature of potential columns in auditory cortex remained uncertain for some time, but there is now an indication that auditory cortex in cats and bats contains columns of neurons with particular responses to binaural stimuli (e.g., Imig and Adrian, 1977).

The mental image that stems from Mountcastle and Powell's work was that the isocortex consists of a large number of cylindrical units extending through the cortical layers normal to its surface. This image changed with the demonstration of "columns" with anatomical techniques. Hubel and Wiesel (1972) were the first to do this. They clarified the anatomical substrate for ocular dominance columns by making restricted lesions of individual laminae of the dorsal lateral geniculate nucleus in monkeys. Since each lamina receives retinal input exclusively from one eye, the resulting degeneration in the primary visual area represented geniculocortical inputs that carried information from either the right or the left eye. Reconstruction of the degeneration in the cortex revealed that the ocular dominance columns consisted of slabs or bands that are about 500 μm wide and extend across the primary visual area. Orientation columns were subsequently visualized using deoxyglucose techniques and turned out to be bands that extend across the visual area in the opposite direction, so that individual ocular dominance and orientation columns typically intersect each other at approximately right angles (Hubel, Wiesel, and Stryker, 1978). It now appears that the same general situation holds for the columns in somatosensory (Sur, Wall, and Kaas, 1981) and auditory areas (Imig and Adrian, 1977). In addition, band-like patterns to the organization of commissural, association, and efferent projections have been identified in a variety of isocortical areas (see Jones, 1981a). The existence of bands defined in terms of the distribution of afferent and efferent connections is apparently a general feature of modality specific areas in isocortex.

The restricted nature of thalamic, commissural, and association projections appears to be one of the anatomical substrates that underlie cortical columns or bands as identified by physiological techniques. However, two additional factors are relevant. The first is the existence of the pyramidal cells whose dendrites extend radially so that an individual cluster of pyramidal cells will have a bundle of dendrites that is restricted to an individual column (e.g., Jones, 1981a). In addition, the tendency for both the pyramidal cells and several varieties of nonpyramidal neurons to have axons that extend radially through the cortex (e.g., Lund, 1981; Jones, 1981a; Gilbert and Wiesel, 1981) results in a general flow of neural information vertically through the cortex, thalamic information that reaches a given layer of the cortex being relayed to supra- and subjacent layers.

Our understanding of ADVR organization is currently that there is some evidence for a radial organization in an auditory area and in nucleus basalis in birds. As in isocortex, electrode penetrations that pass radially through these modality specific areas tend to encounter units with similar properties. There is also anatomical evidence for radially oriented intrinsic connections within ADVR, but the overall geometry of these connections is completely unknown. It is not clear at this time if the radial organization in ADVR is comparable to the columnar organization of isocortex because the idea of columnar organization implies an encoding of some stimulus variable such as right eye versus left eye, orientation, binaural properties, or adaptation properties into discrete units within a modality specific area (Hubel, 1981). There is presently no evidence either way for this type of organization in ADVR. However, Pettigrew (1979) reports that both ocular dominance and orientation columns may be present in the Wulst of owls. This finding is interesting because it indicates that columnar organization is not unique to mammals and that it does not depend on the presence of pyramidal-type neurons.

Despite their ubiquity, the functional significance of columns or bands remains obscure. It is sometimes suggested that ocular dominance columns play some role in stereoscopic vision (e.g., Hubel and Wiesel, 1977). It is also suggested that the existence of columns or bands facilitates the establishment of connections between neurons that are functionally related. However, it is difficult to reconcile either of these suggestions with the variability that is seen in ocular dominance columns between species. Most species of Old World monkeys (Hubel and Wiesel, 1972; Hendrickson, Wilson, and Ogren, 1978) and cats (Shatz, Lindstrom, and Wiesel, 1975) have ocular dominance columns while New World monkeys generally lack ocular dominance columns (Hubel, Wiesel, and LeVay, 1976; Kaas, Lin, and Casagrand, 1976; Tigges, Tigges, and Perachio, 1977; Hendrickson, Wilson, and Ogren, 1978). Tree shrews have orientation columns (Humphrey and Norton, 1980) but not ocular dominance columns (Harting, Diamond, and Hall, 1973; Hubel, 1975). It thus remains to be determined if a columnar organization plays some essential role in the processing of neural information and, if so, what that role might be.

(e) *Nonthalamic Afferents*

It was long believed that the dorsal thalamus is the only source of afferents to the isocortex. The difficulty of demonstrating projections from the dorsal thalamus to the forebrain in reptiles and birds led for a while to the suggestion that these groups lack any structure equivalent to the isocortex of mammals. However, it is now clear not only that the dorsal thalamus does project to the forebrain in reptiles and birds, but that there are additional sources of afferents to the pallium in all three groups.

Both ADVR and isocortex receive projections from several structures in the brainstem. A noradrenergic cell group located in the isthmus is present in reptiles, birds, and mammals (Moore and Bloom, 1979). It gives rise to widespread projections that include ascending projections to the cerebellum and forebrain and descending projections to the spinal cord. The forebrain projections include fibers that terminate in the pallium. These are typically fine caliber axons that bear many varicosities or *terminaux en passant*. Electron microscopic studies (Beaudet and Descarries, 1978; Ouimet, Patrick, and Ebner, 1981) indicate that these varicosities are presynaptic elements, but only a fraction of them contains classical active zones. There is much current interest in the idea that these synapses could release noradrenaline into the extracellular space where it might act as a neuromodulator in addition to forming traditional chemical synapses on specific postsynaptic elements (e.g., Taylor and Stone, 1981). Serotonergic cell groups are present in the raphé nuclei of reptiles, birds, and mammals. They also give rise to extensive ascending and descending projections that involve fine caliber, varicose axons.

In addition to these fine caliber projections, there are additional projections from the brainstem to the forebrain that involve thick caliber axons. Data in reptiles (e.g., Ulinski, 1981) indicate that these include projections from neurons in the midbrain reticular formation. The transmitter substance used by these projections is not known, but is probably not a monoamine. These projections are also extensively collateralized and terminate in the basal forebrain, septum, and cortex as well as ADVR.

The functional role of such widespread or diffuse projections is not certain, although several hypotheses including some role in the modulation of arousal state (e.g., Morgane and Stern, 1974; Amaral and Sinnamon, 1977) are under current investigation. A general feature of all of these systems is that the neurons that give rise to the diffuse projections themselves receive a large variety of afferents including projections from structures in each of the major sensory modalities.

(f) *Efferents: Sensory–Motor Linkages*

Both ADVR and isocortex give rise to efferent projections that terminate in the striatum. These projections arise from pyramidal cells in the case of isocortex and probably from stellate neurons in the case of ADVR. There is some indication that the projections from ADVR to the striatum are at least roughly topographic, but there have not been any detailed studies of the morphology of the axons of ADVR neurons. Degeneration studies of the projections of isocortex to the caudate-putamen in mammals suggested that the projections are topographically organized (Grofova, 1978). However, experiments using autoradiographic tracing techniques showed that the projections are more extensive (Goldman and Nauta, 1977). Injections restricted to particular cortical areas result in silver grains distributed in a network of interlacing bands in the caudate-putamen (Goldman-Rakic, 1982). Thus, the nature of the projections from the pallium to the striatum is poorly understood both in reptiles and birds and in mammals.

The subsequent projections of the striatum involve pathways that lead indirectly to the optic tectum or superior colliculus in all three groups of animals (mammals: Dray, 1979; Harting and Huerta, 1983). The striatum projects to a dopaminergic cell group in the midbrain tegmentum in each case. Cells in this group project in turn to the roof of the midbrain. These projections are of considerable functional significance because the roof of the midbrain gives rise to extensive projections to the brainstem reticular formation, the source of the reticulospinal projections. The result is that the striatum links the pallium to the brainstem reticular formation in all three groups of animals and provides a likely substrate by which sensory information reaching the pallium can modulate movement.

In addition to the sequence of connections between the pallium and tectum that is common to all three groups, there are parallel routes by which the pallium can modulate movements that occur in one group or another. Reptiles and birds have a nucleus at the junction between the pretectum and the caudal thalamus that receives projections from the striatum and sends efferents to the optic tectum. Comparable projections are not known in mammals. Mammals have projections from the motor areas of isocortex that terminate in the brainstem reticular formation and in the direct vicinity of both cranial and spinal motoneurons (Wiesendanger, 1981). Comparable projections have not been seen in reptiles, but there is evidence that the anterior Wulst of the owl *Speotyto cunicularia* contains a topographic representation of the claws and projects to the spinal cord (Karten, 1971; Karten, Konishi, and Pettigrew, 1978). The cortex also projects to the optic tectum in most groups of reptiles (e.g., Elprana, Wouterlood, and Alones, 1980) and the Wulst projects to the tectum in birds (e.g., Bagnoli, Grassi, and Magni, 1980). Similarly, there are projections from widespread areas of the isocortex to the superior colliculus in mammals (e.g., Kawamura, Sprague, and Niimi, 1974).

Descending projections from the striatum are complemented by striatal projections that participate in feedback loops back to the forebrain. One such loop that is common to reptiles, birds, and mammals involves reciprocal projections between the striatum and a dopaminergic cell group in the midbrain tegmentum. This group is variously called the substantia nigra or the pedunculopontine nucleus. A second loop involves structures embedded in the descending striatal efferents. These are the entopeduncular nuclei in reptiles, the nuclei of the ansa lenticularis in birds, and the subthalamic nucleus in mammals. A very significant difference between the three groups in the organization of feedback loops to the forebrain is that only mammals have well-developed striatal projections to thalamic nuclei (the ventral anterior and intralaminar nuclei). Both of these nuclear groups effect connections with the motor cortex and thereby place the striatum in contact with the motor regions of the isocortex. Ulinski (1983) has argued that extensive striatal projections to the thalamus evolved during the therapsid–mammal transition and are characteristic of mammals.

All of these projections must play some role in the modulation of movement, but their specific functions are only beginning to be investigated. The best progress has been made in cases in which it is possible to record from neurons in awake animals performing more or less natural tasks, such as arm movements in monkeys (e.g., Porter, 1975; Fetz, 1981). Such studies indicate that corticospinal neurons can modulate ongoing arm movements in the face of perturbations encountered during the course of a movement. It is conceivable that the anterior Wulst plays a similar role in owls. Since the corticospinal projections are topographically organized, the motor cortex establishes quite specific input–output relationships between sensory inputs from particular regions of the periphery and appropriate groups of motoneurons. The linkage that is established between somatosensory information and the activity of motoneurons is focused specifically on the activities of a small number of motor pools, and the topologically organized ascending and descending projections are the most straightforward means of establishing such a linkage.

By contrast, efferent pathways that issue from the pallium, through the striatum, and to the optic tectum are probably not topologically organized throughout and are likely to modulate the activity of groups of motoneurons rather than specific motor pools. Several of the preceding paragraphs have already pointed out that the organization of the steps in these pathways is inadequately known, so it is not possible to trace in sequence the kinds of transformations occurring at each juncture. However, some general comments on what is known can serve to specify the kinds of questions that remain to be answered.

The fundamental issue here is of course the relation of sensory information to the generation of movement, or what the functional nature of a "sensory–motor" linkage might be. One hypothesis, argued by Sherrington (1906) for example, is that the generation of normal movements is dependent on sensory inputs from the periphery. The opposing hypothesis, suggested at the same time by Graham-Brown (1911), is that the basic units of movement are generated by the central nervous system independent of patterned sensory input from the periphery. This view does not deny peripheral inputs an important role in modulating and fine tuning the activity of those central structures involved in generating movement.

Direct evidence for the existence of such central pattern generators was first attained in invertebrates (Stein, 1978), and attempts to clearly delineate the relative importance of peripheral sensory inputs to the generation of movement in vertebrates were frustrated by technical difficulties for some time. However, there is now clear evidence that spinal neurons can generate patterned output in motoneurons that correspond to the firing patterns that occur in normal movements, even in the absence of peripheral input. This was initially demonstrated in deafferented preparations *in vivo* (e.g., Grillner, 1975) but has now been shown in isolated spinal cords *in vitro* (e.g., Stehouwer and Farel, 1980). The neuronal mechanisms underlying central pattern generators in vertebrates are just beginning to be studied (Wetzel and Howell, 1981).

The current view is that the spinal cord contains a number of pattern generators, one associated with each limb perhaps, and that naturally occurring movements require the coordinated activation of many if not all of the central pattern generators. The task of driving the pattern generators apparently falls on the systems of pathways that descend from the brainstem reticular formation. There is very good evidence in favor of this concept in fishes in the case of identified neurons such as the Mauthner neurons and Müller cells that are closely related to the production of relatively stereotyped swimming and escape behaviors (e.g., Faber and Korn, 1978; Rovainen, 1979). However, the concept can be generalized to a wider range of vertebrate behaviors because electrical or chemical stimulation of the brainstem reticular formation is known to produce relatively natural locomotory movements in a variety of animals including cats, sharks, and turtles (Grillner, 1975; Lennard and Stein, 1977). Similarly, the pontine reticular formation is known to play a role in the generation of coordinated eye movements in mammals (e.g., Carpenter, 1977).

Although the motoneurons, pattern generators, and brainstem systems are probably sufficient to produce the basic sequences of movements involved in many naturally occurring movements, they are probably not adequate to produce movements that represent appropriate responses to environmental stimuli. Some source of sensory information beyond the proprioceptive input needed to modulate the activity of the central pattern generators is required. The optic tectum is a good candidate for the source of this information. It receives receptotopically organized inputs from the visual, auditory, and somatosensory systems and gives rise to extensive projections to the brainstem reticular formation. A substantial body of experimental data indicates that lesions of the optic tectum can interfere with a variety of movements, particularly those involving orientation to sensory stimuli, whereas electrical stimulation of the tectum produces movements that mimic these behaviors (Ingle and Sprague, 1975).

The ability of the tectum to mediate the correct orientation to sensory stimuli implies that it is involved in a sensorimotor transformation. The sensory world is topologically mapped onto the surface of the tectum, and stimuli occurring in a specific locale in the sensory world result in the activation of specific sequences of motor pools and the appropriate orientation of the animal. This could involve direct projections from a region of the tectum that processes information from a given locale to a particular motor pool in special cases. However, most orientation movements will require the coordinated action of a large number of motor pools and imply the existence of divergent projections somewhere between the optic tectum and the motor pools.

It is likely that both the tectoreticular and the reticulospinal projections are at least partially nontopological and involve divergent projections. Both degeneration and autoradiographic studies indicated that the optic tectum and superior colliculus give rise to both ipsilateral and contralateral projections to the brainstem reticular formation (Ulinski, 1977a; Wurtz and Albano, 1980). The contralateral projections arise from neurons situated predominantly in the intermediate layers of the tectum of reptiles (Sereno, 1982) and birds (Reiner and Karten, 1982) and of the superior colliculus (e.g., Holcombe and Hall, 1981b). The ipsilateral projections arise from neurons located throughout the central and deep layers of the tectum (Sereno, 1982; Reiner and Karten, 1982) and colliculus (e.g., Holcombe and Hall, 1981a). The degeneration studies suggested that axons descend from the midbrain roof into the reticular formation, coursing caudally and collateralizing extensively, but did not permit a complete visualization of the morphology of the tectoreticular axons. This has been recently accomplished by Dacey (1982), Sereno (1982), and Grantyn and Grantyn (1982) who used the orthograde transport of HRP to study the morphology of tectoreticular axons. The general result is that individual axons distribute collaterals to several structures in the brainstem reticular formation and collateralize extensively within any one region of the reticular formation. Because several populations of tectal neurons contribute to the tectoreticular pathways, information reaching a particular spot on the tectum will be relayed, through the tectoreticular paths, in a nontopographic fashion to many neurons in the reticular formation. Conversely, any reticular neuron is likely to receive inputs from many tectal neurons distributed over the surface of the tectum.

It has been suspected for some time that the subsequent projections of reticular neurons are highly divergent. This can be seen directly in drawings prepared from Golgi preparations that show axons of reticular neurons bifurcating into ascending and descending branches, each of which bears extensive secondary collateral systems (Scheibel and Scheibel, 1958). Similar conclusions can be drawn from retrograde degeneration studies showing that lesions of specific levels of the spinal cord produce chromatolytic neurons scattered throughout the reticular formation (e.g., Torvik and Brodal, 1957). More recently, it has been shown that reticulospinal neurons have collateralized projections to the spinal cord using double labeling (e.g., Martin et al., 1981) and physiological (Peterson et al., 1975) techniques.

The functional consequence of the organization of the tectoreticular and reticulospinal projections is that sensory information about the visual, auditory, and somatosensory worlds that reaches particular regions of the optic tectum or superior colliculus will be distributed to a variety of motor pools in the brainstem and spinal cord via the divergent tectoreticular and reticulospinal projections. The receptotopically organized visual, auditory, and somatosensory projections to the tectum can provide information on the positions of stimuli in extrapersonal space which is essential to the generation of orientation movements. Similarly, some of the projections from pallial regions, such as modality specific areas of the isocortex, to the tectum can serve a similar purpose. The functional roles of the apparently nontopographic projections from the pallium through the striatum and to the optic tectum are not yet clear. However, the simplest hypothesis is that they provide the tectum with highly processed forms of information necessary to more complicated movements.

Thus, a consideration of the positions that ADVR and isocortex occupy in the functional organization of the brain leads to the suggestion that they form a linkage, through the striatum, between ascending sensory systems and those brainstem structures that modulate coordinated movements. Additional sensory–motor linkages occur in the case of proprioceptive inputs either directly to motoneurons or to interneurons that affect the activity of motoneurons, and in the case of direct projections from the forebrain to motoneuron pools like those that occur in the corticospinal tracts of mammals or the archistriatal projections of birds. These linkages involve relatively specific connections with particular motor pools. By contrast, it appears likely that the sensory–motor linkages effected via ADVR and isocortex via striatal centers involve relatively more complex kinds of sensory information and modulate the activity of many groups of motoneurons, suggesting roles in more complex, naturally occurring behaviors.

(g) Efferents: Sensory–Hypothalamic Linkages

The BDVR and amygdala receive two types of sensory information. There is direct olfactory information from the accessory olfactory system in those species that have a vomeronasal organ and possibly from the main olfactory bulb in species that lack a vomeronasal organ. There is also the likelihood of visual, auditory, and somatosensory information that reaches BDVR and the amygdala from ADVR and isocortex, respectively. Both BDVR and the amygdala (e.g., Eleftheriou, 1972) have subsequent projections to the hypothalamus. Little can be said about their organization, but it seems clear from a functional viewpoint that these connections must establish sensory–hypothalamic linkages that can potentially modulate a wide variety of behaviors, either through the influences that the hypothalamus exerts through the hypothalamohypophyseal pathways or through the projections of the hypothalamus to the autonomic nervous system (e.g., Palkovits and Zabrosky, 1979).

Sensory Linkages in Reptiles, Birds, and Mammals

Having surveyed a number of design features of sensory linkages in reptiles, birds, and mammals, what can be said about the overall functional organization of the forebrain in the three groups? The overriding consideration, and the one that has been emphasized throughout the treatise, is that a component of the pallium participates in sensory linkages with the brainstem reticular formation (Fig. 7.2) and the hypothalamus (Fig. 7.3) in all three groups. This component is ADVR in reptiles and birds and the isocortex in mammals. It receives projections from thalamic sensory nuclei in each group of animals and projects to the underlying striatum. The projections of the striatum include one or more pathways that run through the midbrain tegmentum and terminate in the optic tectum or superior colliculus. The significance of these pathways is that they complete a linkage through the tectoreticular pathways with the brainstem reticular formation and place the pallium in a position to modulate the activity of motoneurons. The behavioral studies discussed above indicate that the sensory information supplied by this linkage does not directly influence the activity of individual pools of motoneurons. It more likely plays a role in the generation or modulation

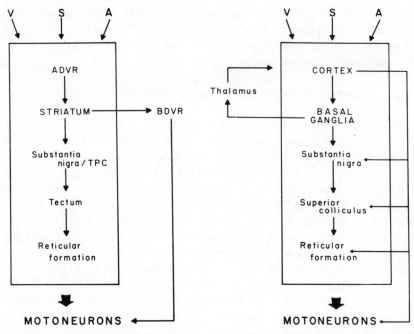

FIGURE 7.2.   Comparisons of sensory–motor linkages in reptiles, birds, and mammals. The basic pattern of linkages between auditory (A), somatosensory (S), and visual (V) inputs through the telencephalon and to motoneurons is shown for reptiles and birds on the left and mammals on the right.

of more complex, species-specific forms of behavior. A second linkage involves projections from the pallium (ADVR or isocortex) to a structure in the caudal telencephalon (BDVR or amygdala). These structures have subsequent projections to the brainstem and to the hypothalamus. The latter projections in particular complete a linkage between the pallium and the pituitary and those forebrain structures that modulate the activity of the autonomic nervous system. This linkage also appears to play a role in the modulation of relatively complex behaviors.

The existence of these linkages in all three groups of animals is a similarity in design that extends across several phylogenetic lineages. Does this similarity reflect a commonality of ancestry (homology) or does it reflect independent and parallel responses to a common functional demand (homoplasy)? The most likely answer is that both factors are involved. There is clearly a general, structural similarity in the layout of the forebrain and upper brainstem in all three groups which includes the presence of a pallial component to the telencephalon, a striatum with fairly conservative connections and histochemistry, and projec-

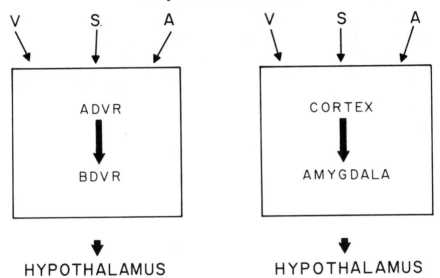

FIGURE 7.3. Comparison of sensory–hypothalamic linkages in reptiles, birds, and mammals. The basic pattern of linkages between auditory (A), somatosensory (S), and visual (V) inputs through the telencephalon and to the hypothalamus is shown for reptiles and birds on the left and mammals on the right.

tions through the mesencephalic tegmentum to the roof of the midbrain. It is reasonable to imagine that these structural features have been present in the various lineages of tetrapod vertebrates throughout much of their evolutionary history. Differences in the more detailed organization of the linkages, on the other hand, hint that some aspects of the linkages have evolved separately and somewhat differently in various lineages. The organization of the pallium is the most striking of these. Although ADVR and the isocortex occupy a similar position in the functional organization of the forebrain, their position, internal organization, and relation to other components of the forebrain are sufficiently different to lend credence to the idea that they evolved independently in reptiles and birds, on one hand, versus mammals, on the other. It may not be possible in that case to establish detailed homologies between pallial components in the three groups.

The idea that homologies may not exist between individual components of the forebrain of reptiles and birds and mammals is a depressing one from the viewpoint of traditional studies in comparative neurology. However it has some interesting implications from a functional viewpoint. The existence of some similarities in the design features of ADVR and isocortex, such as the presence of modality specific areas, modes of vertical or radial organization, and both topologically and nontopologically organized maps, suggests that these are features that have evolved independently in responses to common functional demands. That is, there may be something that is essential about these features to the performance of this particular type of sensory linkages. It is not yet clear why design features of this type are important, but recognizing them opens an avenue of inquiry in which detailed comparisons in design features between groups are likely to help unravel some aspects of their functional significance. This strategy of analyzing design features is not at all a new one, but it has received less of an application to vertebrate neurobiology than it deserves. It is analogous, for example, to a fairly common and productive way in thinking about the function of eyes. Eyes in various groups of invertebrates and vertebrates are recognized as similar, not as homologues but as subserving similar roles in the analysis of visual information, in members of the various groups of animals. This commonality of overall function serves as a satisfactory basis for comparison and leads to the recognition of particular design features, such as the presence of photoreceptors, lenses, ganglion cells, etc. Once the elements of design are known, it is possible to begin determining the specific consequences of various aspects of design and how these variations are related to the particular environmental demands that bear on individual species.

The current situation with regard to DVR, then, is that the efforts of the last two decades of investigation have provided the minimal information needed to define DVR as a component of the pallium in reptiles and birds and to recognize it as one component in a set of sensory linkages that carry visual, auditory, and somatosensory information to centers in the brainstem and hypothalamus that have relatively direct roles in modulating complex, naturally occurring behaviors. Efforts at relating DVR to specific components of the forebrains of mammals on the basis of commonality of ancestry have been unsuccessful for the most part and, in retrospect, may have been somewhat inappropriate. It is possible, however, to use similarity in function to compare the sensory linkages through DVR in reptiles and birds to linkages through the isocortex and amygdala in mammals. These comparisons can provide a framework for more detailed analysis of the design features of such linkages that are likely to improve our understanding of forebrain organization and function in all three groups of animals. Two approaches seem best suited to capitalize on the potentialities of the approach. The first is to continue analytical studies of the roles that DVR plays in specific, naturally occurring behaviors in reptiles and birds. Such studies have the advantage of using an animal's behavior to assure that the variables being investigated have a real, biological significance. The second approach is to seriously begin analytical studies of the organization of DVR using modern physiological and anatomical techniques. There is a pressing need for intensive studies of the physiological properties of DVR in a range of reptiles and birds. It will be particularly interesting to learn more about the properties of maps in modality specific areas, the nature of vertical organization and the response properties of units in various parts of DVR. At the same time, the course of investigations in isocortex during the past 10 years makes it clear that a skillful application of neuroanatomical techniques is necessary to adequately portray the organization of a forebrain structure both at the neuronal level and at the level of the organization of groups of neurons. In some ways, the current situation is that for the first time since John Hunter's dissection in 1861 we know enough about DVR to adequately define and understand the problems that it poses and their significance for vertebrate neurobiology.

REFERENCES

Acheson, D. W. K., S. K. Kemplay, and K. E. Webster (1980). Quantitative analysis of optic terminal profile distribution within the pigeon optic tectum. *Neuroscience*, **5**, 1067–1084.

Adamo, N. J. (1967). Connections of efferent fibers from hyperstriatal areas in chicken, raven, and African lovebird. *J. Comp. Neurol.*, **131**, 337–356.

Adamo, N. J., and R. L. King (1967). Evoked responses in the chicken telencephalon to auditory, visual and tactile stimuli. *Exp. Neurol.*, **17**, 498–504.

Allman, J. (1977). Evolution of the visual system in the early primates. *Prog. Psychobiol. Physiol. Psychol.*, **7**, 1–54.

Altmann, J., and M. B. Carpenter (1961). Fiber projections of the superior colliculus in the cat. *J. Comp. Neurol.*, **116**, 157–178.

Amaral, D. G., and H. M. Sinnamon (1977). The locus coeruleus: Neurobiology of a central noradrenergic nucleus. *Prog. Neurobiol.*, **9**, 147–196.

Anderson, J. A., and C. E. Hinton (1981). "Models of information processing in the Brain." In J. A. Anderson and C. E. Hinton (Eds.), *Parallel Models of Associative Memory*, Erlbaum, Hillsdale, New Jersey, pp. 9–48.

Angevine, J. B., and R. L. Sidman (1961). Autoradiographic study of cell migration during histogenesis of cerebral cortex in the mouse. *Nature (London)*, **192**, 766–768.

Arends, J. J. A., and J. L. Dubbeldam (1982). Exteroceptive and proprioceptive afferents of the trigeminal and facial motor nuclei in the mallard (*Anas platyrhynchos* L.). *J. Comp. Neurol.*, **209**, 313–329.

Ariëns Kappers, C. U. (1921). *Vergleichende Anatomie des Nervensystems*, E. F. Bohn, Haarlem, The Netherlands.

Ariëns Kappers, C. U., G. C. Huber, and E. C. Crosby (1936). *The Comparative Anatomy of the Nervous System of Vertebrates, Including Man.* Republished in 1967 by Hafner, New York.

Armstrong, J. A., H. G. Gamble, and F. Goldby (1953). Observations on the olfactory apparatus and telencephalon of *Anolis*, a microsmatic lizard. *J. Anat. (London)*, **87**, 288–307.

235

Arnold, A. P. (1979). Hormone accumulation in the brain of the zebra finch after injection of various steroids and steroid competitors. *Soc. Neurosci. Abstr.*, **5**, 437.

Arnold, A. P. (1980). Quantitative analysis of sex differences in hormone accumulation in the zebra finch brain: Methodological and theoretical issues. *J. Comp. Neurol.*, **189**, 421–436.

Arnold, A. P., F. Nottebohm, and D. W. Pfaff (1976). Hormone concentrating cells in vocal control and other areas of the brain of the zebra finch (*Poephila guttata*). *J. Comp. Neurol.*, **165**, 487–512.

Arnold, A. P., and A. Saltiel (1978). Sexual differences in pattern of hormone accumulation in the brain of a song bird. *Neurosci. Abstr.*, **4**, 339.

Auffenberg, W. (1978). "Social and feeding behavior in *Varanus komodensis.*" In N. Greenberg and P. D. MacLean (Eds.), *Behavior and Neurology of Lizards*, NIMH, Rockville, Maryland, pp. 301–331.

Bagnoli, P., S. Grassi, and F. Magni (1980). A direct connection between visual Wulst and tectum opticum in the pigeon (*Columba livia*) demonstrated by horseradish peroxidase. *Arch. Ital. Biol.*, **118**, 72–83.

Baker-Cohen, K. F. (1968). Comparative enzyme histochemical observations on submammalian brains. I. Striatal structures in reptiles and birds. II. Basal structures of the brainstem in reptiles and birds. *Ergeb. Anat.*, **40**, 1–70.

Balaban, C. D. (1977). Olfactory projections in Emydid turtles (*Pseudemys scripta elegans* and *Graptemys pseudogeographica*). *Am. Zool.*, **17**, 887.

Balaban, C. D. (1978a). Structure of anterior dorsal ventricular ridge in turtles (*Pseudemys scripta elegans*). *J. Morphol.*, **158**, 291–322.

Balaban, C. D. (1978b). Structure of the pallial thickening in turtles (*Pseudemys scripta elegans*). *Anat. Rec.*, **190**, 330–331.

Balaban, C. D. (1979). Organization of thalamic projections to anterior dorsal ventricular ridge in two species of turtles (*Pseudemys scripta elegans* and *Chrysemys picta belli*). Doctoral Dissertation, University of Chicago.

Balaban, C. D., and P. S. Ulinski (1981a). Organization of thalamic afferents to anterior dorsal ventricular ridge in turtles. I. Projections of thalamic nuclei. *J. Comp. Neurol.*, **200**, 95–130.

Balaban, C. D., and P. S. Ulinski (1981b). Organization of thalamic afferents to anterior dorsal ventricular ridge in turtles. II. Properties of the rotundo-dorsal map. *J. Comp. Neurol.*, **200**, 131–150.

Bass, A. H., and R. G. Northcutt (1981). Retinal recipient nuclei in the painted turtle, *Chrysemys picta:* An autoradiographic and HRP study. *J. Comp. Neurol.*, **199**, 97–112.

Baumgarten, H. G., and H. Braak (1968). Catecholamine im Gehirn der Eidechse (*Lacerta viridis* und *Lacerta muralis*). *Z. Zellforsch.*, **86**, 574–608.

Bayon, A., L. Koda, E. Battenberg, R. Azad, and F. E. Bloom (1980). Regional distribution of endorphin, Met[5]-enkephalin and Leu[5]-enkephalin in the pigeon brain. *Neurosci. Lett.*, **16**, 75–80.

Beaudet, A., and L. Descarries (1978). The monoamine innervation of rat cerebral cortex: Synaptic and nonsynaptic axon terminals. *Neuroscience*, **3**, 851–860.

Belekhova, M. G. (1979). "Neurophysiology of the forebrain." In C. G. Gans, R. G. Northcutt, and P. S. Ulinski (Eds.), *Biology of the Reptilia*, Vol. 10, Academic Press, London, pp. 287–359.

Belekhova, M. G., and M. M. Akulina (1970). The tecto-thalamo telencephalic system of the turtle (electrophysiological study). *Neurofiziologia (Kiev)*, **2**, 296–306.

Belekhova, M. G., and A. A. Kosareva (1971). Organization of the turtle thalamus: Visual, somatic and tectal zones. *Brain Behav. Evol.*, **4**, 337–375.

Belekhova, M. G., A. A. Kosareva, N. P. Veselkin, and T. V. Ermakova (1978). Telencephalic afferent connections in the turtle *Emys orbicularis*: A peroxidase study. *J. Evol. Biochem. Physiol.*, **15**, 97–103.

Benowitz, L. (1980). "Functional organization of the avian telencephalon." In S. O. E. Ebbesson (Ed.), *Comparative Neurology of the Telencephalon*, Plenum, New York, pp. 389–421.

Benowitz, L. I., and H. J. Karten (1976). Organization of the tectofugal visual pathway in the pigeon: A retrograde transport study. *J. Comp. Neurol.*, **167**, 503–520.

Berkhoudt, H. (1980). The morphology and distribution of cutaneous mechano-receptors (Herbst and Grandry corpuscles) in bill and tongue of the mallard (*Anas platyrhynchos* L.). *Neth. J. Zool.*, **30**, 1–34.

Berkhoudt, H., J. L. Dubbeldam, and S. Zeilstra (1981). Studies on the somatotopy of the trigeminal system in the mallard, *Anas platyrhynchos* L. IV. Tactile representation in the nucleus basalis. *J. Comp. Neurol.*, **196**, 407–420.

Berry, M. S., and V. W. Pentreath (1977). The integrative properties of electronic synapses. *Comp. Biochem. Physiol.*, **57A**, 289–295.

Bertler, A., B. Falck, C.-G. Gottfries, L. Ljunggren, and E. Rosengren (1964). Some observations on adrenergic connections between the mesencephalon and the cerebral hemispheres. *Acta Pharmacol. Toxicol.*, **21**, 283–298.

Biederman-Thorson, M. (1967). Auditory responses of neurones in the nucleus (inferior colliculus) of the barbary dove. *J. Physiol. (London)*, **193**, 695–705.

Biederman-Thorson, M. (1970a). Auditory evoked responses in the cerebrum (Field L) and ovoid nucleus of the ring dove. *Brain Res.*, **24**, 235–245.

Biederman-Thorson, M. (1970b). Auditory responses of units in the ovoid nucleus and cerebrum (Field L) of the ring dove. *Brain Res.*, **24**, 247–256.

Bohringer, R. C., and M. J. Rowe (1977). The organization of the sensory and motor areas of cerebral cortex in platypus (*Ornithorhyncus anatinus*). *J. Comp. Neurol.*, **174**, 1–14.

Boiko, V. P., and N. V. Goncharova (1976). Morphological and functional organization of the tectal visual center in the turtles *Agrionemys horsfieldi* and *Emys orbicularis*. *J. Evol. Biochem. Physiol.*, **12**, 399–404.

Bonke, D. A., D. Bonke, and H. Scheich (1979). Connectivity of the auditory forebrain nuclei in the guinea fowl (*Numida meleagris*). *Cell Tiss. Res.*, **200**, 101–121.

Bonke, D., H. Scheich, and G. Langner (1979). Responsiveness of units in the auditory neostriatum of the guinea fowl (*Numida meleagris*) to species-specific calls and synthetic stimuli. I. Tonotopy and functional zones of field L. *J. Comp. Physiol.*, **132A**, 243–255.

Bonke, D., B. A. Bonke, G. Langner, and H. Scheich (1981). "Some aspects of functional organization of the auditory neostriatum (Field L) in the guinea fowl." In J. Syka and L. Aitkin (Eds.), *Neuronal Mechanisms of Hearing*, Plenum, New York, pp. 323–327.

Bonner, J. T. (1980). *The Evolution of Culture in Animals*. Princeton Univ. Press, Princeton, New Jersey.

Boord, R. L. (1968). Ascending projections of the primary cochlear nuclei and nucleus laminaris in the pigeon. *J. Comp. Neurol.*, **133**, 523–542.

Boord, R. L., and G. L. Rasmussen (1963). Projection of the cochlear and lagenar nerves on the cochlear nuclei of the pigeon. *J. Comp. Neurol.*, **120**, 463–475.

Bowling, D. B. (1980). Light responses of ganglion cells in the retina of the turtle. *J. Physiol. (London)*, **299**, 173–196.

Braak, H., H. G. Baumgarten, and B. Falck (1968). 5-Hydroxytryptamine im Gehirn der Eidechse (*Lacerta viridis* und *Lacerta muralis*). *Z. Zellforsch.*, **90**, 161–185.

Braford, M. R., Jr. (1972). Ascending efferent tectal projections in the South American spectacled caiman. *Anat. Rec.*, **172**, 275–276.

Braford, M. R., Jr. (1973). Retinal projections in *Caiman crocodilus*. *Am. Zool.*, **13**, 1345.

Brauth, S. E., and C. A. Kitt (1980). The paleostriatal system of *Caiman crocodilus*. *J. Comp. Neurol.*, **189**, 437–466.

Brauth, S. E., J. L. Ferguson, and C. A. Kitt (1978). Prosencephalic pathways related to the paleostriatum of the pigeon (*Columba livia*). *Brain Res.*, **147**, 205–221.

Brazier, M. A. B. (1978). Architectonics of the cerebral cortex: Research in the 19th century. In M. A. B. Brazier and H. Petsche (Eds.), *Architectonics of the Cerebral Cortex*, Raven, New York, pp. 9–29.

Brecha, N., S. P. Hunt, and H. J. Karten (1976). Relations between the optic tectum and basal ganglia in the pigeon. *Neurosci. Abstr.*, **2**, 1069.

Bremer, F., R. S. Dow, and G. Moruzzi (1939). Physiological analysis of the general cortex in reptiles and birds. *J. Neurophysiol.*, **2**, 473–499.

Brown, J. L. (1971). An exploratory study of vocalization areas in the brain of the red-winged blackbird (*Agelaius phoeniceus*). *Behaviour*, **39**, 91–127.

Brown, J. L. (1973). Behaviour elicited by electrical stimulation of the brain of the Stellar's Jay. *Condor*, **75**, 1–16.

Brown, J. L. (1974). "Brain stimulation parameters affecting vocalizations in birds." In I. J. Goodman and M. W. Schein (Eds.), *Birds: Brain and Behavior*. Academic, New York, pp. 87–99.

Bruce, L. L. (1982). Organization and evolution of the reptilian forebrain: experimental studies of forebrain connections in lizards. Doctoral Dissertation, Georgetown University.

Bruce, L. L., and A. B. Butler (1979). Afferent projections to the anterior dorsal ventricular ridge in the lizard *Iguana iguana*. *Neurosci. Abstr.*, **5**, 140.

Bugbee, N. M., and W. Hodos (1979). The basal ganglia-tectal pathway: Its role in visually guided behavior in the pigeon. *Neurosci. Abstr.*, **5**, 68.

Bullock, T. H. (1977). *Recognition of Complex Acoustic Signals*, Abakon Verlags-Gesellschaft, Berlin.

Burghardt, G. M., and G. H. Pruitt (1975). The role of the tongue and senses in the feeding of naive and experienced garter snakes. *Physiol. Behav.*, **14**, 185–194.

Butler, A. B. (1976). Telencephalon of the lizard *Gekko gecko* (*Linnaeus*): Some connections of the cortex and dorsal ventricular ridge. *Brain Behav. Evol.*, **13**, 396–417.

Butler, A. B. (1978). "Forebrain connections in lizards and the evolution of sensory systems." In N. Greenberg and P. D. MacLean (Eds.), *Behavior and Neurology of Lizards*, NIMH, Rockville, Maryland, pp. 65–78.

Butler, A. B. (1980). "Cytoarchitectonic and connectional organization of the lacertilian telencephalon with comments of vertebrate forebrain evolution." In S. O. E. Ebbesson (Ed.), *Comparative Neurology of the Telencephalon*, Plenum, New York, pp. 297–329.

Butler, A. B., and F. F. Ebner (1972). Thalamotelencephalic projections in the lizard *Iguana iguana. Anat. Rec.*, **172**, 282.

Butler, A. B., and R. G. Northcutt (1971). Ascending tectal efferent projections in the lizard *Iguana iguana. Brain Res.*, **35**, 597–601.

Cairney, J. (1926). A general survey of the forebrain of *Sphenodon punctatum. J. Comp. Neurol.*, **42**, 255–348.

Campbell, C. B. G., and W. Hodos (1970). The concept of homology and the evolution of the nervous system. *Brain Behav. Evol.*, **3**, 353–367.

Canady, R., D. Kroodsma, and F. Nottebohm (1981). Significant differences in volume of song control nuclei is associated with variance in song repertoire in a free ranging bird. *Neurosci. Abstr.*, **7**, 845.

Carey, J. H. (1967). The striatum in the box turtle, *Terrapene c. carolina. Ala. J. Med. Sci.*, **4**, 381–389.

Carey, J. H. (1970). The amygdala of the box turtle, *Terrapene c. carolina. J. Comp. Neurol.*, **138**, 251–264.

Carlson, M., and C. Welt (1981). "The somatic sensory cortex: Sm I in prosimian primates." In C. N. Woolsey (Ed.), *Cortical Sensory Organization, Vol. 1, Multiple Somatic Areas*, Humana, Clifton, New Jersey, pp. 1–28.

Caroll, R. L. (1969). "Origin of Reptiles." In C. Gans, A. d'A. Bellairs, and T. S. Parsons (Eds.), *Biology of the Reptilia*, Academic Press, London, Vol. 1, pp. 1–44.

Carpenter, R. H. S. (1977). *Movements of the Eyes.* Pion, London.

Case, E. C. (1897). On the foramina perforating the cranial cavity of a permian reptile and on a cast of its brain cavity. *Am. J. Sci.*, **3**, 321–326.

Caviness, V. S., and D. O. Frost (1980). Tangential organization of thalamic projections to the neocortex in the mouse. *J. Comp. Neurol.*, **194**, 335–367.

Clark, J. M., and P. J. Ulinski (1982). Structure of the anterior dorsoventricular ridge of *Alligator. Am. Zool.*, **22**, 945.

Clarke, P. G. H., and D. Whitteridge (1976). The projection of the retina, including the "red area," in the pigeon. *Q. J. Exp. Physiol.*, **61**, 351–358.

Cohen, D. H. (1975). Involvement of the avian amygdalar homologue (archistriatum posterior and mediale) in defensively conditioned heart rate change. *J. Comp. Neurol.*, **160**, 13–36.

Cohen, D. H. (1980). "The functional neuroanatomy of a conditioned response." In R. F. Thompson, L. H. Hicks, and V. B. Shvyrkov (Eds.), *Neural Mechanisms of Goal-Directed Behavior and Learning*, Academic Press, New York, pp. 283–302.

Cohen, D. H., and H. J. Karten (1974). "The structural organization of avian brain: An overview." In I. J. Goodman and M. W. Schein (Eds.), *Birds: Brain and Behavior*, Academic Press, New York, pp. 29–73.

Cohen, D. H., and D. A. Trauner (1969). Studies of avian visual pathways involved in cardiac conditioning: Nucleus rotundus and ectostriatum. *Exp. Brain Res.*, **7**, 133–142.

Contestabile, A., and A. DiPardo (1976). Enzymatic patterns in the reptilian brain. Histochemical characterization of the telencephalon. *Monitore Zool. Ital.* (N.S.) **10**, 315–332.

Cooke, J. (1980). Early organization of the central nervous system: Form and pattern. *Curr. Top. Dev. Biol.*, **15**, 373–407.

Cowan, W. M., and M. Cuénod (1975). *The Use of Axonal Transport for Studies of Neuronal Connectivity*, Elsevier, Amsterdam.

Cowey, A. (1981). "Why are there so many visual areas?" In F. O. Schmitt, F. G. Worden, G. Adelman, and S. G. Dennis (Eds.), *The Organization of the Cerebral Cortex*, MIT Press, Cambridge, Massachusetts, pp. 395–413.

Craigie, E. H. (1928). Observations on the brain of the humming bird (*Chrysolampis mosquitus* Linn. and *Chlorostibon caribaeus* Lawr.). *J. Comp. Neurol.*, **45**, 377–481.

Craigie, E. H. (1930). Studies on the brain of the kiwi. *J. Comp. Neurol.*, **49**, 223–357.

Craigie, E. H. (1932). The cell structure of the cerebral hemisphere in the humming bird. *J. Comp. Neurol.*, **56**, 135–168.

Craigie, E. H. (1935a). The cerebral hemispheres of the kiwi and the emu (*Apteryx* and *Dromiceius*). *J. Anat. (London)*, **69**, 380–393.

Craigie, E. H. (1935b). Some features of the pallium of the cassowary (*Casuarius uniappendiculatus*). *Anat. Anz.*, **81**, 16–28.

Craigie, E. H. (1936). The cerebral cortex of the ostrich (*Struthio*). *J. Comp. Neurol.*, **64**, 389–415.

Craigie, E. H. (1939). The cerebral cortex of *Rhea americana*. *J. Comp. Neurol.*, **70**, 331–353.

Crews, D., and N. Greenberg (1981). Function and causation of social signals in lizards. *Am. Zool.*, **21**, 273–294.

Crompton, A. W., and F. A. Jenkins, Jr. (1979). "Origin of mammals." In J. A. Lillegraven, Z. Kielan-Jaworowska, and W. A. Clemens (Eds.), *Mesozoic Mammals*, Univ. California, Berkeley, pp. 59–73.

Crompton, A. W., and P. Parker (1978). Evolution of the mammalian masticatory apparatus. *Am. Sci.*, **66**, 192–201.

Crosby, E. C. (1917). The forebrain of *Alligator mississippiensis*. *J. Comp. Neurol.*, **27**, 325–403.

Crossland, W. J. (1972). Receptive field characteristics of some thalamic visual nuclei of the pigeon (*Columba livia*). Doctoral Dissertation, University of Illinois, Urbana.

Cruce, W. L. R. (1975). Termination of supraspinal descending pathways in the spinal cord of the tegu lizard (*Tupinambis nigropunctatus*). *Brain Behav. Evol.*, **12**, 247–269.

Cruce, W. L. R. (1979). "Spinal cord in lizards." In C. Gans, R. G. Northcutt, and P. S. Ulinski (Eds.), *Biology of the Reptilia*, Academic Press, London, Vol. 10, pp. 111–131.

Cruce, J. A. F., and W. L. R. Cruce (1978). "Analysis of the visual system in a lizard, *Tupinambis nigropunctatus*." In N. Greenberg and P. D. MacLean (Eds.), *Behavior and Neurology of Lizards*, NIMH, Rockville, Maryland, pp. 79–90.

Cruce, W. L. R., and D. B. Newman (1981). Brain stem origins of spinal projections in the lizard *Tupinambis nigropunctatus*. *J. Comp. Neurol.*, **198**, 185–208.

Curwen, A. O. (1938). The telencephalon of *Tupinambis nigropunctatus*. II. Corpus striatum. *J. Comp. Neurol.*, **69**, 229–247.

Dacey, D. M. (1982). The optic tectum in the snake *Thamnophis sirtalis*. Ph.D. Dissertation, University of Chicago.

Dacey, D. M., and P. S. Ulinski (1983). Nucleus rotundus in a snake (*Thamnophis sirtalis*). *J. Comp. Neurol.*, In Press.

De Britto, L. R. G., M. Brunelli, W. Francesconi, and F. Magni (1975). Visual response pattern of thalamic neurons in the pigeon. *Brain Res.*, **97**, 337–343.

DeFina, A. V., and D. B. Webster (1974). Projections of the intraotic ganglion to the medullary nuclei in the tegu lizard, *Tupinambis nigropunctatus*. *Brain Behav. Evol.*, **10**, 197–211.

de Lanerolle, N. C., R. P. Elde, S. B. Sparber, and M. Frick (1981). Distribution of methionine-enkephalin immunoreactivity in the chick brain: An immunohistochemical study. *J. Comp. Neurol.*, **199**, 513–534.

Delius, J. D. (1971). Neural substrates of vocalization in gulls and pigeons. *Exp. Brain Res.*, **12**, 64–80.

Delius, J. D., and K. Bennetto (1972). Cutaneous sensory projections to the avian forebrain. *Brain Res.*, **37**, 205–221.

Delius, J. D., T. E. Runge, and H. Oeckinghaus (1979). Short-latency auditory projection to the frontal telencephalon of the pigeon. *Exp. Neurol.*, **63**, 594–609.

Dendy, A. (1899). Outlines of the development of the tuatara. *Q. J. Micros. Sci., N.S.*, **43**, 1–88.

DeVoogd, T. J., and F. Nottebohm (1981). Sex differences in dendritic morphology of a song control nucleus in the canary: A quantitative Golgi study. *J. Comp. Neurol.*, **196**, 309–316.

Distel, H., and S. O. E. Ebbesson (1975). Connections of the thalamus in the monitor lizard. *Soc. Neurosci. Abstr.*, **1**, 559.

Dobrokhotova, I. (1981). Fine structural morphology of paleostriatum and neostriatum neurons of birds which vary their extrapolative capabilities. *Doklady Biol. Sci.*, **257**, 200–202.

Dray, A. (1979). The striatum and substantia nigra: A commentary on their relationships. *Neuroscience*, **4**, 1407–1439.

Dubbeldam, J. L. (1980). Studies on the somatotopy of the trigeminal system in the mallard, *Anas platyrhynchos* L. II. Morphology of the principal sensory nucleus. *J. Comp. Neurol.*, **191**, 557–571.

Dubbeldam, J. L., C. S. M. Brauch, and A. Don (1981). Studies on the somatotopy of the trigeminal system in the mallard, *Anas platyrhynchos* L. III. Afferents and organization of the nucleus basalis. *J. Comp. Neurol.*, **196**, 391–405.

Dubbeldam, J. L., and H. J. Karten (1978). The trigeminal system in the pigeon (*Columba livia*). I. Projections of the Gasserian ganglion. *J. Comp. Neurol.*, **180**, 661–678.

Dubbeldam, J. L., and C. L. Veenman (1978). Studies on the somatotopy of the trigeminal system in the mallard, *Anas platyrhynchos* L. I. The ganglion trigeminale. *Neth. J. Zool.*, **28**, 150–160.

Dubbeldam, J. L., and J. P. M. Wijsman (1975). The ascending projections of the principal sensory trigeminal nucleus in the mallard (*Anas platyrhynchos*). *Acta Morphol. Neerl.-Scand.*, **13**, 230–231.

Dubbeldam, J. L., E. R. Brus, S. B. J. Menken, and S. Zeilstra (1979). The central projections of the glossopharyngeal and vagus ganglia in the mallard, *Anas platyrhynchos* L. *J. Comp. Neurol.*, **183**, 149–168.

Dubé, L., and A. Parent (1978). Histofluorescence study of the catecholaminergic innervation of the avian forebrain. *Neurosci. Abstr.*, **4**, 271.

Dubé, L., and A. Parent (1981). The monoamine-containing neurons in avian brain: I. A study of the brain stem of the chicken (*Gallus domesticus*) by means of fluorescence and acetylcholinesterase histochemistry. *J. Comp. Neurol.*, **196**, 695–708.

Dünser, K. R., J. H. Maxwell, and A. M. Granda (1981). Motion sensitivity in turtle anterior dorsal ventricular ridge. *Neurosci. Abstr.*, **7**, 461.

Dünser, K. R., A. M. Granda, J. H. Maxwell, and J. E. Fulbrook (1981). Visual properties of cells in anterior dorsal ventricular ridge of turtle. *Neurosci. Lett.*, **25**, 281–285.

Durward, A. (1930). The cell masses in the forebrain of *Sphenodon punctatum. J. Anat. (London)*, **65**, 8–44.

Durward, A. (1932). Observations on the cell masses in the cerebral hemisphere of the New Zealand kiwi (*Apteryx australis*). *J. Anat. (London)*, **66**, 437–477.

Durward, A. (1934). Some observations on the development of the corpus striatum of birds with especial reference to certain stages in the common sparrow (*Passer domesticus*). *J. Anat. (London)*, **68**, 492–497.

Ebbesson, S. O. E. (1967). Ascending axon degeneration following hemisection of the spinal cord in the tegu lizard, *Tupinambis nigropunctatus. Brain Res.*, **5**, 178–206.

Ebbesson, S. O. E. (1969). Brain stem afferents from the spinal cord in a sample of reptilian and amphibian species. *Ann. N.Y. Acad. Sci.*, **167**, 80–101.

Ebbesson, S. O. E. (1970). "The selective silver-impregnation of degenerating axons and their synaptic endings in nonmammalian species." In W. J. H. Nauta and S. O. E. Ebbesson (Eds.), *Contemporary Research Methods in Neuroanatomy*, Springer-Verlag, Berlin, pp. 132–161.

Ebbesson, S. O. E. (1978). "Somatosensory pathways in lizards: The identification of the medial lemniscus and related structures." In N. Greenberg and P. D. MacLean (Eds.), *Behavior and Neurology of Lizards*, NIMH, Rockville, Maryland, pp. 91–104.

Ebbesson, S. O. E., and D. C. Goodman (1981). Organization of ascending spinal projections in *Caiman crocodilus. Cell Tis. Res.*, **215**, 383–396.

Ebbesson, S. O. E., and R. G. Northcutt (1976). "Neurology of anamniotic vertebrates. In R. B. Masterton, C. B. G. Campbell, M. E. Bitterman, and N. Hotton (Eds.), *Evolution of Brain and Behavior in Vertebrates*, Wiley, New York, pp. 115–146.

Ebner, F. F., and M. Colonnier (1975). Synaptic patterns in the visual cortex of turtle: An electron microscopic study. *J. Comp. Neurol.*, **160**, 51–80.

Ebner, F. F., and R. E. Myers (1975). Distribution of corpus callosum and anterior commissure in cat and raccoon. *J. Comp. Neurol.*, **124**, 353–366.

Edinger, L., A. Wallenberg, and G. Holmes (1903). Untersuchungen über die vergleichende Anatomie des Gehirns. 5. Das Vorderhirn der Vogel. *Abhandl. Senckenb. Nat. Gesellsch.*, **20**, 343–426.

Edinger, T. (1956). Objects et résultats de la paleoneurologie. *Ann. Paleontol.*, **42**, 97–116.

Edinger, T. (1964). Midbrain exposure and overlap in mammals. *Am. Zool.*, **4**, 5–19.

Eleftheriou, B. E. (1972). *The Neurobiology of the Amygdala*, Plenum, New York.

Elliot Smith, G. (1919). A preliminary note on the morphology of the corpus striatum and the origin of the neopallium. *J. Anat. (London)*, **53**, 271–291.

Elprana, D. F., G. Wouterlood, and V. E. Alones (1980). A corticotectal projection in the lizard *Agama agama. Neurosci. Lett.*, **18**, 251–256.

Erulkar, D. S. (1955). Tactile and auditory areas of the brain of the pigeon. An experimental study by means of evoked potentials. *J. Comp. Neurol.*, **103**, 421–458.

Evarts, E. V. (1970). Central control of movement. *Neurosci. Res. Prog. Bull.*, **9**, 1–170.

Ewert, J. P. (1982). Advances in vertebrate neuroethology. *Trends Neurosci.*, **5**, 141–143.

Faber, D. S., and H. K. Korn (1978). *Neurobiology of the Mauthner Cell*, Raven, New York.

Faccioli, G., and G. Minelli (1975). Diencephalic degenerations following ablation of a telencephalic hemisphere in *Coturnix coturnix japonica. Boll. Zool.*, **42**, 1–7.

Ferster, D., and S. LeVay (1978). The axonal arborizations of lateral geniculate neurons in the striate cortex of the cat. *J. Comp. Neurol.*, **182**, 923–944.

Fetz, E. E. (1981). "Neuronal activity associated with conditioned limb movements." In A. L. Towe and E. S. Luschei (Eds.), *Handbook of Behavioral Neurobiology*, Vol. 5, *Motor Coordination*, Plenum, New York, pp. 493–526.

Fitzpatrick, K. A., and T. J. Imig (1982). "Organization of auditory connections. The primate auditory cortex." In C. N. Woolsey (Ed.), *Cortical Sensory Organization*, Vol. 3, *Multiple Auditory Areas*, Humana, Clifton, New Jersey, pp. 71–109.

Foster, R. E., and W. C. Hall (1978). The organization of central auditory pathways in a reptile, *Iguana iguana*. *J. Comp. Neurol.*, **178**, 783–832.

Fox, C. A., D. E. Hillman, and K. A. Siegesmund, and L. Sether (1966). "The primate globus pallidus and its feline and avian homologues; a Golgi and electron microscopic study." In R. Hassler and H. Stephan (Eds.), *Evolution of the Forebrain*, Thieme, Stuttgart, pp. 237–248.

Frost, D. O., and V. S. Caviness (1980). Radial organization of thalamic projections to the neocortex in the mouse. *J. Comp. Neurol.*, **194**, 369–393.

Fulbrook, J. E. (1982). Motion sensitivity of optic nerve axons in turtle, *Pseudemys scripta elegans*. Ph.D. Dissertation, University of Delaware.

Fulbrook, J. E., and A. M. Granda (1977). Receptive field properties of retinal ganglion cells in turtle. *Neurosci. Abstr.*, **3**, 560.

Fulbrook, J. E., A. M. Granda, and J. H. Maxwell (1980). Velocity tuning of retinal ganglion cells in turtle (*Pseudemys*). *Neurosci. Abstr.*, **6**, 347.

Fuxe, K., and L. Ljungren (1965). Cellular localization of monoamine in the upper brain stem of the pigeon. *J. Comp. Neurol.*, **125**, 355–382.

Gaidenko, G. V. (1978). Efferent connections of the dorsal cortex in tortoises. *J. Evol. Biochem. Physiol.*, **13**, 268–270.

Galambos, R., and F. G. Worden (1972). Auditory processing of biological significant sounds. *Neurosci. Res. Prog. Bull.*, **10**, 1–119.

Gallistel, C. R. (1980). *The Organization of Action: A New Synthesis*. Erlbaum, Hillsdale, New Jersey.

Gamble, H. J. (1952). An experimental study of the secondary olfactory connections in *Lacerta viridis*. *J. Anat. (London)*, **86**, 180–196.

Gamble, H. J. (1956). An experimental study of the secondary olfactory connexions in *Testudo graeca*. *J. Anat. (London)*, **90**, 15–29.

Gamlin, P. D. R., and D. H. Cohen (1982). A possible second ascending avian tectofugal pathway. *Neurosci. Abstr.*, **8**, 206.

Getting, P. A. (1974). Modification of neuron properties by electrotonic synapses. I. Input resistance, time constant, and integration. *J. Neurophysiol.*, **37**, 846–857.

Getting, P. A., and A. O. D. Willows (1974). Modification of neuron properties by electrotonic synapses. II. Burst formation by electrotonic synapses. *J. Neurophysiol.*, **37**, 858–868.

Ghiselin, M. T. (1976). "The nomenclature of correspondence: A new look at "homology" and "analogy." In R. B. Masterton, W. Hodos, and H. Jerison (Eds.), *Evolution, Brain and Behavior: Persistent Problems*, Erlbaum, Hillsdale, New Jersey, pp. 129–142.

Gilbert, C. D., and J. P. Kelly (1975). The projections of cells in different layers of the cat's visual cortex. *J. Comp. Neurol.*, **163**, 81–106.

Gilbert, C. D., and T. N. Wiesel (1981). "Laminar specialization and intracortical connections in cat primary visual cortex." In F. O. Schmitt, F. G. Worden, G. Adelman, and S. G. Dennis (Eds.), *The Organization of the Cerebral Cortex*, MIT Press, Cambridge, Massachusetts, pp. 163–194.

Gogan, P. (1963). Projections sensorielles au niveau du telencephale chez le pigeon sans anaesthesie general. *J. Physiol. (Paris)*, **55**, 258–269.

Goldby, F. (1934). The cerebral hemispheres of *Lacerta viridis*. *J. Anat. (London)*, **68**, 157–215.

Goldby, F., and L. R. Robinson (1962). The central connections of dorsal spinal nerve roots and the ascending tracts in the spinal cord of *Lacerta viridis*. *J. Anat. (London)*, **96**, 153–170.

Goldman, P. S., and W. J. H. Nauta (1977). An intricately patterned prefronto-caudate projection in the rhesus monkey. *J. Comp. Neurol.*, **171**, 369–386.

Goldman-Rakic, P. S. (1982). Cytoarchitectonic heterogeneity of the primate neostriatum: Subdivision into *Island* and *Matrix* cellular components. *J. Comp. Neurol.*, **205**, 398–413.

Gottschaldt, K. M. (1974). The physiological basis of tactile sensibility in the beak of geese. *J. Comp. Physiol.*, **95**, 29–47.

Gottschaldt, K. M., and S. Lausmann (1974). The peripheral morphological basis of the tactile sensibility in the beak of geese. *Cell Tis. Res.*, **153**, 477–496.

Gottschaldt, K. M., H. Fruhstorfer, W. Schmidt, and I. Kraff (1982). Thermosensitivity and its possible fine-structural basis in mechanoreceptors in the beak skin of geese. *J. Comp. Neurol.*, **205**, 219–245.

Graham Brown, T. (1911). The intrinsic factors in the act of progression in the mammal. *Proc. R. Soc. London, Ser. B*, **84**, 308–319.

Granda, A. M., and S. Yazulla (1971). The spectral sensitivity of single units in the nucleus rotundus of pigeon (*Columba livia*). *J. Gen. Physiol.*, **57**, 363–384.

Grantyn, A., and R. Grantyn (1982). Axonal patterns and sites of termination of cat superior colliculus neurons in the tecto-bulbo-spinal tract. *Exp. Brain Res.*, **46**, 243–256.

Graybiel, A. M., and D. M. Berson (1980). "On the relation between transthalamic and transcortical pathways in the visual system." In F. O. Schmitt, F. G. Worden, G. Adelman, and S. G. Dennis (Eds.), *The Organization of the Cerebral Cortex*, MIT Press, Cambridge, Massachusetts, pp. 286–319.

Greenberg, N. (1977). A neuroethological study of display behavior in the lizard *Anolis carolinensis* (Reptilia, Lacertilia, Iguanidae). *Am. Zool.*, **17**, 191–201.

Greenberg, N. (1978). "Ethological considerations in the experimental study of lizard behavior." In N. Greenberg and P. D. MacLean (Eds.), NIMH, Rockville, Maryland, pp. 203–224.

Greenberg, N., P. D. MacLean, and J. L. Ferguson (1979). Role of the paleostriatum in species-typical display behavior of the lizard (*Anolis carolinensis*). *Brain Res.*, **172**, 229–241.

Gregory, J. E. (1973). An electrophysiological investigation of the receptor apparatus of the duck's bill. *J. Physiol. (London)*, **229**, 151–164.

Grillner, S. (1975). Locomotion in the vertebrates—Central mechanisms and reflex interaction. *Physiol. Rev.*, **55**, 247–304.

Grofova, I. (1978). "Extrinsic connections of the neostriatum." In I. Divac and R. G. E. Oberg (Eds.), *The Neostriatum*, Pergamon, Oxford, pp. 37–51.

Gross, C. G., C. J. Bruce, R. Desimone, J. Flemming, and R. Gattass (1981). "Cortical visual areas of the temporal lobe. Three areas in the *Macaque*." In C. N. Woolsey (Ed.), *Cortical Sensory Organization*, Vol. 2, *Multiple Visual Areas*, Humana, Clifton, New Jersey, pp. 187–216.

Gurney, M. E. (1981). Hormonal control of cell form and number in the zebra finch song system. *J. Neurosci.*, **1**, 658–673.

Gurney, M. E., and M. Konishi (1980). Hormone induced sexual differentiation of brain and behavior in zebra finches. *Science*, **208**, 1380–1382.

Guselnikov, V. I., E. D. Morenkov, and A. S. Pivavarov (1970). On functional organization of the visual system of the tortoise (*Emys orbicularis*). *Fiziol. Zh. SSSR Sechenova*, **56**, 1377–1385.

Haartsen, A. B., and W. J. C. Verhaart (1967). Cortical projections to brain stem and spinal cord in the goat by way of the pyramidal tract and the bundle of Bagley. *J. Comp. Neurol.*, **129**, 189–201.

Haefelfinger, H. R. (1958). *Beitrage zur vergleichenden Ontogenese des Vorderhirns bei Vogeln*, Helbing and Lichtenhahn, Basel.

Hahn, M. E., C. Jensen, and B. C. Dudek (1979). *Development and Evolution of Brain Size*, Academic Press, New York.

Hall, W. C., and F. F. Ebner (1970a). Parallels in the visual afferent projections of the thalamus in the hedgehog (*Paraechinus hypomelas*) and the turtle (*Pseudemys scripta*). *Brain Behav. Evol.*, **3**, 135–154.

Hall, W. C., and F. F. Ebner (1970b). Thalamo telencephalic projections in the turtle (*Pseudemys scripta*). *J. Comp. Neurol.*, **140**, 101–122.

Halpern, M. (1976). The efferent connections of the olfactory bulb and accessory olfactory bulb in the snakes, *Thamnophis sirtalis* and *Thamnophis radix*. *J. Morphol.*, **150**, 553–578.

Halpern, M. (1980). "The telencephalon of snakes." In S. O. E. Ebbesson (Ed.), *Comparative Neurology of the Telencephalon*, Plenum, New York, pp. 257–295.

Halpern, M., and N. Frumin (1973). Retinal projections in a snake, *Thamnophis sirtalis*. *J. Morphol.*, **141**, 359–382.

Halpern, M., and J. L. Kubie (1980). Chemical access to the vomeronasal organs of garter snakes. *Physiol. Behav.*, **24**, 367–371.

Halpern, M., J. I. Morrell, and D. W. Pfaff (1982). Cellular [^{3}H]estradiol and [^{3}H]testosterone localization in the brains of garter snakes: An autoradiographic study. *Gen. Comp. Endocrinol.*, **46**, 211–224.

Halpern, M., and R. Silfen (1974). The efferent connections of the nucleus sphericus in the snake, *Thamnophis sirtalis*. *Anat. Rec.*, **178**, 368.

Hamburger, V., and H. Hamilton (1951). A series of normal stages in the development of the chick embryo. *J. Morphol.*, **88**, 49–92.

Hamdi, F. A., and D. Whitteridge (1954). The representation of the retina on the optic tectum of the pigeon. *Q. J. Exp. Physiol.*, **39**, 111–119.

Harman, A. L., and R. E. Phillips (1967). Responses in the avian midbrain, thalamus and forebrain evoked by click stimuli. *Exp. Neurol.*, **18**, 276–286.

Harting, J. K., I. T. Diamond, and W. C. Hall (1973). Anterograde degeneration study of the cortical projections of the lateral geniculate and pulvinar nuclei in the tree shrew (*Tupaia glis*). *J. Comp. Neurol.*, **150**, 393–440.

Harting, J. K., and M. F. Huerta (1983). "The mammalian superior colliculus: studies of its morphology and connections." In H. Vanegas (Ed.), *The Comparative Neurology of the Optic Tectum*, Plenum, In Press.

Hartline, P. (1971). Physiological basis for detection of sound and vibration in snakes. *J. Exp. Biol.*, **54**, 349–371.

Heimer, L. (1969). The secondary olfactory connections in mammals, reptiles and sharks. *Ann. N.Y. Acad. Sci.*, **167**, 129–146.

Hendrickson, A. E., J. R. Wilson, and M. P. Ogren (1978). The neuroanatomical organization of pathways between the dorsal lateral geniculate nucleus and visual cortex in old world and new world primates. *J. Comp. Neurol.*, **182**, 123–136.

Heric, T. M., and L. Kruger (1965). Organization of the visual projection upon the optic tectum of a reptile (*Alligator mississippiensis*). *J. Comp. Neurol.*, **124**, 101–112.

Herrick, C. J. (1926). *Brains of Rats and Men*. Univ. Chicago Press.

Herrick, C. J. (1948). *The Brain of the Tiger Salamander*. Univ. Chicago Press.

Herrick, C. L. (1892). Embryological notes on the brain of the snake. *J. Comp. Neurol.*, **2**, 160–176.

Hetzel, W. von (1974). Die Ontogenese des Telencephalons bei *Lacerta sicula* (Rafinesque), mit besonderer Berucksichtigung der palliallen Entwicklung. *Zool. Beit. N. S.*, **20**, 361–458.

Hewitt, W. (1967). The basal ganglia of *Testudo graeca*. *J. Comp. Neurol.*, **131**, 605–614.

Hines, M. (1923). The development of the telencephalon in *Sphenodon punctatum*. *J. Comp. Neurol.*, **35**, 483–537.

His, W. (1888). Zur Geschichte des Gehirns, sowie der centralen und peripherischen Nervenbahnen beim menshlichen Embryo. *Abk. K. Sachs. Ges. Wiss. Math.-Phys. Kl.*, **14**, 341–372.

Hodos, W. (1970). "Evolutionary interpretation of neural and behavioral studies of living vertebrates." In F. O. Schmitt (Ed.), *The Neurosciences: Second Study Program*, Rockefeller Univ., New York, pp. 26–38.

Hodos, W. (1976). Vision and the visual system: A bird's-eye view. *Prog. Psychobiol. Physiol. Psychol.*, **6**, 29–62.

Hodos, W., and C. B. G. Campbell (1969). *Scala naturae*: Why there is no theory in comparative psychology. *Psychol. Rev.*, **76**, 337–350.

Holcombe, V., and W. C. Hall (1981a). The laminar origin of ipsilateral tectopontine pathway. *Neuroscience*, **6**, 255–260.

Holcombe, V., and W. C. Hall (1981b). The laminar origin and distribution of the crossed tectoreticular pathways. *J. Neurosci.*, **1**, 1103–1112.

Holmgren, N. (1925). Points of view concerning forebrain morphology in higher vertebrates. *Acta Zool.*, **6**, 415–477.

Hoogland, P. V. (1977). Efferent connections of the striatum in *Tupinambis nigropunctatus*. *J. Morphol.*, **152**, 229–246.

Hoogland, P. V. (1981). Spinothalamic projections in a lizard, *Varanus exanthematicus*: An HRP study. *J. Comp. Neurol.*, **198**, 7–12.

Hoogland, P. V. (1982). Brainstem afferents to the thalamus in a lizard, *Varanus Exanthematicus*. *J. Comp. Neurol.*, **210**, 152–162.

Hoogland, P. V., H. J. ten Donkelaar, and J. A. F. Cruce (1978). Efferent connections of the septal area in a lizard. *Neurosci. Lett.*, **7**, 1–6.

Hopkins, D. A. (1975). Amygdalo-tegmental projections in the rat, cat and monkey. *Neurosci. Lett.*, **1**, 263–270.

Hopkins, D. A., and G. Holstege (1978). Amygdaloid projections to the mesencephalon, pons and medulla oblongata in the cat. *Exp. Brain Res.*, **32**, 529–547.

Hopson, J. A. (1969). The origin and adaptive radiation of mammal-like reptiles and nontherian mammals. *Ann. N.Y. Acad. Sci.*, **167**, 199–216.

Hopson, J. A. (1979). "Paleoneurology." In C. C. Gans, R. G. Northcutt, and P. S. Ulinski (Eds.), *Biology of the Reptilia*, Academic Press, London, Vol. 9, pp. 39–146.

Hopson, J. A. (1980). "Relative brain size in dinosaurs: implications for dinosaurian endothermy." In R. D. K. Thomas, and E. C. Olson (Eds.), *A Cold Look at the Warm-Blooded Dinosaurs*, Westview Press, Boulder, Colorado, pp. 287–310.

Hubel, D. H. (1975). An autoradiographic study of the retino-cortical projections in the tree shrew (*Tupaia glis*). *Brain Res.*, **96**, 41–50.

Hubel, D. H. (1981). "Columns and their function in the primate visual cortex." In W. E. Reichardt and T. Poggio (Eds.), *Theoretical Approaches in Neurobiology*. MIT Press, Cambridge, Massachusetts, pp. 109–115.

Hubel, D. H., and T. N. Wiesel (1962). Receptive fields, binocular interaction and functional architecture in the cat's visual cortex. *J. Physiol. (London)*, **160**, 106–154.

Hubel, D. H., and T. N. Wiesel (1963). Shape and arrangement of columns in cat's striate cortex. *J. Physiol. (London)*, **165**, 559–568.

Hubel, D. H., and T. N. Wiesel (1972). Laminar and columnar distribution of geniculocortical fibers in the macaque monkey. *J. Comp. Neurol.*, **146**, 421–450.

Hubel, D. H., and T. N. Wiesel (1974). Sequence regularity and geometry of orientation columns in the monkey striate cortex. *J. Comp. Neurol.*, **158**, 267–295.

Hubel, D. H., and T. N. Wiesel (1977). Functional architecture of the macaque monkey visual cortex. *Proc. R. Soc. London, Ser. B*, **196**, 1–59.

Hubel, D. H., T. N. Wiesel, and S. LeVay (1976). Functional architecture of area 17 in normal and monocularly deprived macaque monkeys. *Cold Spring Harbor Symp. Quant. Biol.*, **40**, 581–589.

Hubel, D. H., T. N. Wiesel, and M. Stryker (1978). Anatomical demonstration of orientation columns in macaque monkey. *J. Comp. Neurol.*, **177**, 361–379.

Huber, G. C., and E. C. Crosby (1926). On thalamic and tectal nuclei and fiber paths in the brain of the American alligator. *J. Comp. Neurol.*, **40**, 97–227.

Hughes, C. P., and A. L. Pearlman (1974). Single unit receptive fields and the cellular layers of the pigeon optic tectum. *Brain Res.*, **80**, 365–377.

Humphrey, A. L., and T. S. Norton (1980). Topographic organization of the orientation column system in the striate cortex of the tree shrew (*Tupaia glis*). I. Microelectrode recording. *J. Comp. Neurol.*, **192**, 531–547.

Humphrey, O. D. (1894). On the brain of the snapping turtle: *Chelydra serpentina*. *J. Comp. Neurol.*, **4**, 73–116.

Hunt, S. P., and H. Künzle (1976). Observations on the projections and intrinsic organization of the pigeon optic tectum: An autoradiographic study based on anterograde and retrograde axonal and dendritic flow. *J. Comp. Neurol.*, **170**, 153–172.

Hunt, S. P., and K. E. Webster (1975). The projection of the retina upon the optic tectum of the pigeon. *J. Comp. Neurol.*, **162**, 433–466.

Hunter, J. (1861). *Essays and Observations on Natural History, Anatomy, Physiology, Psychology and Geology*, J. VanVoorst, London.

Ikeda, H., and J. Gotoh (1971). Distribution of monoamine-containing cells in the central nervous system of the chicken. *Jpn. J. Pharmacol.*, **21**, 763–784.

Iljtschow, V. D. (1966). Electrophysiological study of the hearing centre of the forebrain of birds. *Z. Vyss. Nerv. Deyat I.P. Pavlova*, **16**, 480–488.

Imig, T. J., and H. O. Adrian (1977). Binaural columns in the primary field (AI) of cat auditory cortex. *Brain Res.*, **138**, 241–257.

Imig, T. J., and J. F. Brugge (1978). Sources and terminations of callosal axons related to binaural and frequency maps in primary auditory cortex of the cat. *J. Comp. Neurol.*, **182**, 637–660.

Ingle, D., and J. M. Sprague (1975). Sensorimotor function of the midbrain tectum. *Neurosci. Res. Prog. Bull.*, **13**, 169–288.

Irvine, D. R. F., and D. P. Phillips (1982). "Polysensory 'association' areas of the cerebral cortex: Organization of acoustic input in the cat." In C. N. Woolsey (Ed.), *Cortical Sensory Organization*, Vol. 3, *Multiple Auditory Areas*, Humana, Clifton, New Jersey, pp. 111–156.

Jacobs, V. L., and R. F. Sis (1980). Ascending projections of the dorsal column in a garter snake (*Thamnophis sirtalis*): A degeneration study. *Anat. Rec.*, **196**, 37–50.

Jacobson, M. (1975). "Development and evolution of Type II neurons: Conjectures a century after Golgi." In M. Santini (Ed.), *Golgi Centennial Symposium*, Raven, New York, pp. 147–152.

Jacobson, M. (1978). *Developmental Neurobiology*, 2nd ed., Plenum, New York.

Jassik-Gershenfeld, D., and J. Guichard (1972). Visual receptive fields of single cells in the pigeon's optic tectum. *Brain Res.*, **40**, 303–317.

Jassik-Gerschenfeld, D., J. Guichard, and Y. Tessier (1975). Localization of directionally selective and movement sensitive cells in the optic tectum of the pigeon. *Vision Res.*, **15**, 1037–1038.

Jassik-Gerschenfeld, D., F. Minois, and F. Conde-Courtine (1970). Receptive field properties of directionally selective units in the pigeon's optic tectum. *Brain Res.*, **24**, 407–421.

Jerison, H. J. (1973). *Evolution of the Brain and Intelligence*. Academic Press, New York.

Jerison, H. J. (1977). The theory of encephalization. *Ann. N.Y. Acad. Sci.*, **299**, 146–160.

Johnston, J. B. (1915). The cell masses in the forebrain of the turtle *Cistudo carolina*. *J. Comp. Neurol.*, **25**, 393–468.

Johnston, J. B. (1916). The development of the dorsal ventricular ridge in turtles. *J. Comp. Neurol.*, **26**, 481–505.

Johnson, J. I., J. A. W. Kirsch, and R. C. Switzer III (1982). Phylogeny through brain traits: fifteen characters which adumbrate mammalian genealogy. *Brain Behav. Evol.*, **20**, 72–83.

Jones, A., and R. Levi-Montalcini (1958). Patterns of differentiation of the nerve centers and fiber tracts in the avian cerebral hemispheres. *Arch. Ital. Biol.*, **96**, 231–284.

Jones, E. G. (1981a). "Anatomy of cerebral cortex: columnar input-output organization." In F. O. Schmitt, F. G. Worden, G. Adelman, and S. G. Dennis (Eds.), *The Organization of the Cerebral Cortex*, MIT Press, Cambridge, Massachusetts, pp. 199–236.

Jones, E. G. (1981b). "Development of connectivity in the cerebral cortex." In W. M. Cowan (Ed.), *Studies in Developmental Neurobiology*, Oxford Univ. Press, New York, pp. 354–394.

Jones, E. G., J. D. Coulter, and S. H. C. Hendry (1978). Intracortical connectivity of architectonic fields in the somatic sensory, motor and parietal cortex of monkeys. *J. Comp. Neurol.*, **181**, 291–348.

Jones, E. G., J. D. Coulter, and S. P. Wise (1979). Commissural columns in the sensory-motor cortex of monkeys. *J. Comp. Neurol.*, **188**, 113–136.

Jones, E. G., and S. P. Wise (1977). Size, laminar and columnar distribution of efferent cells in the somatic sensory cortex of monkeys. *J. Comp. Neurol.*, **175**, 391–438.

Joseph, B. S., and D. G. Whitlock (1968). Central projections of brachial and lumbar dorsal roots in reptiles. *J. Comp. Neurol.*, **132**, 469–484.

Juorio, A. V. (1969). The distribution of dopamine in the brain of a tortoise, *Geochelone chilensis* (Gray). *J. Physiol. (London)*, **204**, 503–529.

Juorio, A. V., and M. Vogt (1967). Monoamines and their metabolites in the avian brain. *J. Physiol. (London)*, **189**, 489–518.

Kaas, J. H., C. S. Lin, and V. A. Casagrande (1976). The relay of ipsilateral and contralateral retinal input from the lateral geniculate nucleus to striate cortex in the owl monkey: A transneuronal transport study. *Brain Res.*, **106**, 371–378.

Kaas, J. H., R. J. Nelson, M. Sur, and M. M. Merzenich (1981a). "Organization of somatosensory cortex in primates." In F. O. Schmitt, F. G. Worden, G. Adelman, and S. G. Dennis (Eds.), *The Organization of the Cerebral Cortex*, MIT Press, Cambridge, Massachusetts, pp. 237–261.

Kaas, J. H., M. Sur, R. J. Nelson, and M. M. Merzenich (1981b). "The postcentral somatosensory cortex. Multiple representations of the body in primates." In C. N. Woolsey (Ed.), *Cortical Sensory Organization*, Vol. 1, *Multiple Somatic Areas*, Humana, Clifton, New Jersey, pp. 29–45.

Kalischer, O. (1905). Das Grosshirn der Papageien in anatomischer und physiologischer Beziehung. *Abh. Kon. Press. Akad. Wiss. IV*, **1**, 1–105.

Källén, B. (1951). On the ontogeny of the reptilian forebrain. Nuclear structures and ventricular sulci. *J. Comp. Neurol.*, **95**, 307–347.

Källén, B. (1953). On the nuclear differentiation during ontogenesis of the avian forebrain and some notes on the amniote strio-amygdaloid complex. *Acta Anat.*, **17**, 72–83.

Källén, B. (1956). Notes on the mode of formation of brain nuclei during ontogenesis. *C. R. Assoc. Anat. Reun.*, **42**, 747–756.

Källén, B. (1962). Embryogenesis of brain nuclei in the chick telencephalon. *Ergebn. Anat. Entwicklkungsgesch.*, **36**, 62–82.

Kamon, K. (1906). Zur Entwicklungsgeschicte des Gehirns des Hunchens. *Anat. Hefte*, **30**, 562–650.

Karten, H. J. (1963). Ascending pathways from the spinal cord in the pigeon. *Proc. 16th Int. Congr. Zool.*, **2**, 23.

Karten, H. J. (1965). Projections of the optic tectum of the pigeon (*Columba livia*). *Anat. Rec.*, **151**, 369.

Karten, H. J. (1967). The organization of the avian ascending auditory pathway in the pigeon (*Columba livia*). I. Diencephalic projections of the inferior colliculus (Nucleus mesencephalicus lateralis, pars dorsalis). *Brain Res.*, **6**, 409–427.

Karten, H. J. (1968). The ascending auditory pathway in the pigeon (*Columba livia*). II. Telencephalic projections of the nucleus ovoidalis thalami. *Brain Res.*, **11**, 134–153.

Karten, H. J. (1969). The organization of the avian telencephalon and some speculations on the phylogeny of the amniote telencephalon. *Ann. N.Y. Acad. Sci.*, **167**, 164–180.

Karten, H. J. (1971). Efferent projections of the Wulst of the owl. *Anat. Rec.*, **169**, 353.

Karten, H. J., and J. L. Dubbeldam (1973). The organization and projections of the paleo-striatal complex in the pigeon (*Columba livia*). *J. Comp. Neurol.*, **148**, 61–80.

Karten, H. J., and W. Hodos (1967). *A Stereotaxic Atlas of the Brain of the Pigeon.* Johns Hopkins Press, Baltimore, Maryland.

Karten, H. J., and W. Hodos (1970). Telencephalic projections of the nucleus rotundus in the pigeon (*Columba livia*). *J. Comp. Neurol.,* **140,** 35–52.

Karten, H. J., M. Konishi, and J. Pettigrew (1978). Somatosensory representation in the anterior Wulst of the owl (*Speotyto cunicularia*). *Neurosci. Abstr.,* **4,** 554.

Karten, H. J., and A. M. Revzin (1966). The afferent connections of the nucleus rotundus in the pigeon. *Brain Res.,* **2,** 368–377.

Karten, H. J., W. Hodos, W. J. H. Nauta, and A. M. Revzin (1973). Neural connections of the "visual Wulst" of the avian telencephalon. Experimental studies in the pigeon and owl. *J. Comp. Neurol.,* **150,** 253–278.

Katz, L. C. (1982). The avian motor system for song has multiple sizes and types of auditory input. *Neurosci. Abstr.,* **8,** 1020.

Katz, L. C., and M. E. Gurney (1981). Auditory responses in the zebra finch's motor system for song. *Brain Res.,* **221,** 192–197.

Kawamura, S., J. M. Sprague, and K. Niimi (1974). Corticofugal projections from the visual cortices to the thalamus, pretectum and superior colliculus in the cat. *J. Comp. Neurol.,* **158,** 339–362.

Kelley, D. B., and F. Nottebohm (1976). Projections of field L in the canary, *Serinus canarius*—An autoradiographic study. *Neurosci. Abstr.,* **2,** 21.

Kelley, D. B., and F. Nottebohm (1979). Projections of a telencephalic auditory nucleus—field L—in the canary. *J. Comp. Neurol.,* **183,** 455–470.

Kelly, J. P., and D. Wong (1981). Laminar connections of the cat's auditory cortex. *Brain Res.,* **212,** 1–15.

Kim, Y. S., W. E. Stumpf, and M. Sar (1981). Anatomical distribution of estrogen target neurons in turtle brain. *Brain Res.,* **230,** 195–204.

Kimberly, R. P., A. L. Holden, and P. Bambrough (1971). Response characteristics of pigeon forebrain cells to visual stimulation. *Vision Res.,* **11,** 475–478.

Kirsch, M., R. B. Coles, and H. J. Leppelsack (1980). Unit recordings from a new auditory area in the frontal neostriatum of the awake starling (*Sturnus vulgaris*). *Exp. Brain Res.,* **38,** 375–380.

Kirsche, W. (1972). Die Entwicklung des Telencephalons der Reptilien und deren Beziehung zur hirn-Bauplanlehre. *Nova Acta Leopoldina,* **37,** 1–78.

Kitt, C. A., and S. E. Brauth (1978). Neural connections of the avian lateral corticoid areas. *Neurosci. Abstr.,* **4,** 45.

Kitt, C. A., and S. E. Brauth (1980). Telencephalic projections from catecholamine cell groups in the pigeon. *Neurosci. Abstr.,* **6,** 630.

Kitt, C. A., and S. E. Brauth (1981a). Projections of the paleostriatum upon the midbrain tegmentum in the pigeon. *Neuroscience,* **6,** 1551–1556.

Kitt, C. A., and S. E. Brauth (1981b). A basal ganglia-thalamic-telencephalic pathway in pigeons. *Neurosci. Abstr.,* **7,** 194.

Knudsen, E. I., and M. Konishi (1978). Space and frequency are represented separately in the auditory midbrain of the owl. *J. Neurophysiol.,* **41,** 870–884.

Knudsen, E. I., M. Konishi, and J. D. Pettigrew (1977). Receptive fields of auditory neurons in the owl. *Science,* **198,** 1278–1280.

Konishi, M. (1970). Comparative neurophysiological studies of hearing and vocalizations in song birds. *Z. Vergl. Physiol.*, **66**, 257–272.

Kosareva, A. A. (1974). Afferent and efferent connections of the nucleus rotundus in the tortoise *Emys orbicularis*. *Zn. Evol. Biokhim. Fiziol.*, **10**, 395–399.

Kosareva, A. A., E. V. Ozirskaya, N. L. Tumanova, and G. V. Gaidenko (1973). Structural organization of nucleus rotundus in the brain of the tortoise *Emys orbicularis*. *J. Evol. Biochem. Physiol.*, **9**, 195–201.

Kowell, A. P. (1974). The olfactory and accessory olfactory bulbs in constricting snakes: neuroanatomic and behavioral considerations. Ph.D. Dissertation, The University of Pennsylvania.

Kruger, L., and E. C. Berkowitz (1960). The main afferent connections of the reptilian telencephalon as determined by degeneration and electrophysiological methods. *J. Comp. Neurol.*, **115**, 125–141.

Kruger, L., and P. Witkovsky (1961). A functional analysis of neurons in the dorsal column nuclei and spinal nucleus of the trigeminal in the reptile (*Alligator mississippiensis*). *J. Comp. Neurol.*, **117**, 97–106.

Kubie, J. L. (1977). The role of the vomeronasal organ in garter snake prey trailing and courtship. Ph.D. Dissertation, State Univ. New York, Downstate Medical Center.

Kubie, J. L., and T. O. Allen (1978). Deoxyglucose mapping of the visual system in the garter snake. *Neurosci. Abstr.*, **4**, 100.

Kubie, J. L., and M. Halpern (1978). Garter snake trailing behavior: Effects of varying prey-extract concentration and mode of prey-extract presentation. *J. Comp. Physiol. Psychol.*, **92**, 362–373.

Kubie, J. L., and M. Halpern (1979). Chemical senses involved in garter snake prey trailing. *J. Comp. Physiol. Psychol.*, **93**, 648–667.

Kubie, J. L., A. Vagvolgyi, and M. Halpern (1978). Roles of the vomeronasal and olfactory systems in courtship behavior of male garter snakes. *J. Comp. Physiol. Psychol.*, **92**, 627–641.

Kuhlenbeck, H. (1938). The ontogenetic development and phylogenetic significance of the cortex telencephali in the chick. *J. Comp. Neurol.*, **69**, 273–301.

Kusuma, A., and H. J. ten Donkelaar (1980). Dorsal root projections in various types of reptiles. *Brain Behav. Evol.*, **17**, 291–309.

Kusunoki, T. (1969). The chemoarchitectonics of the avian brain. *J. Hirnforsch.*, **11**, 477–497.

Kusunoki, T. (1971). The chemoarchitectonics of the turtle brain. *Yokohama Med. Bull.*, **22**, 1–29.

Landry, P., and M. Deschenes (1981). Intracortical arborization and receptive fields of identified ventrobasal thalamocortical afferents to the primary somatic sensory cortex in the cat. *J. Comp. Neurol.*, **199**, 345–371.

Langner, G., D. Bonke, and H. Scheich (1981a). Neuronal discrimination of natural and synthetic vowels in field L of the trained mynah bird. *Brain Res.*, **43**, 11–24.

Langner, G., D. Bonke, and H. Scheich (1981b). "Selectivity of auditory neurons for vowels and consonants in the forebrain of the mynah bird." In J. Syka and L. Aitkin (Eds.), *Neuronal Mechanisms of Hearing*, Plenum, New York, pp. 317–321.

Lashley, K. S., and G. Clark (1946). The cytoarchitecture of the cerebral cortex of *Ateles*: A critical examination of architectonic studies. *J. Comp. Neurol.*, **85**, 223–306.

Leake, P. A. (1974). Central projections of the statoacoustic nerve in *Caiman crocodilus*. *Brain Behav. Evol.*, **10**, 170–196.

Leitner, L. M., and M. Roumy (1974). Mechanosensitive units in the upper bill and in the tongue of the domestic duck. *Pflügers Arch.*, **346**, 414–450.

Lende, R. A. (1964). Representation in the cerebral cortex of a primitive mammal. *J. Neurophysiol.*, **27**, 37–48.

Lennard, P. R., and P. S. G. Stein (1977). Swimming movements elicited by electrical stimulation of turtle spinal cord. I. Low spinal and intact preparations. *J. Neurophysiol.*, **40**, 768–778.

Leonard, R. B., and D. H. Cohen (1975). Spinal terminal fields of dorsal root fibers in the pigeon (*Columba livia*). *J. Comp. Neurol.*, **163**, 181–192.

Leppelsack, H. (1974). Funktionelle Eigenschaften der Horbahn im Feld L des Neostriatum caudale des Staren (*Sturnus vulgaris* L., Aves). *J. Comp. Physiol.*, **88**, 271–320.

Leppelsack, H.-J. (1978). Unit responses to species-specific sounds in the auditory forebrain center of birds. *Fed. Proc. Fed. Am. Soc. Exp. Biol.*, **37**, 2336–2341.

Leppelsack, H.-J. (1981). Effects of song learning on auditory neurons in the forebrain of an awake bird. *Neurosci. Abstr.*, **7**, 391.

Leppelsack, H.-J., and J. Schwartzkopf (1972). Eigenschaften von akustichen Neuronen im kaudalen Neostriatum von Vogeln. *J. Comp. Physiol.*, **80**, 127–140.

Leppelsack, H.-J., and M. Vogt (1976). Responses of auditory neurons in the forebrain of a songbird to stimulation with species-specific sounds. *J. Comp. Physiol.*, **107**, 263–274.

LeVay, S., and H. Sherk (1981). The visual claustrum of the cat. I. Structure and connections. *J. Neurosci.*, **1**, 956–980.

Levine, R. R., and H. P. Zeigler (1981). Extratelencephalic pathways and feeding behavior in the pigeon (*Columba livia*). *Brain Behav. Evol.*, **19**, 56–92.

Lewis, J. W., S. M. Ryan, A. P. Arnold, and L. L. Butcher (1981). Evidence for a catecholaminergic projection to area X in the zebra finch. *J. Comp. Neurol.*, **196**, 347–354.

Lipetz, L. E., and R. M. Hill (1970). Discrimination characteristics of the turtle's retinal ganglion cells. *Experentia*, **26**, 373–374.

Lippe, W. R., and R. B. Masterton (1980). The distribution of activity in the avian auditory system to monoaural sound stimulation examined with ^{14}C-2-deoxy-D-glucose autoradiography. *Neurosci. Abstr.*, **6**, 555.

Lohman, A. H. M., and G. M. Mentink (1972). Some cortical connections of the tegu lizard (*Tupinambis teguixin*). *Brain Res.*, **45**, 325–344.

Lohman, A. H. M., and I. van Woerden-Verkley (1976). Further studies on the cortical connections of the tegu lizard. *Brain Res.*, **103**, 9–28.

Lohman, A. H. M., and I. van Woerden-Verkley (1978). Ascending connections to the forebrain in the tegu lizard. *J. Comp. Neurol.*, **182**, 555–594.

Lorente de Nó, R. (1938). "The cerebral cortex." In J. F. Fulton, *Physiology of the Nervous System*, Oxford Univ. Press, London.

Lorenz, K. Z. (1981). *The Foundations of Ethology*. Springer, New York.

Lovejoy, A. O. (1960). *The Great Chain of Being*. Harper, New York.

Lund, J. S. (1981). "Intrinsic organization of the primate visual cortex, area 17, as seen in Golgi preparations." In F. O. Schmitt, F. G. Worden, G. Adelman, and S. G. Dennis (Eds.), *The Organization of the Cerebral Cortex*, MIT Press, Cambridge, Massachusetts, pp. 105–124.

Lund, R. D. (1978). *Development and Plasticity of the Brain*. Oxford Univ. Press, New York.

MacDonald, R. L., and D. H. Cohen (1973). Heart rate and blood pressure responds to electrical stimulation of the central nervous system in the pigeon. *J. Comp. Neurol.*, **150**, 109–136.

Macko, K., and W. Hodos (1979). Near field visual acuity in pigeons following lesions of thalamic visual nuclei. *Neurosci. Abstr.*, **5**, 144.

Manley, G. (1970). Frequency sensitivity of auditory neurons in the *Caiman* cochlear nucleus. *Z. Vergl. Physiol.*, **60**, 251–256.

Manley, J. A. (1971). Single unit studies in the midbrain auditory area of *Caiman*. *Z. Vergl. Physiol.*, **71**, 255–261.

Manogue, K. R., and F. Nottebohm (1982). Relation of medullary motor nuclei to nerves supplying the vocal tract of the budgerigar (*Melopsittacus undulatus*). *J. Comp. Neurol.*, **204**, 384–391.

Manogue, K. R., J. A. Paton and F. Nottebohm (1982). Bilateral interactions within the vocal control pathway of birds. *Neurosci. Abstr.*, **8**, 610.

Marchiafava, P. L., and H. G. Wagner (1981). Interactions leading to colour opponency in ganglion cells of the turtle retina. *Proc. R. Soc. London, Ser. B*, **211**, 261–267.

Marchiafava, P. L., and R. Weiler (1980). Intracellular analysis and structural correlates of the organization of inputs to ganglion cells in the retina of the turtle. *Proc. R. Soc. London, Ser. B*, **208**, 103–113.

Margoliash, D. (1982). Specificity and selectivity of neuronal responses to song in a vocal control nucleus of white-crowned sparrows (*Zonotrichia leucophrys*). *Neurosci. Abstr.*, **8**, 1022.

Martin, G. F., T. Cabana, A. O. Humbertson, Jr., L. C. Laxson, and W. M. Panneton (1981). Spinal projections from the medullary reticular formation of the North American opossum: Evidence for connectional heterogeneity. *J. Comp. Neurol.*, **196**, 663–682.

Martinez-Vargas, M. C., D. A. Keefer, and W. E. Stumpf (1978). Estrogen localization in the brain of the lizard, *Anolis carolinensis*. *J. Exp. Zool.*, **205**, 141–147.

Masai, H., K. Takatsuji, and Y. Sato (1980). Comparative morphology of the telencephalon of the Japanese colubrid snakes under consideration of habit. *Z. Zool. Systematik., Evolutionforsch.*, **18**, 310–314.

Maturana, H. R., and S. Frenk (1963). Directional movement and horizontal edge detectors in the pigeon retina. *Science*, **150**, 977–979.

Maxwell, J. H., and A. M. Granda (1979). "Receptive fields of movement-sensitive cells in the pigeon thalamus." In A. M. Granda and J. H. Maxwell (Eds.), *Neural Mechanisms of Behavior in the Pigeon*, Plenum, New York, pp. 177–198.

Meyer, A. (1893). Über das Vorderhirn einiger Reptilien. *Z. Wiss. Zool.*, **55**, 63–133.

Miceli, D., J. Peyrichoux, and J. Repérant (1975). The retino-thalamo-hyperstriatal pathway in the pigeon (*Columba livia*). *Brain Res.*, **100**, 125–131.

Miceli, D., J. Peyrichoux, J. Repérant, and C. Weidner (1980). Etude anatomique des afferences du telencephale rostral chez le poussin de *Gallus domesticus* L. *J. Hirnforsch.*, **21**, 627–646.

Miles, F. A. (1972). Centrifugal control of the avian retina. I. Receptive field properties of retinal ganglion cells. *Brain Res.*, **48**, 65–92.

Miller, M. R. (1975). The cochlear nuclei of lizards. *J. Comp. Neurol.*, **159**, 375–406.

Miller, M. R. (1980). The cochlear nuclei of snakes. *J. Comp. Neurol.*, **192**, 717–736.

Miller, M. R., and M. Kasahara (1979). The cochlear nuclei of some turtles. *J. Comp. Neurol.*, **185**, 221–236.

Minelli, G. (1970). Histochemical studies on certain enzymatic activities on the encephalon of *Testudo graeca* and *Coturnix coturnix*. *Riv. Biol.*, **63**, 61–86.

Minelli, G., G. Faccioli, and M. DeLiberali (1979). Experimental study on the nervous connections of some diencephalic and mesencephalic nuclei in *Coturnix coturnix japonica*. *J. Hirnforsch.*, **20**, 217–232.

Molenaar, G. J. (1974). An additional trigeminal system in certain snakes possessing infrared receptors. *Brain Res.*, **78**, 340–344.

Molenaar, G. J. (1978a). The sensory trigeminal system of a snake in the possession of infrared receptors. I. The sensory trigeminal nuclei. *J. Comp. Neurol.*, **179**, 123–136.

Molenaar, G. J. (1978b). The sensory trigeminal system of a snake in the possession of infrared receptors. II. The central projections of the trigeminal nerve. *J. Comp. Neurol.*, **179**, 137–152.

Molenaar, G. J., and J. L. F. P. Fizaan-Oostven (1980). Ascending projections from the lateral descending and common sensory trigeminal nuclei in python. *J. Comp. Neurol.*, **189**, 555–572.

Moore, G. P., and R. D. Tschirigi (1962). Non-specific responses of reptilian cortex to sensory stimuli. *Exp. Neurol.*, **5**, 196–209.

Moore, R. Y., and F. E. Bloom (1979). Central catecholamine neuron systems: Anatomy and physiology of the norepinephrine and epinephrine systems. *Annu. Rev. Neurosci.*, **2**, 113–168.

Morenkov, E. D., and A. S. Pivavarov (1973). "Peculiarities of the organization of the visual system in reptiles." In V. I. Guselnikov (Ed.), *Functional Organization and Evolution of the Vertebrate Visual System*, Nauka, Leningrad, pp. 95–107.

Morenkov, E. D., and A. S. Pivavarov (1975). Peculiarities of cell reactions in turtle dorsal and ventral thalamus to visual stimuli. *Zh. Evol. Biokhim. Fiziol.*, **11**, 70–75.

Morgane, P. J., and W. C. Stern (1974). Chemical anatomy of brain circuits in relation to sleep and wakefulness. *Adv. Sleep Res.*, **1**, 1–131.

Morrell, J. I., D. Crews, A. Ballin, A. Morgentaler, and D. W. Pfaff (1979). ^{3}H-Estradiol, ^{3}H-dihydrotestosterone localization in the brain of the lizard *Anolis carolinensis*: An autoradiographic study. *J. Comp. Neurol.*, **188**, 201–224.

Mountcastle, V. B. (1979). "An organizing principle for cerebral function: the unit module and the distributed system." In F. O. Schmitt and F. G. Worden (Eds.), *The Neurosciences Fourth Study Program*, MIT Press, Cambridge, Massachusetts, pp. 21–42.

Mulvanny, P. (1979). "Discrimination of line orientation by pigeons after lesions of thalamic visual nuclei." In A. M. Granda and J. H. Maxwell (Eds.), *Neural Mechanisms of Behavior in the Pigeon*, Plenum, New York, pp. 199–222.

Munger, B. L. (1971). "Patterns of organization in peripheral sensory receptors." In W. R. Lowenstein (Ed.), *Handbook of Sensory Physiology*, Vol. 1, Springer-Verlag, Berlin, pp. 523–556.

Naik, D. R., M. Sar, and W. E. Stumpf (1981). Immunohistochemical localization of enkephalin in the central nervous system and pituitary of the lizard, *Anolis carolinensis*. *J. Comp. Neurol.*, **198**, 583–602.

Naumon, N. P., and W. D. Iljitschow (1964). Klang analyse im Grosshirn der Vogel. *Naturwissenschaften*, **51**, 644.

Nauta, W. J. H., and H. J. Karten (1970). "A general profile of the vertebrate brain, with sidelights on the ancestry of cerebral cortex." In F. O. Schmitt (Éd.), *The Neurosciences Second Study Program*, Rockefeller Univ., New York, pp. 7–26.

Necker, R. (1973). Temperature sensitivity of thermoreceptors and mechanoreceptors in the beak of pigeons. *J. Comp. Physiol.*, **87**, 379–391.

Necker, R. (1974). Dependence of mechanoreceptor activity on skin temperature in sauropsids. II. Pigeon and duck. *J. Comp. Physiol.*, **92**, 75–83.

Neumayer, L. (1914). "Zur Morphology des Zentralnervensystems der Chelonier und Crokodilier." In A. Voeltzkow, *Reise in Ostafrika*, Vol. 4, Schweizerarbeit, Stuttgart.

Nicoll, R. A., C. Schenker, and S. E. Leeman (1980). Substance P as a transmitter candidate. *Annu. Rev. Neurosci.*, **3**, 227–268.

Nieuwenhuys, R. (1974). Topological analysis of the brain stem: A general introduction. *J. Comp. Neurol.*, **156**, 255–276.

Nieuwenhuys, R. (1982). An overview of the organization of the brain of actinopterygian fishes. *Am. Zool.*, **22**, 287–310.

Northcutt, R. G. (1967). Architectonic studies of the telencephalon of *Iguana iguana*. *J. Comp. Neurol.*, **130**, 109–147.

Northcutt, R. G. (1970). The telencephalon of the western painted turtle (*Chrysemys picta belli*). III. Biol. Mon. No. 43, Univ. Illinois Press, Urbana.

Northcutt, R. G. (1972). The teiid prosencephalon and its bearing on squamate systematics. Program and abstracts of American Society of Ichthyologists and Herpetologists, 75–76.

Northcutt, R. G. (1977). Elasmobranch central nervous system organization and its possible evolutionary significance. *Am. Zool.*, **17**, 411–429.

Northcutt, R. G. (1978a). "Forebrain and midbrain organization in lizards and its evolutionary significance." In N. Greenberg and P. D. MacLean (Eds.), *The Behavior and Neurology of Lizards*, NIMH, Rockville, Maryland, pp. 11–64.

Northcutt, R. G. (1978b). "Brain organization in cartilaginous fishes." In E. S. Hodgson and R. F. Mathewson (Eds.), *Sensory Biology of Sharks, Skates and Rays*, Office of Naval Research, Arlington, Virginia, pp. 117–194.

Northcutt, R. G. (1981). Evolution of the telencephalon in nonmammals. *Annu. Rev. Neurosci.*, **4**, 301–350.

Northcutt, R. G., and M. R. Braford, Jr. (1980). "New observations on the organization and evolution of the telencephalon of actinopterygian fishes." In S. O. E. Ebbesson (Ed.), *Comparative Neurology of the Telencephalon*, Plenum, New York, pp. 41–98.

Northcutt, R. G., and A. B. Butler (1974). Retinal projections in the northern water snake *Natrix sipedon sipedon* (L.). *J. Morphol.*, **142**, 117–136.

Northcutt, R. G., and E. Kicliter (1980). "Organization of the amphibian telencephalon." In S. O. E. Ebbesson (Ed.), *Comparative Neurology of the Telencephalon*, Plenum, New York, pp. 203–255.

Northcutt, R. G., M. R. Braford, Jr., and G. E. Landreth (1974). Retinal projections in the tuatara, *Sphenodon punctatus*. An autoradiographic study. *Anat. Rec.*, **178**, 428.

Nottebohm, F. (1980a). Brain pathways for vocal learning in birds: A review of the first 10 years. *Prog. Psychobiol. Physiol. Psychol.*, **9**, 85–124.

Nottebohm, F. (1980b). A significant correlation between size of canary brain nuclei controlling song and size of song repertoire. *Neurosci. Abstr.*, **6**, 587.

Nottebohm, F. (1981). Laterality, seasons and space govern the learning of a motor skill. *Trends Neurosci.*, **4**, 104–106.

Nottebohm, F., and A. P. Arnold (1976). Sexual dimorphism in vocal control areas of the songbird brain. *Science*, **194**, 211–213.

Nottebohm, F., and D. B. Kelley (1978). Projections to efferent vocal control nuclei of the canary telencephalon. *Neurosci. Abstr.*, **4**, 101.

Nottebohm, F., D. B. Kelly, and J. A. Paton (1982). Connections of vocal control nuclei in the canary telencephalon. *J. Comp. Neurol.*, **207**, 344–357.

Nottebohm, F., T. M. Stokes, and C. M. Leonard (1976). Central control of song in the canary, *Serinus canarius*. *J. Comp. Neurol.*, **165**, 457–486.

O'Neill, W. E., and N. Suga (1982). Encoding target range and its representation in the auditory cortex of the mustache bat. *J. Neurosci.*, **2**, 17–31.

Ostrom, J. H. (1976). *Archaeopteryx* and the origin of birds. *J. Linn. Soc.*, **8**, 91–182.

Ouimet, C. C., R. L. Patrick, and F. F. Ebner (1981). An ultrastructural and biochemical analysis of norepinephrine-containing varicosities in the cerebral cortex of the turtle *Pseudemys*. *J. Comp. Neurol.*, **195**, 289–304.

Owen, R. (1866). *On the Anatomy of Vertebrates*, Vol. 1, *Fishes and Reptiles*, Longmans, Green, London.

Palacios, E. (1976). Golgi studies of the telencephalon of the domestic chicken (*Gallus domesticus*). *Anat. Rec.*, **184**, 495.

Palkovits, M., and L. Zabrovsky (1979). "Neural connections of the hypothalamus." In P. J. Morgane and J. Panskepp (Eds.), *Handbook of the Hypothalamus*, Vol. 1, *Anatomy of the Hypothalamus*, Dekker, New York, pp. 379–510.

Parent, A. (1973a). Distribution of monoamine-containing nerve terminals in the brain of the painted turtle, *Chrysemys picta*. *J. Comp. Neurol.*, **148**, 153–166.

Parent, A. (1973b). Demonstration of catecholaminergic pathway from the midbrain to the strio-amygdaloid complex in the turtle (*Chrysemys picta*). *J. Anat. (London)*, **114**, 379–387.

Parent, A. (1976). Striatal afferent connections in the turtle (*Chrysemys picta*) as revealed by retrograde axonal transport of horseradish peroxidase. *Brain Res.*, **108**, 25–36.

Parent, A. (1979). "Monoaminergic systems in reptile brains." In C. Gans, R. G. Northcutt, and P. S. Ulinski (Eds.), *Biology of the Reptilia*, Academic Press, London, Vol. 10, pp. 247–285.

Parent, A., and A. Olivier (1970/1971). Comparative histochemical study of the corpus striatum. *J. Hirnforsch.*, **12**, 73–81.

Parent, A., and L. J. Poirer (1971). Occurrence and distribution of monoamine-containing neurons in the brain of the painted turtle (*Chrysemys picta*), *J. Anat. (London)*, **110**, 81–89.

Parent, A., and D. Poitras (1974). The origin and distribution of catecholaminergic axon terminals in the cerebral cortex of the turtle (*Chrysemys picta*). *Brain Res.*, **78**, 345–358.

Parker, D. M., and J. D. Delius (1972). Visual evoked potentials in the forebrain of the pigeon. *Exp. Brain Res.*, **14**, 198–209.

Parsons, T. S. (1970). "The nose and Jacobson's organ." In C. Gans and T. S. Parsons (Eds.), *Biology of the Reptilia*, Academic Press, London, Vol. 2, pp. 99–192.

Paton, J. A., and K. R. Manogue (1982). Respiratory gating activity in the avian control pathway. *Neurosci. Abstr.*, **8**, 611.

Paton, J. A., K. R. Manogue, and F. Nottebohm (1980). Telencephalic efferent pathways for vocal control in parakeets. *Neurosci. Abstr.*, **6**, 587.

Paton, J. A., K. R. Manogue, and F. Nottebohm (1981). Bilateral organization of the vocal control pathway in the budgerigar, *Melopsittacus undulatus*. *J. Neurosci.*, **1**, 1279–1288.

Pearlman, A. L., and C. P. Hughes (1976). Functional role of afferents to the avian retina. I. Analysis of retinal ganglion cell receptive fields. *J. Comp. Neurol.*, **166**, 111–122.

Pearson, R. (1972). *The Avian Brain*, Academic Press, New York.

Pedersen, R. (1973). Ascending spinal projections in three species of side-necked turtle: *Podocnemis unifilis, Pelusios subniger*, and *Pelomedusa subrufa*. *Anat. Rec.*, **175**, 409.

Peters, A., and J. Regidor (1981). A reassessment of the forms of non-pyramidal neurons in area 17 of cat visual cortex. *J. Comp. Neurol.*, **203**, 685–716.

Peterson, B. W., R. A. Maunz, N. G. Pitts, and R. G. Mackel (1975). Patterns of projections and branching of reticulospinal neurons. *Exp. Brain Res.*, **23**, 333–351.

Peterson, E. H. (1978). Size classes of ganglion cells which project to the optic tectum in the turtle, *Pseudemys scripta*. *Anat. Rec.*, **190**, 509.

Peterson, E. H. (1980). "Behavioral studies of telencephalic function in reptiles." In S. O. E. Ebbesson (Ed.), *Comparative Neurology of the Telencephalon*, Plenum, New York, pp. 343–388.

Peterson, E. H., and M. Rowe (1976). Electrophysiological evidence for a visual projection to the dorsal ventricular ridge in a lizard, *Dipsosaurus dorsalis*. *Anat. Rec.*, **184**, 500.

Peterson, E. H., and P. S. Ulinski (1979). Quantitative studies of retinal ganglion cells in a turtle, *Pseudemys scripta elegans*. I. Number and distribution of ganglion cells. *J. Comp. Neurol.*, **186**, 17–42.

Peterson, E. H., and P. S. Ulinski (1982). Quantitative studies of retinal ganglion cells in a turtle, *Pseudemys scripta elegans*. II. Size spectrum of ganglion cells and its regional variation. *J. Comp. Neurol.*, **208**, 157–168.

Petras, J. M. (1976). "Comparative anatomy of the tetrapod spinal cord: Dorsal root connections." In R. B. Masterton, C. B. G. Campbell, M. E. Bitterman, and N. Hotton (Eds.), *Evolution of Brain and Behavior in Vertebrates*, Erlbaum, Hillsdale, New Jersey, pp. 345–381.

Pettigrew, J. D. (1979). Binocular visual processing in the owl's telencephalon. *Proc. R. Soc. London, Ser. B*, **204**, 435–454.

Phillips, C. G., and R. Porter (1977). *Corticospinal Neurones*. Academic Press, London.

Phillips, R. E. (1964). "Wildness" in the mallard duck. Effects of brain lesions and stimulation on escape behaviour and reproduction. *J. Comp. Neurol.*, **122**, 139–155.

Phillips, R. E., and A. van Tienhoven (1960). Endocrine factors involved in the failure of pintail ducks, *Anas acuta*, to reproduce in captivity. *J. Endocrinol.*, **21**, 253–261.

Platel, R. (1972). Etude cytoarchitecturale qualitative et quantitative des aires basales d'un saurien scincidae: *Scincus scincus* (L.). I. Etude cytoarchitecturale qualitative. *J. Hirnforsch.*, **13**, 65–87.

Platel, R. (1979). "Brain weight-body weight relationships." In C. Gans, R. G. Northcutt, and P. S. Ulinski (Eds.), *Biology of the Reptilia*, Vol. 9, Academic Press, London, pp. 147–244.

Platel, R. (1980a). Analyse volumetrique compareé des principales subdivisions encéphaliques chez les reptiles sauriens. *J. Hirnforsch.*, **17**, 513–537.

Platel, R. (1980b). Analyse volumetrique compareé des principales subdivisions telencéphaliques chez les reptiles sauriens. *J. Hirnforsch.*, **21**, 271–291.

Popper, A. N., and R. R. Fay (1980). *Comparative Studies of Hearing in Vertebrates.* Springer-Verlag, New York.

Porter, R. (1975). "The neurophysiology of movement performance." In C. C. Hunt (Ed.), *MTP International Review of Science*, Physiology Series One, University Park Press, Baltimore, Maryland, Vol. 3, pp. 151–183.

Portmann, A., and W. Stingelin (1961). "The central nervous system." In A. J. Marshall (Ed.), *Biology and Comparative Physiology of Birds*, Academic Press, New York, Vol. 2, pp. 1–36.

Powell, T. P. S., and W. M. Cowan (1961). The thalamic projection upon the telencephalon in the pigeon (*Columba livia*). *J. Anat. (London)*, **95**, 78–109.

Powell, T. P. S., and L. Kruger (1960). The thalamic projection upon the telencephalon in *Lacerta viridis*. *J. Anat. (London)*, **94**, 528–542.

Powell, T. P. S., and V. B. Mountcastle (1959). Some aspects of the functional organization of the postcentral gyrus of the monkey: A correlation of findings obtained in a single unit analysis with cytoarchitecture. *Bull. Johns Hopkins Hosp.*, **105**, 133–162.

Price, J. L., and D. G. Amaral (1981). An autoradiographic study of the projections of the central nucleus of the monkey amygdala. *J. Neurosci.*, **1**, 1242–1259.

Pritz, M. B. (1974a). Ascending connections of a midbrain auditory area in a crocodile, *Caiman crocodilus*. *J. Comp. Neurol.*, **153**, 179–198.

Pritz, M. B. (1974b). Ascending connections of a thalamic auditory area in a crocodile, *Caiman crocodilus*. *J. Comp. Neurol.*, **153**, 199–214.

Pritz, M. B. (1975). Anatomical identification of a telencephalic visual area in crocodiles: ascending connections of nucleus rotundus in *Caiman crocodilus*. *J. Comp. Neurol.*, **164**, 323–338.

Pritz, M. B., and R. G. Northcutt (1977). Succinate dehydrogenase activity in the telencephalon of crocodiles correlates with the projection areas of sensory thalamic nuclei. *Brain Res.*, **124**, 357–360.

Pritz, M. B., and R. G. Northcutt (1980). Anatomical evidence for an ascending somatosensory pathway to the telencephalon in crocodiles, *Caiman crocodilus*. *Exp. Brain Res.*, **40**, 342–345.

Quiroga, J. C. (1979a). The brain of two mammal-like reptiles (Cynodontia-Therapsida). *J. Hirnforsch.*, **20**, 341–350.

Quiroga, J. C. (1979b). The cell masses in the diencephalon of *Amphisbaena darwinii heterozonata* Burmeister (Amphisbaenia, Squamata, Reptilia). *Acta Anat.*, **104**, 198–210.

Quiroga, J. C. (1980a). The brain of the mammal-like reptile *Probainognathus jensini* (Therapsida, Cynodontia). A correlative paleo-neoneurological approach to the neocortex at the reptile-mammal transition. *J. Hirnforsch.*, **21**, 299–336.

Quiroga, J. C. (1980b). Sobre un molde endocraneano del cinodonte *Probainognathus, jensini* Romer, 1970 (Reptilia, Therapsida) de la Formacion Ischichuca (Triasico medio), La Rioja, Argentina. *Ameghiniana*, **17**, 181–190.

Radinsky, L. (1975a). Evolution of the felid brain. *Brain Behav. Evol.*, **11**, 214–254.

Radinsky, L. (1975b). Primate brain evolution. *Am. Sci.*, **63**, 656–663.

Radinsky, L. (1977). Brains of early carnivores. *Paleobiology*, **3**, 333–349.

Radinsky, L. (1982). "Some cautionary notes on making inferences about relative brain size." In E. Armstrong and D. Falk (Eds.), *Primate Brain Evolution: Methods and Concepts*, Plenum, New York, pp. 29–37.

Rainey, W. T. (1979). Organization of nucleus rotundus, a tectofugal thalamic nucleus in turtles. I. Nissl and Golgi analyses. *J. Morphol.*, **160**, 121–142.

Rainey, W. T., and P. S. Ulinski (1982a). Organization of nucleus rotundus, a tectofugal thalamic nucleus in turtles. II. The tectorotundal projection. *J. Comp. Neurol.*, **209**, 187–207.

Rainey, W. T., and P. S. Ulinski (1982b). Organization of nucleus rotundus, a tectofugal thalamic nucleus in turtles. III. Ultrastructural analyses. *J. Comp. Neurol.*, **209**, 208–223.

Rakic, P., and R. L. Sidman (1969). Telencephalic origin of pulvinar neurons in the fetal human brain. *Z. Anat. Entwicklungsgesch.*, **129**, 53–82.

Ramón, P. (1896). Estructura del encefalo del camaleon. *Rev. Trim. Micrografica*, **1**, 146–182.

Ramón y Cajal, S. (1955). *Histologie du Systeme Nerveux de l'Homme et des Vertebres*, Consejo superior de Investigaciones Cientificas, Instituto Ramón y Cajal, Madrid.

Reese, A. M. (1910). The development of the brain of the American alligator. *Smithsonian Misc. Coll.*, **54**, No. 21922.

Reiner, A., N. C. Brecha, and H. J. Karten (1982). Basal ganglia pathways to the tectum: The afferent and efferent connections of the lateral spiriform nucleus of birds. *J. Comp. Neurol.*, **208**, 16–36.

Reiner, A., and H. J. Karten (1978). A bisynaptic retinocerebellar pathway in the turtle. *Brain Res.*, **150**, 163–169.

Reiner, A., and H. J. Karten (1982). Laminar distribution of the cells of origin of the descending tectofugal pathways in the pigeon (*Columba livia*). *J. Comp. Neurol.*, **204**, 165–187.

Reiner, A., H. J. Karten, and N. C. Brecha (1982). Enkephalin-mediated basal ganglia influences over the optic tectum: Immunohistochemistry of the tectum and the lateral spiriform nucleus in birds. *J. Comp. Neurol.*, **208**, 37–53.

Reiner, A., H. J. Karten, and G. E. Korte (1980). Substance P: Localization within paleostriatal-tegmental pathways in birds and reptiles. *Neurosci. Abstr.*, **6**, 810.

Reiner, A., S. E. Brauth, C. A. Kitt, and H. J. Karten (1980). Basal ganglionic pathways to the tectum: Studies in reptiles. *J. Comp. Neurol.*, **193**, 565–589.

Repérant, J. (1973). Nouvelles donnees sur les projections visuelles chez le pigeon (*Columba livia*). *J. Hirnforsch.*, **14**, 152–287.

Repérant, J. (1975). Nouvelles donneés sur les projections retinese chez *Caïman sclerops*. Étude radio-autographique. *C. R. Acad. Sci. Paris*, **280**, 2881–2884.

Repérant, J., J.-P. Raffin, and D. Miceli (1974). La voie retino-thalamo-hyperstriatale chez le pouissin (*Gallus domesticus*). *C. R. Acad. Sci. Paris*, **279**, 279–281.

Repérant, J., and J.-P. Rio (1976). Retinal projections in *Vipera aspis*. A reinvestigation using light radioautographic and electron microscopic degeneration techniques. *Brain Res.*, **107**, 603–609.

Repérant, J., J.-P. Rio, D. Miceli, and M. Lemire (1978). A radioautographic study of retinal projections in type I and type II lizards. *Brain Res.*, **142**, 401–411.

Revzin, A. M. (1970). Some characteristics of wide-field units in the brain of the pigeon. *Brain Behav. Evol.*, **3**, 195–204.

Revzin, A. M. (1979). "Functional localization in the nucleus rotundus." In A. M. Granda and J. H. Maxwell (Eds.), *Neural Mechanisms of Behavior in the Pigeon*, Plenum, New York, pp. 165–176.

Revzin, A. M., and H. J. Karten (1967). Rostral projections of the optic tectum and the nucleus rotundus in the pigeon. *Brain Res.*, **3**, 264–276.

Rieke, G. K., and B. M. Wenzel (1978). Forebrain projections of the pigeon olfactory bulb. *J. Morphol.*, **158**, 41–56.

Riss, W., M. Halpern, and F. Scalia (1969). The quest for clues to forebrain evolution—the study of reptiles. *Brain Behav. Evol.*, **2**, 1–50.

Ritchie, T. C., and D. H. Cohen (1977). The avian tectofugal visual pathway: Projections of its telencephalic target, the ectostriatal complex. *Neurosci. Abstr.*, **3**, 94.

Robbins, D. O. (1972). Coding of intensity and wavelength in optic tectal cells of the turtle. *Brain Behav. Evol.*, **5**, 124–142.

Robinson, L. R. (1969). Bulbospinal fibers and their nuclei of origin in *Lacerta viridis* demonstrated by axonal degeneration and chromatolysis, respectively. *J. Anat. (London)*, **105**, 59–88.

Rodieck, R. W. (1979). Visual pathways. *Annu. Rev. Neurosci.*, **2**, 193–226.

Rogers, K. T. (1960). Studies on the chick brain of biochemical differentiation related to morphological differentiation. I. Morphological development. *J. Exp. Zool.*, **144**, 77–87.

Rolon, R. R., and L. C. Skeen (1980). Afferent and efferent connections of the olfactory bulb in the soft-shell turtle (*Trionyx spinifer spinifer*). *Neurosci. Abstr.*, **6**, 305.

Romer, A. S. (1956). *Osteology of the Reptiles*. Univ. Chicago Press.

Roney, K.-J., A. B. Scheibel, and G. L. Shaw (1979). Dendritic bundles: A survey of anatomical experiments and physiological theories. *Brain Res. Rev.*, **1**, 225–271.

Rose, M. (1914). Über die Cytoarchitektonische Gliederung des Vorderhirns der Vögel. *J. Psychol. Neurol. Lpz.*, **21**, 278–352.

Rose, M. (1923). Histologische Lokalization des Vorderhirns der Reptilien. *J. Psychol. Neurol. Lpz.*, **29**, 219–272.

Rovainen, C. M. (1979). Neurobiology of lampreys. *Physiol. Rev.*, **59**, 1008–1077.

Rubel, E. W., and T. N. Parks (1975). Organization and development of brain stem auditory nuclei of the chicken: Tonotopic organization of N. magnocellularis and N. laminaris. *J. Comp. Neurol.*, **164**, 411–434.

Rudin, W. (1974). Untersuchungen am olfaktorischen system der Reptilien III. Differenzierungsformen eniger olfaktorischer Zentren bei Reptilien. *Acta Anat.*, **89**, 481–515.

Sachs, M. B., and J. M. Sinnett (1978). Responses to tones of single cells in nucleus magnocellularis and nucleus angularis of the redwing blackbird (*Agelaius phoeniceus*). *J. Comp. Physiol.*, **126**, 347–361.

Saini, K. D., and H.-J. Leppelsack (1977). Neuronal arrangement in the auditory field L of the neostriatum of the starling. *Cell Tissue Res.*, **176**, 309–316.

Saini, K. D., and H.-J. Leppelsack (1981). Cell types of the auditory caudomedial neostriatum of the starling (*Sturnus vulgaris*). *J. Comp. Neurol.*, **198**, 209–230.

Scalia, F., M. Halpern, and W. Riss (1969). Olfactory bulb projections in the South American Caiman. *Brain Behav. Evol.*, **2**, 238–262.

Scalia, F., and S. S. Winans (1975). The differential projections of the olfactory bulb and accessory olfactory bulb in mammals. *J. Comp. Neurol.*, **161**, 31–56.

Schapiro, H. (1964). Motor functions and their anatomical basis in the forebrain and tectum of the alligator. Doctoral Dissertation, Univ. Florida.

Scheibel, M. E., and A. B. Scheibel (1958). "Structural substrates for integrative patterns in the brainstem reticular core." In H. H. Jasper, L. D. Proctor, et al. (Eds.), *Reticular Formation of the Brain*, Little, Brown, Boston, pp. 31–55.

Scheich, H., G. Langner, and D. Bonke (1979). Responsiveness of units in the auditory neostriatum of the guinea fowl (*Numida meleagris*) to species-specific calls and synthetic stimuli. II. Discrimination of Iambus-like calls. *J. Comp. Physiol.*, **132**, 257–276.

Scheich, H., and V. Maier (1981). "^{14}C-Deoxyglucose labeling of the auditory neostriatum in young and adult guinea fowl." In J. Syka and L. Aitkin (Eds.), *Neuronal Mechanisms of Hearing*, Plenum, New York, pp. 329–334.

Scheich, H., V. Maier, and B. A. Bonke (1980). Deoxyglucose labeling of auditory forebrain areas in adult and newly hatched guinea fowl. *Neurosci. Abstr.*, **6**, 819.

Scheich, H., B. A. Bonke, D. Bonke, and G. Langner (1979). Functional organization of some auditory nuclei in the guinea fowl demonstrated by the 2-deoxyglucose technique. *Cell Tissue Res.*, **204**, 17–27.

Schneider, G. E. (1969). Two visual systems. *Science*, **163**, 895–902.

Schroeder, D. M. (1981). Tectal projections of an infrared sensitive snake, *Crotalus viridis*. *J. Comp. Neurol.*, **195**, 477–500.

Schroeder, D. M., and M. S. Loop (1976). Trigeminal projections in snakes possessing infrared sensitivity. *J. Comp. Neurol.*, **169**, 1–14.

Schwartz, E. A. (1973). Organization of on-off cells in the retina of the turtle. *J. Physiol.* (*London*), **230**, 1–14.

Senn, D. G. (1969). The saurian and ophidian colliculi posteriores of the midbrain. *Acta Anat.*, **74**, 114–120.

Senn, D. G. (1970). Die Zusammenhange von Grosshirnstriatum, dorsalem Thalamus und Tectum Opticum bei Echsen. *Verhandl. Naturf. Ges. Basel*, **80**, 209–225.

Senn, D. G. (1974). Notes on the amphibian and reptilian thalamus. *Acta Anat.*, **87**, 555–596.

Senn, D. G. (1979). "Embryonic development of the central nervous system." In C. Gans, R. G. Northcutt and P. S. Ulinski (Eds.), *Biology of the Reptilia*, Vol. 9, Academic, London, pp. 173–244.

Senn, D. G., and R. G. Northcutt (1973). The forebrain and midbrain of some squamates and their bearing on the origin of snakes. *J. Morphol.*, **140**, 135–152.

Sereno, M. (1982). Axonal and dendritic morphology of tectoreticular cells in a turtle, *Pseudemys scripta*. *Neurosci. Abstr.*, **8**, 951.

Shanklin, W. M. (1930). The central nervous system of *Chameleon vulgaris*. *Acta Zool.*, **11**, 425–490.

Shatz, C., S. Lindstrom, and T. Wiesel (1975). Ocular dominance columns in the cat's visual cortex. *Neurosci. Abstr.*, **5**, 56.

Sherrington, C. (1906). *The Integrative Action of the Nervous System*. Cambridge Univ. Press.

Shiosaka, S., K. Takatsuki, S. Inagaki, M. Sakavaka, H. Takagi, E. Senaba, T. Matsuzaki, and M. Tohyama (1981). Topographic atlas of somatostatin-containing neuron system in the avian brain in relation to catecholamine-containing neuron system. II. Mesencephalon, rhombencephalon, and spinal cord. *J. Comp. Neurol.*, **202**, 115–124.

Sidman, R. L., and P. Rakic (1973). Neuronal migration, with special reference to developing human brain: A review. *Brain Res.*, **62**, 1–35.

Simpson, G. G. (1927). Mesozoic mammalia. IX. The brains of Jurassic mammals. *Am. J. Sci.*, **14**, 259–268.

Simpson, G. G. (1937). Skull structure of the multituberculata. *Bull. Am. Mus. Nat. Hist.*, **73**, 727–763.

Simpson, G. G. (1961). *Principles of Animal Taxonomy.* Columbia Univ. Press, New York.

Snyder, S. H., and S. R. Childers (1979). Opiate receptors and opioid peptides. *Annu. Rev. Neurosci.*, **2**, 35–112.

Stehouwer, D. J., and P. B. Farel (1980). Central and peripheral controls of swimming in anuran larvae. *Brain Res.*, **195**, 323–335.

Stein, B. E., and N. S. Gaither (1981). Sensory representation in reptilian optic tectum: Some comparisons with mammals. *J. Comp. Neurol.*, **202**, 69–87.

Stein, P. S. G. (1978). Motor systems, with specific reference to the control of locomotion. *Annu. Rev. Neurosci.*, **1**, 61–82.

Stingelin, W. (1958). *Vergleichend morphologische Untersuchungen am Vorderhirn der Vögel auf cytologischer und cytoarchitektonischer Grundlage*, Helbing and Lichtenhahn, Basel, 123 pp.

Stingelin, W. (1961). Grossenunterschiede des sensiblen Trigeminuskerns bei verschiedenen Vogeln. *Rev. Suisse Zool.*, **68**, 247–251.

Stokes, T. M., C. M. Leonard, and F. Nottebohm (1974). The telencephalon, diencephalon, and mesencephalon of the canary, *Serinus canaria*, in stereotaxic coordinates. *J. Comp. Neurol.*, **156**, 337–374.

Stone, J., B. Dreher, and A. Leventhal (1979). Hierarchical and parallel mechanisms in the organization of visual cortex. *Brain Res. Rev.*, **1**, 345–394.

Streit, P., A. Burkhalter, M. Stella, and M. Cuénod (1980). Patterns of activity in pigeon brain's visual relays as revealed by the [^{14}C]2-deoxyglucose method. *Neuroscience*, **5**, 1053–1066.

Suga, N. (1982). "Functional organization of the auditory cortex: representation beyond tonotopy in the bat." In C. N. Woolsey (Ed.), *Cortical Sensory Organization*, Vol. 3, *Multiple Auditory Areas*, Humana, Clifton, New Jersey, pp. 157–218.

Sur, M., M. M. Merzenich, and J. H. Kaas (1980). Magnification, receptive-field area, and "hypercolumn" size in areas 3b and 1 of somatosensory cortex in owl monkeys. *J. Neurophysiol.*, **44**, 295–311.

Sur, M., J. T. Wall, and J. H. Kaas (1981). Modular segregation of functional cell classes within the post-central somatosensory cortex of monkeys. *Science*, **212**, 1059–1061.

Switzer, R. C., III, J. A. W. Kirsch, and J. I. Johnson, Jr. (1980). Phylogeny through brain traits. Relation of lateral olfactory tract fibers to the accessory olfactory formation as a palimpset of mammalian descent. *Brain Behav. Evol.*, **17**, 339–363.

Tandler, J., and H. Kantor (1907). Die Entwicklungsgeschicte des Geckogehirnes. *Anat. Hefte*, **33**, 553–665.

Taylor, D. A., and T. W. Stone (1981). "Neurotransmodulatory control of cerebral cortical neuron activity." In F. O. Schmitt, F. G. Worden, G. Adelman, and S. G. Dennis (Eds.), *The Organization of the Cerebral Cortex*, MIT Press, Cambridge, Massachusetts, pp. 347–356.

ten Donkelaar, H. J. (1976a). Descending pathways from the brain stem to the spinal cord in some reptiles I. Origin. *J. Comp. Neurol.*, **167**, 421–442.

ten Donkelaar, H. J. (1976b). Descending pathways from the brain stem to the spinal cord in some reptiles II. Course and site of termination. *J. Comp. Neurol.*, **167**, 443–464.

ten Donkelaar, H. J., and R. De Boer-van Huizen (1978). Cells of origin of pathways descending to the spinal cord in a lizard (*Lacerta galloti*). *Neurosci. Lett.*, **9**, 123–128.

ten Donkelaar, H. J., and R. De Boer-van Huizen (1981a). Basal ganglia projections to the brainstem in the lizard *Varanus exanthematicus* as demonstrated by the retrograde transport of horseradish peroxidase. *Neuroscience*, **6**, 1567–1590.

ten Donkelaar, H. J., and R. De Boer-van Huizen (1981b). Ascending projections of the brain stem reticular formation in a nonmammalian vertebrate (the lizard *Varanus exanthematicus*), with notes on the afferent connections of the forebrain. *J. Comp. Neurol.*, **200**, 501–528.

Terashima, S., and R. C. Goris (1975). Tectal organization of pit viper infrared reception. *Brain Res.*, **83**, 490–494.

Tigges, J., M. Tigges, and A. A. Perachio (1977). Complementary laminar terminations of afferents to area 17 originating in area 18 and in the lateral geniculate nucleus in squirrel monkey. *J. Comp. Neurol.*, **176**, 87–100.

Tohyama, M., M. Toshihiro, J. Hashimoto, G. R. Shrestha, O. Tamura, and N. Shimizu (1974). Comparative anatomy of the locus coeruleus I. Organizations and ascending projections of the catecholamine containing neurons in the pontine region of the bird, *Melopsittacus undulatus*. *J. Hirnforsch.*, **15**, 319–330.

Torvik, A., and A. Brodal (1957). The origin of reticulospinal fibers in the cat. An experimental study. *Anat. Rec.*, **128**, 113–137.

Tsai, H. M. (1977). An autoradiographic analysis of histogenesis in the developing chick telencephalon in situ and in vitro. Doctoral Dissertation, University of Chicago.

Tsai, H. M., B. B. Garber, and L. M. H. Larramendi (1981a). Thymidine autoradiographic analysis of telencephalic histogenesis in the chick embryo: I. Neuronal birthdates of telencephalic compartments *in situ*. *J. Comp. Neurol.*, **198**, 275–292.

Tsai, H. M., B. B. Garber, and L. M. H. Larramendi (1981b). Thymidine autoradiographic analysis of telencephalic histogenesis in the chick embryo: II. Dynamics of neuronal migration, displacement, and aggregation. *J. Comp. Neurol.*, **198**, 293–306.

Tucker, D., and J. C. Smith (1976). "Vertebrate olfaction." In R. B. Masterton, M. E. Bitterman, C. B. G. Campbell, and N. Hotton (Eds.), *Evolution of Brain and Behavior in Vertebrates*, Erlbaum, Hillsdale, New Jersey, pp. 25–52.

Tumanova, N. L., and E. V. Ozirskaya (1973). Electron microscopic studies on degenerative changes in the nucleus rotundus of the tortoise *Emys orbicularis* after tectotomy. *Zhurn. Evol. Biokhim. Fiziolog.*, **10**, 315–317.

Turner, B. H., M. Mishkin, and M. Knapp (1980). Organization of the amygdalopetal projection from modality-specific cortical association areas in the monkey. *J. Comp. Neurol.*, **191**, 515–543.

Tusa, R. J., L. A. Palmer, and A. C. Rosenquist (1978). The retinotopic organization of area 17 (striate cortex) in the cat. *J. Comp. Neurol.*, **177**, 213–236.

Ulinski, P. S. (1976). Structure of anterior dorsal ventricular ridge in snakes. *J. Morphol.*, **148**, 1–22.

Ulinski, P. S. (1977a). Tectal efferents in the banded water snake, *Natrix sipedon*. *J. Comp. Neurol.*, **173**, 251–274.

Ulinski, P. S. (1977b). Efferent projections of the posterior colliculus in the garter snake (*Thamnophis sirtalis*). *Anat. Rec.*, **187**, 735.

Ulinski, P. S. (1978a). Organization of anterior dorsal ventricular ridge in snakes. *J. Comp. Neurol.*, **178**, 411–450.

Ulinski, P. S. (1978b). Distribution of neurons in the optic tectum of the turtle, *Pseudemys scripta*. *Anat. Rec.*, **190**, 562.

Ulinski, P. S. (1980). Organization of the retinogeniculate projection in pond turtles, *Pseudemys* and *Chrysemys*. *Neurosci. Abstr.*, **6**, 748.

Ulinski, P. S. (1981). Thick caliber projections from brainstem to cerebral cortex in the snakes *Thamnophis sirtalis* and *Natrix sipedon*. *Neuroscience*, **6**, 1725–1743.

Ulinski, P. S. (1982). "Neurobiology of the therapsid-mammal transition." In J. J. Roth, E. C. Roth, P. D. MacLean, and N. Hotton III (Eds.), *The Ecology and Biology of Mammal-Like Reptiles*, Smithsonian Institution, Washington, D.C. In Press.

Ulinski, P. S., and D. A. Kanarek (1973). Cytoarchitecture of nucleus sphericus in the common boa, *Constrictor constrictor*. *J. Comp. Neurol.*, **151**, 159–174.

Ulinski, P. S., and E. H. Peterson (1981). Patterns of olfactory projections in the desert iguana, *Dipsosaurus dorsalis*. *J. Morphol.*, **168**, 189–228.

Underwood, G. (1967). *A Contribution to the Classification of Snakes*. British Museum (Nat. Hist.), London.

Underwood, G. (1970). "The Eye." In C. Gans and T. S. Parsons, (Eds.), *The Biology of the Reptilia*, Academic Press, London, Vol. 2, pp. 1–98.

Van Essen, D. C. (1979). Visual areas of the mammalian cerebral cortex. *Annu. Rev. Neurosci.*, **2**, 227–263.

Van Essen, D. C., W. T. Newsome, and J. L. Bixby (1982). The pattern of interhemispheric connections and its relationship to extrastriate visual areas in the macaque monkey. *J. Neurosci.*, **2**, 265–283.

van Tienhoven, A., and L. P. Juhasz (1962). The chicken telencephalon, diencephalon and mesencephalon in stereotaxic coordinates. *J. Comp. Neurol.*, **118**, 185–197.

Voneida, T. J., and C. M. Sligar (1979). Efferent projections of the dorsal ventricular ridge and the striatum in the tegu lizard, *Tupinambis nigropunctatus*. *J. Comp. Neurol.*, **186**, 43–64.

Wallenberg, A. (1903). Der Ursprung des Tractus isthmostriatus (oder bulbostriatus) der Taube. *Neurol. Zbl.*, **22**, 98–101.

Walls, G. L. (1942). *The Vertebrate Eye and Its Adaptive Radiation*. Hafner Reprints, New York.

Wang, R. T., and M. Halpern (1977). Afferent and efferent connections of thalamic nuclei of the visual system of garter snakes. *Anat. Rec.*, **187**, 741–742.

Warner, F. J. (1946). The development of the forebrain of the American watersnake (*Natrix sipedon*). *J. Comp. Neurol.*, **84**, 385–418.

Webster, K. E. (1979). "Some aspects of the comparative study of the corpus striatum. In I. Divac and R. G. E. Oberg (Eds.), *The Neostriatum*, Pergamon, New York, pp. 107–126.

Weisbach, W., and J. Schwartzkopf (1967). Nervose Antworten auf Schallreiz im Grosshirn von Krokodilen. *Naturwissenschaften*, **54**, 650.

Weiss, J. C. (1982). Ultrastructural analysis of dorsal area of turtle dorsal ventricular ridge, including comments on cell clusters. *Neurosci. Abstr.*, **8**, 716.

Wetzel, M. C., and L. G. Howell (1981). "Properties and mechanisms of locomotion." In A. L. Towe and E. S. Luschei (Eds.), *Handbook of Behavioral Neurobiology*, Vol. 5, *Motor Coordination*, Plenum, New York, pp. 567–625.

White, E. L. (1979). Thalamocortical synaptic relations: A review with emphasis on the projections of specific thalamic nuclei to the primary sensory areas of the neocortex. *Brain Res.*, **1**, 275–312.

Wiesendanger, M. (1981). "The pyramidal tract. Its structure and function." In A. L. Towe and E. S. Luschei (Eds.), *Handbook of Behavioral Neurobiology*, Vol. 5, *Motor Coordination*, Plenum, New York, pp. 401–491.

Wild, J. M., and H. P. Zeigler (1982). Central control of eating in the pigeon: a sensorimotor chain from grain through brain. *Neurosci. Abstr.*, **8**, 612.

Witkovsky, P., H. P. Zeigler, and R. Silver (1973). The nucleus basalis of the pigeon: A single-unit analysis. *J. Comp. Neurol.*, **147**, 119–128.

Woolsey, C. N. (1981a). *Cortical Sensory Organization*, Vol. 1, *Multiple Somatic Areas*, Humana, Clifton, New Jersey.

Woolsey, C. N. (1981b). *Cortical Sensory Organization*, Vol. 2, *Multiple Visual Areas*, Humana, Clifton, New Jersey.

Woolsey, C. N. (1982). *Cortical Auditory Organization*, Vol. 3, *Multiple Auditory Visual Areas*, Humana, Clifton, New Jersey.

Wurtz, R., and J. E. Albano (1980). Visual-motor function of the primate superior colliculus. *Annu. Rev. Neurosci.*, **3**, 189–226.

Wyeth, F. J. (1924). The development and neuromery of the forebrain in *Sphenodon punctatum*. *Proc. Zool. Soc. London*, **2**, 923–959.

Yamamoto, K., M. Tohyama, and N. Shimizu (1977). Comparative anatomy of the topography of catecholamine containing neuron systems in the brain stem from birds to teleosts. *J. Hirnforsch.*, **18**, 229–240.

Yazulla, S., and A. M. Granda (1973). Opponent-color units in the thalamus of the pigeon (*Columba livia*). *Vision Res.*, **13**, 1555–1563.

Zaretsky, M. D. (1978). A new auditory area of the songbird forebrain. *Exp. Brain Res.*, **32**, 267–273.

Zaretsky, M. D., and M. Konishi (1976). Tonotopic organization in the avian telencephalon. *Brain Res.*, **111**, 167–171.

Zeier, H., and H. J. Karten (1971). The archistriatum of the pigeon: Organization of afferent and efferent connections. *Brain Res.*, **31**, 313–326.

Zeier, H., and H. J. Karten (1973). Connections of the anterior commissure in the pigeon (*Columba livia*). *J. Comp. Neurol.*, **150**, 201–216.

Zeigler, H. P. (1974). "Feeding behavior in the pigeon: A neurobehavioral analysis." In I. J. Goodman and M. W. Schein (Eds.), *Birds: Brain and Behavior*, Academic Press, New York, pp. 101–132.

Zeigler, H. P. (1976). Feeding behavior of the pigeon. *Adv. Study Behav.*, **7**, 285–398.

Zeigler, H. P., and H. J. Karten (1973a). Brain mechanisms and feeding behavior in the pigeon (*Columba livia*). I. Quinto-frontal structures. *J. Comp. Neurol.*, **152**, 59–82.

Zeigler, H. P., and H. J. Karten (1973b). Brain mechanism and feeding behavior in the pigeon (*Columba livia*). II. Analysis of feeding behavior deficits after lesions of the quintofrontal structures. *J. Comp. Neurol.*, **152**, 83–102.

Zeigler, H. P., P. W. Levitt, and R. R. Levine (1980). Eating in the pigeon (*Columba livia*): Movement patterns, stereotypy, and stimulus control. *J. Comp. Physiol. Psychol.*, **94**, 783–794.

Zeigler, H. P., and P. Witkovsky (1968). The main sensory trigeminal nucleus in the pigeon: A single-unit analysis. *J. Comp. Neurol.*, **134**, 255–264.

AUTHOR INDEX

Acheson, D.W.K., 110
Adamo, N.J., 123, 143
Adrian, H.O., 221
Akulina, M.M., 105
Albano, J.E., 188, 227
Allen, T.O., 97
Allman, J., 218
Alones, V.E., 224
Altman, J., 208
Amaral, D.G., 211, 223
Anderson, J.A., 189
Angevine, J.B., 210
Arends, J.J.A., 177, 179
Ariens Kappers, C.U., 6, 23, 29, 86, 206–208
Armstrong, J.A., 56, 145
Arnold, A.P., 85
Auffenberg, W., 56
Azad, R., 88

Bagnoli, P., 224
Baker-Cohen, K.F., 52, 68, 75, 83
Balaban, C.D., 2, 6, 60, 61, 65–68, 70, 72, 73,
    91, 92, 100, 105, 107–109, 140–144, 146,
    154, 158, 166, 184, 185, 216, 217
Bambrough, P., 118
Bass, A.H., 92, 93, 101
Battenberg, E., 88
Baumgarten, H.G., 152, 153
Bayon, A., 88
Beaudet, A., 223
Belekhova, M.G., 91, 105, 106, 131, 142, 154,
    166

Benetto, K., 132, 134
Benowitz, L.I., 113–115, 195, 199
Berkhoudt H., 134, 135, 137-140,187
Berkowitz, E.C., 6
Berry, M.S., 185
Berson, D.M., 208
Bertler, A., 153, 154
Biederman-Thorson, M., 123, 125, 127
Bixby, J.L., 219
Bloom, F.E., 88, 222
Bohringer, R.C., 217
Boiko, V.P., 101
Bonke, B.A., 83, 84, 123–128, 169, 175
Bonke, D., 83, 84, 123–128, 169, 175
Bonner, J.T., 35
Boord, R.L., 118
Bowling, D.B., 101
Braak, H., 152, 153
Braford, M.R., Jr., 35, 92, 93, 110, 112
Brauch, C.S.M., 79, 80, 136, 137
Brauth, S.E., 76, 142, 152, 154, 156, 157,
    166–168, 172, 173, 175, 176
Brazier, M.A.B., 217
Brecha, N., 175, 176
Bremer, F., 117
Brodal, A., 228
Brown, J.L., 84, 196
Bruce, C.J., 218
Bruce, L.L., 49, 56, 91, 93, 99, 119, 131, 132,
    142, 158, 164
Brugge, J.F., 214, 219
Brunelli, M., 114, 116, 117

Bugbee, N.M., 195
Bullock, T.H., 127
Burghardt, G.M., 198
Butcher, L.L., 154
Butler, A.B., 56, 91–93, 97, 99, 119, 142, 143, 158, 163, 164

Cabana, T., 228
Cairney, J., 60
Campbell, C.B.G., 202
Canady, R., 86
Carey, J.H., 68, 70
Carlson, M., 218
Carpenter, M.B., 208
Carpenter, R.H.S., 226
Carroll, R.L., 193, 194, 203
Case, E.C., 205
Caviness, V.S., 216
Childers, S.R., 52
Clark, G., 217
Clark, J.M., 75
Clarke, P.G.H., 92, 110
Cohen, D.H., 82, 118, 137, 199
Coles, R.B., 130
Colonnier, M., 209
Conde-Courtine, F., 110
Contestabile, A., 60, 68, 70, 75, 77, 152
Cooke, J., 14
Coulter, J.D., 214
Cowan, W.M., 6
Cowey, A., 218
Craigie, E.H., 78
Crews, D., 99
Crompton, A.W., 201, 202
Crosby, E.C., 6, 23, 29, 75, 76, 86, 110, 112, 132, 147, 206, 207, 208
Crossland, W.J., 114
Cruce, J.A.F., 93
Cruce, W.L.R., 93, 142, 191, 192
Cuénod, M., 6
Curwen, A.O., 49, 58

Dacey, D.M., 93, 95, 188, 227
De Boer-van Huizen, R., 91, 119, 132, 142, 152, 153, 158, 171, 192
De Britto, L.R.G., 114, 116, 117
De Fina, A.V., 118
de Lanerolle, N.C., 88
De Liberaldi, M., 176
Delius, J.D., 117, 130, 132, 134, 196

Dendy, A., 17, 18
Descarries, L., 223
Deschenes, M., 216
Desimone, R., 218
De Voogd, T.J., 84, 86
Diamond, I.T., 222
Di Pardo, A., 60, 68, 70, 75, 77, 152
Distel, H., 99, 119, 209
Dobrokhatova, I., 80
Don, A., 79, 80, 136, 137
Dow, R.S., 117
Dray, A., 224
Dreher, B., 215
Dubbeldam, J.L., 79, 80, 86, 87, 132, 135–140, 154, 166, 168, 173, 175, 177, 179, 187
Dubé, L., 87, 152, 154
Dudek, B.C., 35
Dünser, K.R., 106, 110, 188
Durward, A., 28, 60, 78

Ebbesson, S.O.E., 6, 33, 99, 119, 131, 132, 209
Ebner, F.F., 6, 93, 99, 100, 101, 105, 119, 158, 209, 219, 223
Edinger, T., 86, 205
Elde, R.P., 88
Eleftheriou, B.E., 229
Elliot Smith, G., 207
Elprava, D.F., 224
Erulkar, D.S., 123, 134
Evarts, E.V., 192
Ewert, J.P., vii

Faber, D.S., 226
Faccioli, G., 116, 176
Falck, B., 152, 153
Farel, P.B., 226
Fay, R.R., 118
Ferguson, J.L., 173, 195
Ferster, D., 216
Fetz, E.E., 225
Fitzpatrick, K.A., 214
Fizaan-Oostven, J.L.F.P., 132
Flemming, J., 218
Foster, R.E., 118–120
Fox, C.A., 87
Francesconi, W., 114, 116, 117
Frenk, S., 110
Frick, M., 88

Frost, D.O., 216
Frumin, N., 92–93
Fulbrook, J.E., 101
Fuxe, K., 152

Gaidenko, G.V., 143
Gaither, P.S.G., 92
Galambos, R., 127, 198
Gallistel, C.R., 198
Gamble, H.G., 56, 145, 146
Gamlin, P.D.R., 118
Garber, B.B., 21–23, 26–29, 93
Gatlass, R., 218
Getting, P.A., 185
Ghiselin, M.T., 200
Gilbert, C.D., 214, 221
Gogan, P., 117
Goldby, F., 6, 55, 56, 131, 145
Goldman, P.S., 223
Goncharova, N.V., 101
Goodman, D.C., 131, 132
Goris, R.C., 92
Gotoh, J., 152
Gottfries, C.G., 153, 154
Gottschaldt, K.M., 134, 135
Graham-Brown, T., 225
Granda, A.M., 101, 110, 114, 116, 189
Grantyn, A., 227
Grantyn, R., 227
Grassi, S., 224
Graybiel, A.M., 208
Greenberg, N., 6, 99, 195
Gregory, J.E., 134
Grillner, S., 226
Grofova, F., 223
Gross, C.G., 218
Guichard, J., 110, 111
Gurney, M.E., 80, 82–86, 130, 169, 177
Guselnikov, V.I., 92

Haartsen, A.B., 211
Haefelfinger, H.R., 28
Hahn, M.E., 35
Hall, W.C., 6, 93, 100, 101, 105, 118–120, 158, 209, 222, 227
Halpern, M., 45, 60, 75, 76, 92, 93, 119, 145–148, 176, 198
Hamburger, V., 21
Hamdi, F.A., 92, 110
Hamilton, H., 21

Harman, A.L., 123
Harting, J.K., 222, 224
Hartline, P., 145
Hendrickson, A.E., 222
Hendry, S.H., 214
Heric, T.M., 92
Herrick, C.J., 208
Herrick, C.L., 11
Hetzel, W. von, 11, 14, 15, 17
Hewitt, W., 68, 70
Hill, R.M., 101
Hillman, D.E., 87
Hines, M., 14, 17, 18, 60
Hinton, C.E., 189
His, W., 206
Hodos, W., 6, 23, 113, 116, 188, 195, 202, 209
Holcombe, V., 227
Holden, A.L., 118
Holmes, G., 86
Holmgren, N., 11, 14, 18, 19
Holstege, G., 211
Hoogland, P.V., 49, 58, 97, 131, 142, 162, 163, 171
Hopkins, D.A., 211
Hopson, J.A., 203–205
Howell, L.G., 226
Hubel, D.H., 215, 220–222
Huber, G.C., 6, 23, 29, 86, 110, 132, 206, 208
Huerta, M.F., 224
Hughes, C.P., 110
Humbertson, A.O., Jr., 228
Humphrey, A.L., 70, 222
Hunt, S.P., 110, 113, 114, 176
Hunter, J., 6

Ikeda, H., 152
Iljitschow, W.D., 123, 130
Imig, T.J., 214, 219, 220, 221
Inagaki, S., 152
Ingle, D., 227
Irvine, D.R.F., 219

Jacobs, V.L., 132
Jacobson, M., 14, 35
Jassik-Gerschenfeld, D., 110, 111
Jenkins, F.A., 202
Jensen, C., 35
Jerison, H.J., 33, 35, 205
Johnson, J.I., Jr., 193, 201
Johnston, J.B., 6, 14, 19, 68, 70, 207

Jones, A., 14, 21, 29
Jones, E.G., 7, 28, 210, 214, 221
Joseph, B.S., 131
Juhasz, L.P., 23
Jurio, A.V., 54, 157

Kaas, J.H., 218, 221, 222
Kalischer, O., 196
Källen, B., 11, 14, 15, 18, 19, 21, 28, 207
Kamon, K., 11
Kanareck, D.A., 45, 47
Kantor, H., 11
Karten, H.J., 6, 23, 71, 81, 83, 86, 87,
    113–117, 119, 122, 123, 131, 132, 135, 137,
    142, 143, 154, 166, 168, 169, 173, 175–177,
    179, 197, 207, 209, 210, 224, 227
Kasahara, M., 118
Katz, L.C., 80, 82, 83, 130
Kawamura, S., 224
Keefer, D.A., 57
Kelly, D.B., 83, 123, 169
Kelly, J.P., 214
Kemplay, S.K., 110
Kicliter, E., 3
Kim, Y.S., 68
Kimberly, R.P., 118
King, R.L., 123
Kirsch, A.W., 193, 201
Kirsch, M., 130
Kirsche, W., 11, 14, 19, 20
Kitt, C.A., 76, 130, 142, 152, 154, 156, 157,
    166–168, 172, 173, 175, 176
Knapp, M., 7, 219
Knudsen, E.I., 119, 125, 189
Koda, L., 88
Konishi, M., 86, 118, 119, 125, 189, 224
Korn, H.J., 226
Korte, G.E., 71, 175
Kosareva, A.A., 103, 105, 131
Kowell, A.P., 145
Kroodsma, D., 86
Kruger, L., 6, 92, 132
Kubie, J.L., 97, 198
Kuhlenbeck, H., 14, 21, 23, 86
Künzle, H., 113, 114
Kusunaki, T., 70, 83, 87, 131, 157

Landreth, G.E., 92, 93
Landry, P., 216

Langner, G., 125, 126, 128
Larramendi, L.M.H., 21, 23, 26–29, 93
Lashley, K.S., 217
Lausmann, S., 134
Laxson, L.C., 228
Leake, P.A., 118
Leeman, S.E., 70
Leitner, L.M., 134
Lende, R.A., 217
Lennard, P.R., 226
Leonard, C.M., 23, 83, 87, 123, 169, 170, 173,
    175, 177, 181, 196, 197
Leonard, R.B., 131
Leppelsack, H.J., 80, 83, 123, 125, 127, 128,
    130
Le Vay, S., 214, 216, 222
Leventhal, A., 215
Levi-Montalcini, R., 14, 21, 28, 29, 210
Levine, R.R., 197
Levitt, P.W., 197
Lewis, J.W., 154
Lindstrom, S., 222
Lipetz, L.E., 101
Lippe, W.R., 123
Ljungren, L., 152–154
Lohman, A.H.M., 93, 99, 119, 142, 143,
    158
Loop, M.S., 132
Lorente de No', R., 7, 215, 216
Lorentz, K.Z., vii
Lovejoy, A.O., 202
Lund, J., 7, 214, 221
Lund, R., 14

MacDonald, R.L., 199
Macko, K., 188
MacLean, P.D., 195
Magni, F., 114, 116, 117, 224
Maier, V., 127
Manley, J.A., 118, 119
Manogue, K.R., 166, 177, 196
Marchiafava, P.L., 99
Margoliash, D., 128
Martin, G.F., 288
Martinez-Vargas, M.C., 57
Masai, H.K., 36
Masterton, R.B., 123
Matsuzaki, T., 152
Maturana, H.R., 110
Maxwell, J.H., 101, 110, 114, 189

Mentink, G.M., 143
Merzenich, M.M., 218
Meyer, A., 49
Miceli, D., 93, 157
Miller, M.R., 118
Minelli, G., 83, 87, 116, 157, 176
Minois, F., 110
Mishkin, M., 7, 219
Molenaar, G.J., 132
Moore, G.P., 219
Moore, R.Y., 222
Morell, J.I., 45, 57
Morenkov, E.D., 92, 105, 188
Morgane, P.J., 223
Moruzzi, G., 117
Mountcastle, V.B., 7, 220
Mulvanny, P., 188
Munger, B.L., 134
Myers, R.E., 219

Naik, D.R., 52, 60
Naumon, N.P., 123
Nauta, W.T.H., 210, 223
Necker, R., 134
Nelson, J., 218
Neumayer, L., 11
Newman, D.B., 192
Newsome, L.W.T., 219
Nicoll, R.A., 70
Nieuwenhuys, R., 13, 206
Niimi, K., 224
Northcutt, R.G., 3, 4, 6, 33, 35, 44, 48, 49,
    51–53, 56, 60, 61, 65, 68, 70, 76, 92, 93,
    97, 101, 131, 132, 143, 146, 164, 165,
    193, 203, 207
Norton, T.S., 222
Nottebohm, F., 23, 83–87, 123, 166, 169,
    170, 173, 175, 177, 181, 196, 199

Oeckinghaus, H., 130
Ogren, M.P., 222
Olivier, A., 70, 87, 154
O'Neill, W.E., 189
Ostrom, J.H., 194, 203
Ouimet, C.C., 223
Owen, R., 6
Ozirskaya, E.V., 103
Palacios, E., 6, 80, 87, 184
Palkovits, M., 229
Palmer, L.A., 218

Panneton, W.M., 228
Parent, A., 70, 87, 105, 142, 152–154
Parker, D.M., 117, 201
Parks, T.N., 118
Parsons, T.S., 145
Paton, J.A., 166, 169, 177, 196
Patrick, R.L., 223
Pearlman, A.L., 110
Pearson, R., 23, 78, 195, 199
Pederson, R., 131
Pentreath, V.W., 185
Perachio, A.A., 222
Peters, A., 7, 214
Peterson, E.H., 48, 56, 58, 60, 99, 101,
    106, 145, 188, 195, 228
Petras, J.M., 131
Pettigrew, J.D., 93, 125, 209, 222, 224
Peyrichoux, J., 93
Pfaff, D.W., 45, 85
Phillips, C.G., 7, 199
Phillips, D.P., 219
Phillips, R.E., 123
Pivavarov, A.S., 92, 105, 188
Platel, R., 33, 49, 52, 57, 205
Poirer, L.J., 53
Poitras, D., 154
Popper, A.N., 118
Porter, R., 7, 225
Portmann, A., 33
Powell, T.P.S., 6, 220
Price, J.L., 211
Pritz, M.B., 51, 76, 110, 112, 119, 121, 131,
    132
Pruitt, G.H., 198

Quiroga, J.C., 97, 204, 205

Radinsky, L., 35, 205
Raffin, J.-P., 93
Rainey, W.T., 100, 101, 103, 104, 106
Rakic, P., 7, 210
Ramón, P., 53, 55, 97
Ramón y Cajal, S., 80, 81
Rasmussen, G.L., 118
Reese, A.M., 11
Regidor, J., 214
Reiner, A.H., 71, 114, 167, 171–173, 175,
    176, 227
Repérant, J., 92, 93
Revzin, A.M., 111, 114, 116, 117, 142, 189

Rieke, G.K., 147
Rio, J.-P., 92
Riss, W., 60, 75, 76, 119, 147, 148
Ritchie, T.C., 82
Robbins, D.O., 101
Robinson, L.R., 131, 191
Rodieck, R.W., 208
Rogers, K.T., 11
Rolon, R.R., 146
Romer, A.S., 193
Roney, K.-J., 215
Rose, M., 23, 75, 86, 119, 123, 125
Rosengren, E., 153, 154
Rosenquist, A.C., 218
Roumy, M., 134
Rovainen, C.M., 226
Rowe, M., 99
Rowe, M.J., 217
Rubel, E.W., 118
Rudin, W., 56
Runge, T.E., 130
Ryan, J.M., 154

Sachs, M.B., 118
Saini, K.O., 78, 80, 83
Sakavaka, M., 152
Saltiel A., 85
Sar, M., 52, 68
Sato, Y., 36
Scalia, F., 60, 75, 76, 119, 147, 148, 219
Schapiro, H., 166, 167
Scheich, H., 83, 84, 123–129, 169, 175
Schenker, C., 70
Schiebel, A.B., 215, 228
Schiebel, M.E., 228
Schneider, G.E., 208
Schroeder, D.M., 93, 132
Schwartz, E.A., 101
Schwartzkopf, J., 119, 123
Senaba, E., 152
Senn, D.G., 11, 12, 35, 44, 48, 52, 56, 119
Sereno, M., 227
Sether, L., 87
Shanklin, W.M., 49
Shatz, C., 222
Shaw, G.L., 215
Sherk, H., 214
Sherrington, C., 225
Shimizu, N., 152, 153
Shiosaka, S., 152

Sidman, R.L., 7, 210
Siegesmond, K.A., 87
Silfen, R., 176
Silver, R., 134, 137, 140
Simpson, G.G., 200, 205, 208
Sinnamon, H.M., 223
Sinnett, J.M., 118
Sis, R.F., 132
Skeen, L.C., 146
Sligar, C.M., 163, 171
Smith, J.C., 145
Snyder, S.H., 52
Sparber, S.P., 88
Sprague, J.M., 224, 227
Stehouwer, D.J., 226
Stein, P.S.G., 226
Stern, W.C., 223
Stingelin, W., 33, 78, 79, 134
Stokes, T.M., 23, 83, 87, 123, 169, 170, 173,
  175, 177, 181, 196, 197
Stone, J., 215
Stone, T.W., 223
Stryker, M., 221
Stumpf, W.E., 52, 57, 60, 68
Suga, N., 189, 218
Sur, N., 218, 221
Switzer, R.C. III, 193, 201

Takagi, H., 152
Takatsuji, K., 36
Takatsuki, K., 152
Tandler, J., 11
Taylor, D.A., 223
ten Donkelaar, H.J., 91, 119, 131, 132, 142,
  152, 153, 158, 171, 191, 192
Terashima, S., 92
Tessier, Y., 111
Tigges, J., 222
Tigges, M., 222
Tohyama, M., 152–154, 157
Torvik, A., 228
Trainer, D.A., 199
Tsai, H.M., 21–23, 26–29, 93, 210
Tschirigi, R.D., 219
Tucker, D., 145
Tumanova, N.L., 103
Turner, B.H., 7, 219
Tusa, R.J., 218

Ulinski, P.S., 36, 37, 40–45, 47–49, 56, 58, 60,

67, 70, 75, 91–93, 95, 96, 99–101, 103–109,
119, 140–142, 145, 154, 157–159, 162, 166,
184, 185, 188, 191, 216, 219, 223, 225, 227
Underwood, G., 37, 212

Vagvolgyi, A., 198
Van Essen, D.C., 217, 219
van Tienhoven, A., 23, 199
van Woerden-Verkley, I., 93, 99, 142, 143,
    158
Veenman, C.L., 135
Verhaart, W.J.C., 27
Vogt, M., 127, 154, 157
Voneida, T.J., 163, 171

Wagner, H.G., 101
Wall, J.T., 221
Wallenberg, A., 86, 137, 169
Walls, G.L., 212
Wang, R.T., 93
Warner, F.J., 14–16, 44
Webster, D.B., 118
Webster, K.E., 110, 211
Weidner, C., 157
Weiler, R., 99
Weisbach, W., 119
Weiss, J.C., 62
Welt, C., 218
Wenzel, M.B., 147

Wetzel, M.C., 226
White, E.L., 7, 214, 215
Whitlock, D.G., 131
Whitteridge, D., 92, 110
Wiesel, T., 215, 220–222
Wiesendanger, M., 224
Wijsman, J.P.M., 137
Wild, J.M., 169
Willows, A.O.D., 185
Wilson, J.R., 222
Winans, S.S., 219
Wise, S.P., 7, 214
Witkovsky, P., 132, 134, 135, 137, 140
Wong, D., 214
Woolsey, C.M., 7, 217
Worden, F.G., 127, 198
Wouterlood, G., 224
Wurtz, R., 188, 227
Wyeth, F.J., 11

Yamamoto, K., 152, 153
Yazulla, S., 114, 116

Zabrosky, L., 229
Zaretsky, M.D., 125, 127
Zeier, H., 20, 83, 166, 168, 169, 177, 179
Zeigler, H.P., 134, 135, 137, 140, 169,
    197
Zeilstra, S., 137–140, 187

SUBJECT INDEX

Acetylcholinesterase, 60, 61, 70,77,87,160
Acuity, 188
ADVR, *see* Anterior dorsal ventricular ridge
Aetosaurid, 205
Agamidae, 48
Agelaius phoeniceus, 83
Agkistrodon piscivorous, 15
Agrionemys, 101
Alligator, 78,79,92, 132, 207, 219
    mississippiensis, 19, 21, 75, 76, 155
Alligatoridae, 75
Alligator lizard, *see Gerrhonottus*
    multicarinatus
Allometry, 49, 52
    -methyl-p-tyrosine, 157
Amphibian, 3, 4, 204, 207
Amphisbaenia darwinii, 97
Amphisbaenian, 97
Amygdala, 7, 207, 211, 213, 219, 220, 229,
    231, 232
Anas platyrhynchos, 79, 83, 132, 134, 137, 138,
    140, 157, 177, 187–190, 199
Androgen, 86
Anguidae, 48, 53
Anole, *see Anolis carolinensis*
Anolis carolinensis, 52, 56, 57, 60, 99, 145,
    195, 196
Ansa lenticularis, 84, 124, 174, 175, 179
Anterior dorsal ventricular ridge, 1–3, 23,
    25, 35–37, 39–41, 43, 48–50, 54, 55–57,
    59–63, 65, 67–73, 75–82, 88, 91–94, 96,
    97–100, 105, 107, 109, 116, 119, 124,

125, 134, 140, 142–144, 146–149, 151,
    153, 154, 157, 158, 160–168, 170, 174,
    179, 181, 182, 184–186, 190, 192, 194,
    195, 200, 209, 213, 217, 220, 223, 228,
    230, 231
First pattern, 35, 71, 88, 192
Second pattern, 35, 88
Aphagia, 197
Archistriatum, 1, 23–25, 82–85, 88, 122, 124,
    148, 161, 166, 168–170, 173, 177, 179,
    191, 192, 196–199, 207, 210, 211, 220
    intermediale, 84, 166, 168, 177
    See also Nucleus, robustus archistriaticus
Archosaur, 194, 203–206, *See also*
    Crocodilian; Dinosaur
Area:
    caudolateral, 49, 56
    central, 67, 70, 144
    corticoid, 26
    cytoarchitectonic, 217
    dorsal, 18, 62, 66, 69–71, 100, 105, 107,
        110, 141–144
    dorsolateral, 75, 77, 112, 119, 121, 133,
        166
    dorsomedial, 75
    epibasalis, 131
    hippocampus, 26, 179
    intercollicular, 170
    intermediolateral, 75, 166
    lateroventral, 75
    medial, 49, 56, 66, 67, 70, 72, 107, 141–144,
        154

modality specific, 148, 149, 186, 191, 217,
    218, 221, 231, 232
parahippocampal, 26, 179
preoptic, 24, 173
rostrolateral, 49, 56
temporo-parietal-occipital, 23, 29, 83, 166,
    168
ventral, 18, 66, 67, 70, 73, 107, 141, 142,
    144
ventral tegmental, 152, 154, 156, 171, 173,
    192
ventrolateral, 76, 77, 110, 154, 172, 192
ventromedial, 147
x, 85, 87, 169, 170, 173, 192
Autonomic nervous system, 199, 229, 230
Autoradiography, 140, 142
Axon:
    geniculocortical, 143
    rotundal, 108
Axonal transport, 6

Band, 7
Basal dorsal ventricular ridge, 1–3, 23, 35,
    42, 45, 56, 57, 60, 68, 71, 73, 74, 83, 88,
    91, 98–100, 120, 140, 141, 145–148,
    150, 161, 162, 176, 181, 183, 184, 191,
    198, 199, 213, 219, 229–231
Basal ganglia, 4, 6, 7, 206, 208, 214, 230. See
    also Amygdala; Caudate-putamem;
    Claustrum; Globus pallidus
Bat, 189
BDVR, see Basal dorsal ventricular ridge
Beak, 134
Belt, periectostriatal, 82, 83, 144, 193
Bill, 135, 137, 138, 140
    tip organ, 139
Binocular overlap, 92
Bird, 4, 6–8, 11, 14, 15, 21, 22, 24, 29, 30, 33,
    35, 75, 77, 83, 86–89, 92, 93, 110, 119,
    131, 132, 143, 147, 148, 152, 154, 161,
    166, 171, 173, 176, 177, 183–186, 188,
    190–195, 199, 200, 209–213, 217, 222,
    224, 229–231
    carinate, 78
    ratite, 78
    song, 85, 169, 181, 192, 196
    See also Agelaius phoeniceus; Anas
        platyrhynohos; Apteryx australis;
        Chrysolampis mosquitus; Cistothorus
        palustris; Columba livia; Coturnix
        coturnix; Cyanocitta stelleri; Gallus

domesticus; Lampornis mango; Lonchura
    puntulata; Love bird; Melopsittacus
    undulatus; Mynah bird; Numidia
    meleagris; Passer domestica; Petrel;
    Peophilla guttata; Raven; Serinus
    canarius; Speotyto cunicularia;
    Streptopelia risoria; Sturnus vulgaris;
    Turkey vulture; Tyto alba; Uroloncha
    domestica; Zonotrichia leucophrys
Birthdates, 26
Blackbird, see Agelaius phoeniceus
Blue racer, see Coluber constrictor
Boa constrictor, see Constrictor constrictor
Bone, jaw, 201
Brainstem, 151, 162, 179
Brain weight-body weight ratio, 33, 36, 205.
    See also Allometry
Bundle, dendritic, 221
    lateral forebrain, 15, 25, 46, 53, 59, 67, 70,
        77, 83, 84, 86, 87, 95, 96, 98–101, 105,
        112, 119–121, 123, 124, 133, 137, 142,
        158, 159, 164, 166, 171, 172, 175, 176,
        179, 181, 186, 192

Caenophidia, 37
Caiman, see Caiman
Caiman, 51, 75–77, 93, 110–112, 118, 120,
    131–133, 147–149, 152, 166, 167, 171,
    186, 192, 217
    sclerops, 35, 111
    crocodilus, 110, 119
Call:
    Iambus, 128, 129
    species specific, 127, 128
Canary, see Serinus canarius
Cardiac function, 199
Casual apposition, 65
Cat, 209, 226
Catecholamine, 152, 157. See also Dopamine;
    Noradrenalin
Caudate-Putamen, 5, 207, 223
Cell:
    aspiny stellate, 55, 62, 68, 75, 81, 214
    dorsal root ganglion, 131, 132
    double pyramidal, 49
    juxtaependymal, 37, 40, 43, 61, 64, 72, 75,
        78, 184, 185, 192
    Mauthner, 226
    Müller, 226
    nonpyramidal, 7

pyramidal, 7, 68, 209, 211, 214, 215, 218, 221–223
retinal ganglion, 99, 101, 106, 110, 187, 211
spiny stellate, 40–43, 55, 61, 62, 65–67, 75, 79, 81, 214
stellate, 37, 49, 68, 73, 75, 80, 83, 84, 101, 184, 191, 193, 210, 214, 215
Central pattern generator, 226
Cerebellum, 13, 222
Chamaeleo, 15
Chameleon, *see Chamaeleo*
Chamaeleonidae, 48
Chelydra serpentina, 70
Chick, *see Gallus domesticus*
Chicken, *see Gallus domesticus*
Chrysemys, 19, 65, 70, 99, 140, 142, 146, 153, 154, 164, 165, 171
  marginata, 18
  picta, 18, 60, 68
  scripta, *see Pseudemys scripta*
Chrysolampis mosquitus, 78
Cistothorus palustris, 86
Cistudo carolina, *see Terrapene carolina*
Claustrum, 214
Clusters, neuronal, 37, 39, 41, 43, 49, 51, 52, 55, 60, 61, 64–66, 69, 72, 75, 77, 78, 80, 88, 93, 154, 184, 185, 215
Colliculus:
  posterior, 119
  superior, 7, 188, 208, 214, 224, 227–230
Coluber constrictor, 35, 37
Columba livia, 6, 23–25, 28, 35, 80, 84, 92, 110, 113–115, 122, 123, 130–132, 134, 137, 140, 145, 147, 149, 154, 156–168, 173–177, 187, 188, 195, 197, 209, 210
Commissure:
  anterior, 23, 24, 83, 84, 94, 96, 100, 123, 124, 154, 158, 159, 163, 166, 176, 177, 179
  posterior, 84, 95, 104
Column, 7
  binaural, 219
  ocular dominance, 209, 220–222
  orientation, 209, 220–222
Complex, epithelial cell-neurite, 134
  perifascicular, 46, 48, 162
  principal optic, 93
Cone, 212
Constrictor constrictor, 36, 37, 45, 47, 145
Corpus callosum, 5
Corpuscle:

Herbst, 134, 135, 140
Grandry, 134, 140
Pacinian, 134
Cortex:
  auditory, 189
  dorsal, 53, 61, 62, 93, 140, 141, 143, 146, 147, 153, 158, 163, 209, 210
  dorsomedial, 140, 141, 209
  lateral, 15, 17, 18, 30, 53, 61, 62, 107, 141, 146, 147
  medial, 53, 61, 62, 141, 146
  motor, 211
  peristriate, 209, 210
  pyriform, 26
Coturnix coturnix, 83, 116, 176
Crocodilian, 11, 14, 19, 21, 34, 35, 75, 76, 88, 92, 110, 111, 119, 132, 142, 145, 147, 148, 152, 154, 166, 172, 188, 193, 194, 203, 205. *See also Alligator; Caiman; Crocodilus*
Crocodilidae, 75
Crocodilus palustris, 75
Crotalus, 93
Cumulative labeling, 21
Curve;
  isofrequency, 127
  tuning, 125, 127, 131, 187
Cyanocitta stelleri, 84
Cynodont, 202, 205

Deoxyglucose, 97, 99, 117, 123, 127, 221
Desert iguana, *see Dipsosaurus dorsalis*
Desmatosuchus, 205
Develop, 195
Diadectes, 204
Diencephalon, 13, 154
Dihydrosterone, 86
Dinosaur, 203
Dipsosaurus dorsalis, 35, 49, 56–58, 60, 99, 145
Display, 195
Dopamine, 151, 153, 154, 156, 157, 179, 190
Duck, *see Anas platyrhynchos*

Ear, inner, 201
Echolocation, 218
Ectostriatum, 22–27, 29, 81–83, 89, 113, 116–118, 124, 142, 143, 166, 168, 181, 185, 187, 193
Emys, 99, 101
  orbicularis, 105, 142
Endocast, 203–205

Enkephalin, 52, 60, 87, 160, 176
Enzyme, 60. *See also* Acetylcholinesterase;
    Monoamine oxidase; Succinic
    dehydrogenase
Ep. *see* Belt, periectostriatal
Ependyma, 38
Epiphysis, 13
Epistriatum, 19
Estradiol, 45, 57, 68, 86
Evagination, 11
Eye, 213

Fasciculus, medial longitudinal, 181
Feeding, 197
Field G, 119, 130, 131
    L, 23, 24, 26, 28, 29, 78, 81, 83–85, 89, 122,
        123, 125–128, 130, 131, 166, 168–170,
        181, 185, 187, 190, 192, 196, 210
    prerubral, 171
Finch, *see Uroloncha domestica*
Fink-Heimer preparation, 45, 49, 96, 107,
    132, 140, 147, 158, 159, 163, 171
Fish:
    actinopterygian, 4
    bony, 3, 33, 211
    chondrostean, 4
    crossopterygian, 4
    dipnoan, 3, 4, 204
    holostean, 4,
    polypteriform, 4
    sarcopterygian, 4, 207
    teleostean, 4
    See also Shark
Foramen, interventricular, 11
Forebrain, 101
Formant, 128
Fornix, 61

Gallus domesticus, 21–23, 28, 85, 87, 93, 143,
    157, 184
Ganglion:
    acoustic
    trigeminal, 135, 136
Garter snake, *see Thamnophis*
Gecko, 212. *See also Gekko gecko; Tarentola
    mauretanica*
Gekko gecko, 52, 54, 55, 97–99, 132, 143, 158,
    163
Gekkonidae, 48
Gerrhonottus multicarinattus, 35, 51, 53
Gila monster, *see Heloderma*

Globus pallidus, 70, 207
Golgi technique, 6, 28, 37, 40, 41, 44, 47, 53,
    55, 56, 58, 61, 64–68, 72, 73, 75, 79, 81,
    87, 103, 108, 191
Graecian tortoise, *see Testudo graeca*
Guinea fowl, *see Numidia meleagris*

Habenula, 45, 95, 102, 104, 115, 147, 173
Heloderma, 56
Hippocampus, 206
Histofluorescence, 152
Homology, viii, 8, 200, 202, 203, 208–212,
    230, 231
Homoplasy, 201, 209–211, 230
Horned toad, *see Phrynosoma cornutum*
Horseradish peroxidase, 82, 83, 91, 93,
    103–106, 109, 114–116, 118, 132, 142,
    144, 146, 152–154, 164, 166, 169,
    171–173, 175–177, 214, 216
Hummingbird, *see Chrysolampis mosquitus;
    Lampornis mango*
HVc, *see* Hyperstriatum ventrale
Hyperstriatum, 23, 29, 117, 143, 166
    accessorium, 23–27, 113, 124, 136, 157
    anterius, 48
    dorsale, 23, 29, 124
    intercalatus, 23, 26, 27, 29
    intercalatus superioris, 24, 124
    ventrale, 23–27, 29, 82–87, 89, 113, 116,
        123, 124, 127, 130, 136, 156, 157, 166,
        168–170, 179, 181, 185, 191, 197
Hypopallium, 207
Hypophysis, 13
Hypothalamus, 3, 4, 7, 8, 95, 115, 140,
    161–163, 171, 176, 177, 179, 181, 183,
    199, 200, 210, 211, 213, 229–232

Iguana, *see Iguana iguana*
Iguana iguana, 49, 51–53, 55, 56, 60, 61, 92,
    93, 97–99, 119, 120, 132, 142, 149, 158
Iguanidae, 48
Immunocytochemistry, 52
Intelligence, 35
Isocortex, 4, 7, 200, 206, 208, 210–212,
    214–217, 220, 221, 223–225, 228,
    230–232

Jay, *see Cyanocitta stelleri*
Junction, gap, 37

King snake, *see Lampropeltis getulus floridanus*

Kiwi, *see Apteryx australis*

Lacerta, 15, 55, 97, 145, 153
  muralis, 60, 152
  sicula 12, 17
  viridis, 152
Lacertidae, 48, 49, 52
Lamina, archistriatalis dorsalis, 179
  dorsal medullary, 22–25, 27, 28, 84, 86, 87,
    179
  frontalis suprema, 23, 27
  frontal medullary, 22–24
  hyperstriatica, 22–25, 27, 71, 84, 181, 193
Lampornis mango, 78
Lampropeltis getulus floridanus, 145
Learning, 35
Lepidosaur, 193, 203, 205. *See also*
    Amphisbaenian; Lizard; Snake;
    Rhynchocephalian
Lialis burtoni, 52
Linkage, 1, 179, 183, 194, 199, 212, 213, 223,
    225, 229, 232
Lizard, 8, 11, 14, 15, 33–35, 48, 56–58, 71, 73,
    75, 91–93, 97, 118, 119, 131, 142, 143,
    145, 150, 152, 158, 162, 171, 184, 185,
    187, 191, 195, 196, 209, 212, 219
  Dracomorph, *see* Lizard, Type II
  Lacertomorph, *See* Lizard, Type I
  Type I, 34, 48, 51–55, 88, 163, 193, 194
  Type II, 34, 48–52, 88, 193, 194
  *See also Anolis carolinensis, Chamaeleo,
    Dipsosaurus dorsalis, Gekko gecko,
    Gerrhonottus multicarinattus,
    Heloderma, Iguana iguana, Lacerta,
    Phrynosoma cornutum, Tarentola
    maurentanica, Tupinambis, Varanus,
    Xantusia vigilis*
Lobe:
  parolfactory, 24–26, 28, 29, 85–87, 136,
    154, 156, 157, 166, 168–170, 175, 176,
    192
  pyriform, 206
Locus coeruleus, 152, 154, 157, 160, 173, 177,
    190
Lonchura punctulata, 157
Love bird, 143
LPO, *see* Lobe, paraolfactory

Magnification, 218
Mammal, 5, 6, 35, 104, 108, 184, 200, 201, 203,
    210–213, 218, 224, 229–232

Mesozoic, 206
  prototherian, 204
  monotreme, 217
  marsupial, 217
  placental, 217
Mandibulation, 197
Marchi technique, 137
Massetognathus, 205
Mechanoreceptor, 134
Medulla, 11
Melopsittacus undulats, 28, 83, 166, 177, 196
Microneuron, 81
Migration
  c_i 18
  c^I, 21, 28
  c^{II}, 21, 28
  d_i 18
  $d^{I + II}$, 18
  d^I 19, 21, 28
  d^{II}, 19, 21, 28
  d^{III}, 19, 21, 28
  d^{IV}, 19
  radial, 7
Minimum convex polygon, 205
Mitochondrion, 51
MLD, *see* Nucleus, mesencephalicus
    lateralis pars dorsalis
Monitor lizard, *see* Varanus
Monoamine, 151, 157
  oxidase, 152
  system, 152
Moorish gecko, *see Tarentola maurentanica*
Motoneurons, 2, 4, 7, 183, 224, 225, 228–230
  hypoglossal, 192
Mouth, 137
Multituberculate, 205
Mynah bird, 128

Natrix sipedon, 15, 16, 35, 36, 38, 39, 45, 48,
    93, 94, 158, 159, 162,
Neostriatum, 15, 17, 22–24, 26, 27, 29, 48, 80,
    81, 83–85, 87, 113, 117, 136, 143, 156,
    157, 166, 168, 174, 179, 181, 193, 207
  caudale, 23, 80, 82, 83, 122–124, 134, 140,
    169, 171, 181
  dorsale, 84
  frontale, 23, 24, 130
  intermediale, 23–25, 82, 118, 176
Nerodia sipedon, see Natrix sipedon
Nerve:
  glossopharyngeal, 135, 139

oculomotor, 153
optic, 159
trigeminal, 132, 135, 139, 185
Neural tube, 3, 11
Neuroblast, 14, 15, 18, 21, 30
Neuroepithelium, 11, 14–16, 18, 20, 21, 23, 28, 30
Neuroethology, vii, 6
Neuromodulator, 223
Neurotransmitter, 60. *see also* Dopamine; Noradrenalin; Serotonin
NI, *see* Neostriatum, intermediale
Night lizard, *see* Xantusia vigilis
Noradrenalin, 151, 152, 154, 157, 190, 222
Norepinephrine, *see* Noradrenalin
Nucleus:
    accumbens, 24, 48, 53, 54, 59–62, 146, 152, 157, 163
    angularis, 181
    ansa lenticularis of, 182, 192, 224
    basalis, 23, 24, 26, 29, 79, 130, 132, 134–140, 166, 169, 185–188, 190, 193, 197, 221
    caudalis, 70, 104, 106, 141
    central, 3
    dorsal column, 133, 177, 186
    dorsalis-intermedius posterior, 174–176
    dorsal lateral geniculate, 46, 81, 92, 93, 95, 102, 104, 106, 141, 159, 208, 209, 215, 220
    dorsal nucleus of posterior commissure, 165, 167, 171, 172, 179, 181, 191
    dorsolateralis anterior, 115, 140, 142, 173, 186
    dorsolateralis lateralis, 115
    dorsolateralis posterior, 84, 118, 134, 177
    dorsomedial, 95
    dorsomedial anterior, 102, 104, 106, 115, 140–142, 186
    entopeduncular, 164, 167, 171, 172, 175, 182, 192, 224
    facial, 179, 181
    hypoglossal, 85, 170, 177, 181
    intercollicularis, 177, 181
    interpenduncular, 153
    intralaminar, 216, 225
    intrapeduncular, 24, 46, 48, 58–60, 63, 86, 87, 156, 162–164, 166, 173, 175, 177
    isthmi, 115
    laminaris, 181
    lateral amygdaloid, 163

lateral cerebellar, 164, 171, 176
lateral olfactory tract of, 53, 60–62, 75, 147
lateral pontine, 177
lateral posterior, 208, 210
lentiformis mesencephali, 70, 94, 95
lentiformis thalami, 94, 95, 104, 106, 119
magnocellularis, 181
medial geniculate, 216
medialis, 97–99, 119, 120
medialis posterior, 111, 132, 133
medial striatal, 45, 48, 59, 162, 163
mesencephalicus lateralis pars dorsalis, 118, 119, 122, 181
motor, 136, 179
oculomotor, 122, 155
ovalis, 104, 106, 141
ovoidalis, 24, 84, 117, 119, 122–124, 175, 185, 192
parovoidalis, 123
perirotundal, 140–142, 186
periventricularis magnocellularis, 124
posterocentralis, 132
posterodorsal, 95
preoptic, 61
pretectal, 96, 104
principal, 135–137, 140, 186
profundus mesencephali, 158, 165, 172
pulvinar, 208, 210
red, 156
reticularis superior, 84, 124
reuniens, 51, 70, 111, 119, 121, 133
robustus archistriaticus, 83–86, 102, 103, 169, 170, 175, 177, 181, 196
rotundus, 24, 51, 78, 84, 92, 94, 95, 97–101, 104, 105, 107–114, 116, 118, 120–122, 124, 133, 141, 147, 164, 166, 174, 179, 181, 185, 186, 188, 189, 192, 195, 209, 210
sphericus, 42, 44–47, 53, 56–58, 60, 61, 73, 98, 99, 120, 145, 146, 150, 159, 163, 176, 198, 219
spinal, 135
spiriformis lateralis, 84, 115, 174, 175, 179, 181, 191, 195
spiriformis medialis, 84
subpretectalis, 115
subrotundus, 84, 124
subthalamic, 224
superficialis parvocellularis, 134, 137, 140
taeniae, 179
trigeminal, 132, 137, 177
trochlear, 137

umbonate, 141
ventral, 104, 106
ventral anterior, 225
ventral lateral geniculate, 94, 124, 179, 216
ventrobasal, 216
ventrolateral, 147
ventromedial, 42, 45, 57, 60, 62, 147
Numidia meleagris, 83, 84, 123–127, 168, 175

Olfactory:
    accessory bulb, 45, 46, 56, 73, 145, 146,
        150, 176, 198, 201, 219, 229
    bulb, 2, 13, 147
    main bulb, 145, 150, 229
    system, 7
    tract, accessory, 45, 46, 58, 96, 150, 159,
        163, 198
    tract, lateral, 58, 146, 150, 201
    tubercle, 5, 26, 61, 146, 152, 163, 171
Optic chiasm, 96, 98–100, 120, 146, 148, 159,
    163, 170, 174, 179
Organ, vomeronasal, 45, 198, 219, 229
Oxybelis aeneus, 36, 37
Owl, 145, 189, 225. *See also Speotyto
    cuniculara; Tyto alba*

PA, *see* Paleostriatum augmentatum
Paleostriatum, 207
Paleostriatum augmentatum, 15, 22, 24–28,
    83–87, 113, 115, 123, 124, 136, 143,
    154, 156, 157, 166, 168–170, 173–175,
    179, 181
    primitivum, 24, 26–28, 83, 86, 87, 115, 123,
        124, 136, 156, 166, 168, 173, 176, 177,
        179, 181
Pallial thickening, 141, 143, 144
Pallium, 14, 16, 17, 18, 21, 23, 30, 93, 206,
    207, 209, 212, 213, 217, 222, 228, 230,
    231
Parakeet, *see Melopsittacus undulatus*
Parrot, 196
Passer domesticus, 28
Path:
    auditory, 118, 120–122, 124
    catecholaminergic, 153
    dorsal archistriatal, 166, 169, 179
    dorsal column, 132
    frontoarchistriatal, 26, 124, 169, 179
    hypothalamo-hypophyseal, 229
    quinto-frontal, 136, 137, 179, 197
    reticulospinal, 192, 224, 227, 228

somatosensory, 131, 133
spinothalamic, 131
tectofugal, 100, 112, 113, 209
visual, 92
Pecking, 195, 197
Pelycosaur, 202, 206
Peptide, 52. *See also* Enkephalin; Substance
    P
Petrel, 148
Pheromone, 198
Phylogenetic tree, 202
Phrynosoma cornutum, 52
Pigeon, *see Columbia livia*
Plate:
    alar, 206
    basal, 206
Podocnemis unifilis, 60
Poephila guttata, 82, 84–86, 127, 130, 157,
    169, 177, 196
Polysensory input, 219
Posterior dorsal ventricular ridge, 53, 62,
    162
PP, *see* Paleostriatum primitivum
Pretectum, 84, 115, 165, 174, 175, 179, 191
Prey odor, 198
    tracking, 198
Probainognathus, 204, 205
Probelesodon, 205
Projection:
    association, 214
    commissural, 214, 218, 219
    nontopological, 232
    retinogeniculate, 93
    retinotectal, 92, 93, 110
    serotonergic, 153
    tectorotundal, 104, 106, 110, 115
    tectoreticular, 191, 227, 228
    thalamostriate, 142
    thalamotelencephalic, 148, 185
Pseudemys scripta, 2, 6, 35, 60, 62–68, 70,
    72–74, 100–109, 140–142, 144, 146,
    147, 149, 154, 158, 165
Pseudosuchian, 205
Psychology, experimental, 6
Psychophysics, 6
Ptilodus, 204, 205
Pygopodidae, 52
Python, *see Python reticulatus*
Python reticulatus, 46, 132

Quail, *see Coturnix coturnix*

RA, *see* Nucleus, robustus archistriaticus
Raphé, 152, 153, 160, 190, 223
Rattlesnake, *see Crotalus*
Raven, 143
Red-eared turtle, *see Pseudemys scripta*
Representation, distributed, 189
Reptile, 4, 6–8, 14, 15, 22, 29, 30, 33, 152,
        183–185, 190, 191, 193–195, 200, 201,
        204, 208–210, 212, 213, 217, 222, 224,
        229–231
    see also Amphisbaenian; Crocodilian;
        Lizard; Rhynchocephalian; Snake;
        Turtle
Reticular Formation, 1, 161, 162, 171, 174,
        179, 181, 183, 190, 200, 223, 224, 226,
        227, 229, 230
    paramedial pontine, 188
    parvocellular, 177
    pontine, 192, 226
Retinotopy, 188
Ring dove, *see Streptopelia risoria*
Rod, 212
Rhynchocephalian, 17, 60, 193. *See also*
        Sphenodon
Scala naturae, 202
Schema, 197
Scincidae, 48
Septum, 5, 16, 17, 20, 24–26, 30, 36, 50, 53,
        54, 57–59, 61, 62, 87, 96, 112, 120, 121,
        133, 136, 141, 142, 144, 146, 158, 159,
        163, 181, 186, 207, 212
Serinus canarius, 23, 83, 85, 86, 123, 127, 168,
        170, 177, 192, 196
Serotonin, 151, 152, 157, 190, 223
Sex hormone, 45. *See also* Androgen;
        Dihydrosterone; Estradiol;
        Testosterone
Sexual dimorphism, 85
Shark, 3, 33, 226
Snake, 11, 14, 15, 34–36, 38–40, 42, 43, 45,
        46, 48, 49, 71, 73, 88, 92–94, 96, 118,
        119, 131, 132, 145, 158, 162, 163, 176,
        184, 187, 191, 193, 219
    boid, 36, 37
    colubrid, 35
    *see also Agkistrodon piscivorous; Coluber
        constrictor; Constrictor constrictor;
        Crotalus; Lampropeltus getulus
        floridanus; Natrix sipedon; Oxybelis
        aeneus; Python reticulatus; Thamnophis
        sirtalis; Tupinambis*

Snapping turtle, *see Chelydra serpentina*
Soft shelled turtle, *see Trionyx s. spinifer*
Somatotopy, 139
Space map, 189
Sparrow, *see Passer domesticus*
Speotyto cunicularia, 224
Sphenodon, 11, 14, 17, 18, 34, 35, 60, 62, 71,
        88, 92, 93, 185, 193
Spice finch, *see Lonchura punctulata*
Spinal cord, 7, 13, 133, 179, 185, 191, 214
    gray matter, 131
Spine, dendritic, 37, 42, 49, 62
SPL, *see* Nucleus, spiriformis lateralis
Starling, *see Sturnus vulgaris*
Stratum:
    album centrale, 115
    fibrosum et griseum superficiale, 101,
        104, 115
    griseum centrale, 104, 110, 114, 115, 118
    griseum periventriculare, 101, 104, 115
    opticum, 104, 115
Streak, visual, 106, 188
Streptopelia risoria, 123, 127
Stria medullaris, 124, 147, 148
    terminalis, 163, 179
Striatum, 2, 3, 6, 8, 14–18, 20–22, 28, 36, 37,
        40, 41, 48, 50, 53–55, 57–63, 70, 71, 76,
        85–87, 98–100, 112, 121, 133, 140–142,
        144, 147, 151–154, 156, 157, 160–162,
        164–168, 170, 171, 174, 179, 181, 183,
        185, 190–192, 195, 206, 207, 212, 213,
        223–225, 228, 230
Sturnus vulgaris, 78, 80, 123, 127
Synapse, electrotonic, 37, 185
Substance P, 70, 71, 160, 175
Substantia nigra, 152, 164, 165, 171, 172,
        179, 181, 182, 191, 192, 224, 230
Succinic dehydrogenase, 51, 53, 68, 75, 83,
        187
Sulcus, 14
    a, 19
    d, 19
    dorsal ventricular, 15–17, 19–21, 29, 30,
        207
    interstriaticus, *see* Sulcus, middle
        ventricular
    middle ventricular, 14–21, 28–30, 207
    superstriaticus, *see* Sulcus, dorsal
        ventricular
    terminalis, *see* Sulcus, middle ventricular
    ventral ventricular, 14

Synaptic vesicle, 37
Syrinx, 177, 196

Tanycyte, 40
Tarentola maurentanica, 35
Tectum, optic, 3, 13, 24, 92, 95, 97–101, 103,
      104, 112–115, 120–122, 124, 133, 153,
      161, 162, 164, 165, 167, 168, 171, 172,
      174, 176, 177, 179, 181, 186, 191, 192,
      195, 208–210, 224, 227–230
Tegu lizard, *see Tupinambis*
Teidae
Telencephalon, 4, 5, 13, 21, 154
Template, 198
Terrapene carolina, 6, 70
Terrapin, *see Terrapene carolina*
Testosterone, 45, 57, 85, 86
Testudo hermannii, 19, 20
    graeca, 68, 70, 146
Tetrabenazine, 157
Thalamus, 3, 7, 94, 97, 102, 111, 113, 124,
      146, 162
    afferents from, 51, 67, 70, 92, 96, 185, 215,
      216
Thamnophis sirtalis, 35, 45, 93, 94, 96, 145,
      146, 158, 162, 163, 176, 184, 198
    radix, 145
Therapsid, 202, 205, 206, 225
Thick caliber systems, 159, 223
Tongue, 135
    flicking, 198
Tonotopy, 125–127, 189
Topological organization, 218, 231, 232
Torus semicircularis, 118–121, 155, 185, 189
TPO, *see* Area, temporo-parietal-occipital
Tract:
    corticospinal, 228
    habenulopeduncular, 102
    optic, 53, 58, 61, 62, 84, 92, 95, 96, 106,
      115, 122, 124, 147, 159, 163
    occipitomesencephalic, 84, 124, 177, 179,
      181, 192, 197, 199, 211
    pyramidal, 211
    tectothalamic, 95, 104, 106
Triconodon, 204, 205
Trirachodon, 204
Trionyx s. spinifer
Tritiated thymidine, 21, 211
Tupinambis, 35, 49, 51, 57–59, 93, 99, 119,
      142, 143, 145, 158, 162–164, 171, 185,
      192

nigropunctatus, 49
    teguixin, 49
Turkey vulture, 148
Turtle, 11, 14, 18, 20, 34, 35, 60, 63, 70, 71,
      88, 91–93, 100, 102, 103, 108, 110, 114,
      131, 140, 143–146, 152, 153, 158, 164,
      171, 184, 185, 192, 193, 203, 206, 209,
      212, 226
    cryptodiran, 60, 131, 152, 187
    pleurodiran, 60, 131
    see also Agrionemys; Chelydra serpentina;
            Chrysemys; Emys; Podocnemis unifilis;
            Pseudemys scripta; Terrapene carolina;
            Testudo; Trionyx s. spinifer
Tyto alba, 125

Unit, wide field, 189
Uroloncha domestica, 83

Varanidae, 48
Varanus, 35, 50, 56, 99, 153, 158, 171
    benegalensis, 99, 119, 132
    exanthematicus, 97, 119, 131, 132, 142, 152
Varicosity, 37, 223
Ventricle, lateral, 4, 11, 15, 29, 36, 37, 77, 78,
      84, 86
Vine snake, *see Oxybelis aeneus*

Wall lizard, *see Lacerta*
Water moccasin, *see Agkistrodon piscivorus*
Water snake, *see Natrix sipedon*
White crowned sparrow, *see Zonotrichia*
            leucophrys
Wildness, 199
Wren, longbilled marsh, *see Cistothorus*
            palustris
Wulst, 23, 25, 29, 30, 93, 144, 209, 210, 222
    anterior, 224, 225

Xantusia vigilis, 52
Xantusidae, 52

Zebra finch, *see Poephilla guttata*
Zona limitans, 15–20, 30
Zone, 38, 64, 88
    A, 38, 40–43, 93, 162, 219
    B, 38, 40–43, 93, 96, 158, 162, 219
    C, 38, 40–44, 158, 162, 219
    L_1, 123, 124, 190
    L_2, 123, 124, 190
    L_3, 123, 124, 190

284   Subject Index

1, 64, 65
2, 50, 56, 64–66, 142, 143, 185
3, 50, 64, 65, 142, 143
4, 56, 64, 65, 67, 105, 110, 142, 143

8, 119
active, 37
Zonotrichia leucophrys, 128

Date Due

			UML 735